PHYSIOLOGICAL PROBLEMS IN SPACE EXPLORATION

Publication Number 561
AMERICAN LECTURE SERIES®

A Monograph in
The BANNERSTONE DIVISION *of*
AMERICAN LECTURES IN PHYSIOLOGY

PHYSIOLOGICAL PROBLEMS IN SPACE EXPLORATION

Edited by

JAMES D. HARDY, PH.D.

Director, John B. Pierce Foundation Laboratory
Professor of Physiology, Yale University Medical School
New Haven, Connecticut

Formerly
Director of Research
U. S. Naval Aviation Medical Acceleration Laboratory
Johnsville, Pennsylvania

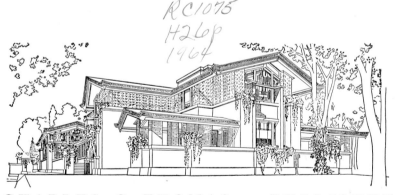

CHARLES C THOMAS • PUBLISHER

Springfield • Illinois • U.S.A.

Published and Distributed Throughout the World by

CHARLES C THOMAS • PUBLISHER

BANNERSTONE HOUSE

301-327 East Lawrence Avenue, Springfield, Illinois, U.S.A.

NATCHEZ PLANTATION HOUSE

735 North Atlantic Boulevard, Fort Lauderdale, Florida, U.S.A.

© *1964,* by CHARLES C THOMAS • PUBLISHER

Library of Congress Catalog Card Number: 63-19579

With THOMAS BOOKS careful attention is given to all details of manufacturing and design. It is the Publisher's desire to present books that are satisfactory as to their physical qualities and artistic possibilities and appropriate for their particular use. THOMAS BOOKS will be true to those laws of quality that assure a good name and good will.

Printed in the United States of America

M-1

CONTRIBUTORS

JOHN R. BROBECK, M.D.: *Professor of Physiology*
School of Medicine, University of Pennsylvania,
Philadelphia, Pennsylvania.

JOHN LOTT BROWN, PH.D.: *Associate Professor of Physiology,*
School of Medicine, University of Pennsylvania,
Philadelphia, Pennsylvania.

RANDALL M. CHAMBERS, PH.D.: *Head, Human Factors Division,*
Aviation Medical Acceleration Laboratory,
U. S. Naval Air Development Center,
Johnsville, Pennsylvania.

CARL C. CLARK, PH.D.: *Manager, Life Sciences Department,*
Martin Company,
Baltimore, Maryland.

FRANZ HALBERG, M.D.: *Professor of Pathology,*
Medical School, University of Minnesota,
Minneapolis, Minnesota.

JAMES D. HARDY, PH.D.: *Director, John B. Pierce Foundation Laboratory,*
and Professor of Physiology,
Yale University School of Medicine,
New Haven, Connecticut.

EDWIN HENDLER, PH.D.: *Manager, Life Sciences Research Group,*
Aerospace Crew Equipment Laboratory,
U. S. Naval Air Engineering Center,
Philadelphia, Pennsylvania.

FOREWORD

The physiological problems which have challenged students and investigators in their attempts to adapt man for space explorations have been those associated with environmental extremes. The high vacuum of inter-stellar and inter-planetary space, marked alterations in acceleration due to high velocities of space craft, inter-stellar dust and atomic nuclei, extremes of heat and cold, and long periods of loneliness in a limited space, are factors which mean stress to the astronaut. Thus, in a real sense space physiology is the physiology of stress. For this reason there has been from the beginning of the space adventure a deepseated conflict between those who have maintained that engineering skills should be strained to provide the same environment for the astronaut in space as he has on Earth and those who would extend man's capabilities for survival by physiological means. In the first instance, therefore, there is no space physiology, only space engineering of the environment. However, the long experience in aviation medicine and physiology has shown that danger and death lie in this direction and unless physiologists and psychologists can provide the data which show the safe and the dangerous limits for human performance and survival, the engineering profession will proceed with designs of aircraft and spacecraft based on their own best guesses. The good fortune which has attended the few space flights to date are examples of the great benefits which have been derived from the somewhat painful but beneficent cooperation between engineering and biological scientists. Space travel is still a most dangerous venture and thus many problems remain to be solved. Rescue operations in space and emergency escape are not practical during most of a space voyage at present. However, progress in space biology up to date is such as to encourage us to approach this and other challenges with optimism. It is the intent of this volume to present background information and our state of knowledge in the several aspects of space psychophysiology for the use of students and the interested general reader.

JAMES D. HARDY, PH.D., *Editor*

New Haven, Connecticut

vii

CONTENTS

PHYSIOLOGICAL PROBLEMS IN SPACE EXPLORATION

1

TEMPERATURE PROBLEMS IN SPACE TRAVEL

JAMES D. HARDY, PH.D.

Man and his progenitors have been born and had their being under the protective envelope of the Earth's atmosphere and near the stabilizing influences of the great water masses—lakes, rivers and oceans. These many protections are apparent to us when we study with great telescopes the harsh and scarred surface of our nearest cellestial neighbor, the Moon, and make plans to explore this landscape in person. Without an atmosphere and with no liquid water surfaces, an astronaut will be exposed to the full radiation from the sun during the lunar day and to the extreme cold of outer space during the night. As we look beyond the moon towards our nearest planetary neighbors, Venus and Mars, and possibly Jupiter and Mercury, with an idea of sending manned expeditions to study their surfaces at close hand, the thermal threats (which set the final limits to the existence of all life) are major problems in the planning. In many areas our information concerning the planets is insufficient to evaluate the extent of the dangers from excessive heat or cold and it will be necessary to send instrumented probes to study conditions before a man actually ventures into the face of the fiery blasts of solar radiation or the silent deep spaces where the cold is such that the molecular motions are almost ceased. It is thus the purpose of this chapter to examine the thermal environment of interest to the astronaut and to describe the physiological

3

limitations of man and his temperature regulatory capacities. It is not enough to say that man will have to be protected in space because, although this is unquestioned, it is necessary to determine for a particular mission how much and for how long. Weight is of overriding importance in space travel and protective equipment will be limited.

THERMAL ENVIRONMENTS IN SPACE

The Earth: The extremes of temperature on the Earth's surface are included in the range of +50° and −75°C, and with proper dress man has found it possible to live for extended periods in regions in which such temperatures are occasionally recorded. However, large land areas have average yearly tempera-

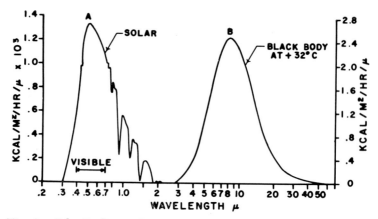

Fig. 1. Solar Radiation Spectrum A; Low Temperature Radiator, B.

tures near +20°C with seasonal means of +10° and +30°C. Day to night variations of temperature in most localities may be less than temperature changes due to the local weather, thus indicating the great stability of temperature provided by the influences of the atmosphere and the large water areas. The sun's radiation which reaches the Earth's surface (see Figure 1) is filtered by atmospheric absorption of the infrared radiation (beyond 3μ) and the ultraviolet and x-radiation. The visible and near

infrared radiation which is absorbed at the Earth's surface is converted largely into heat and a part of this heat is re-radiated back
to space as infrared radiation with a maximum near 10μ.   However, as the water vapor and CO_2 in the atmosphere absorb
strongly in the far infrared, most of this heat is retained during the
night when sun is not shining This "greenhouse" effect tends to
prevent large temperature swings from day to night except in very

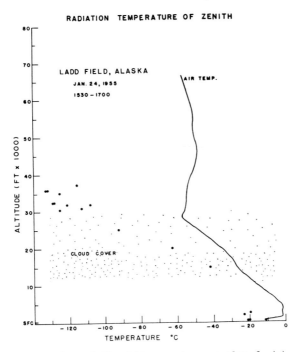

Fig. 2.   Sky and Cloud Temperatures at Altitude ($\cdot$).

arid regions or at high altitude where water vapor content of the
air is reduced.   The effects of cloud layers in reducing radiation
heat loss are seen in Figure 2.   The radiant temperature (equivalent black body temperature) of the Earth's surface, the clouds
and the sky were measured with a radiometer as the aircraft
climbed to 40,000 ft.   The dry bulb temperature recorded by radio
sonde balloon is shown for comparison.   In general the thermal

environment on the Earth is characterized by the water vapor and winds, although in very arid areas such as dry deserts, radiations from the sun and to the sky become important and give one an impression of what it may be like without the protection of the Earth's atmosphere. For example, the climate of San Francisco may be compared to that of Death Valley, or Oslo with Fairbanks.

Space: It has been estimated that the temperature of interstellar dust and hydrogen in equilibrium with the dilute interstellar radiation is of the order of 100°K.[1] Knowledge of this temperature is not complete and temperature lower than this estimated value is possible. In space near the Earth, the sun's radiation is the important heat source. The sun has an irradiance of 2.00 gm cal/sec/cm² outside the Earth's atmosphere,[1a] and this intense radiant-heat falling on the skin is about that which will stimulate pain sensation.[2] Thus, even if it were not for the requirement to protect man from the effects of the high vacuum of the space environment, the radiant heat load would necessitate protection. The radiant heat load will be almost twice this great outside of the Venusian atmosphere and near the planet Mercury about seven times as great as that near the Earth. Thermal radiation from the sun in the neighborhood of Mercury falling on the unprotected skin would cause a skin burn in

TABLE I

Planet	Mean Distance from Sun (millions of miles)	Heat Load Kgcal/m²/hr	Basal Metabolic Rates*
Mercury	36	7950	199
Venus	67	2280	57
Earth	93	1190	30
Earth's surface	—	0–956**	24
Mars	142	510	13
Jupiter	483	42	1

* BMR = 40 kgcal/m²/hr (figures have been rounded to nearest whole number).
** Death Valley during August.

less than a minute. The magnitude of the radiant heat load for the nearby planets in terms of the energy received on a totally absorbing surface normal to the sun's rays is given in Table I.

It is seen that shading or cooling will have to be provided for the astronaut in the space environment near the Earth or Moon and that this problem will be greater as one goes nearer the sun. Of course, the astronaut will be surrounded by the very low radiant temperature of outer space and thus there is a heat sink into which he can pour a great deal of the heat that he absorbs.

Moon: The surface temperature of the moon on the dark side has been estimated at $-125°C$ and on the sunny side at $+100°C$. This latter temperature together with the direct and reflected radiation from the sun will pose a heat problem of major but not impossible proportions. The moon has no water surfaces or atmosphere and thus the radiation to the sky from the moon will assist in the heat loss problem but there will be no cooling by convection currents of air and temperature changes will occur very rapidly with changes in sunlight.

The Planets: In the foreseeable future the Earth Astronaut will not penetrate further than the planets Mars and Venus. The temperature on Venus has been reported as near $800°C$ based on measurements in the radio-frequency spectrum. If this should turn out to be the case, manned exploration of the planet's surface will be most difficult because of the heat. Manned expeditions to Mercury are probably excluded because of heat loads. The Martian icecaps which change with the season may be of carbon dioxide ($-78°C$) and crystals of CO_2 may be responsible for the bluish haze which is sometimes observed. Mars appears to have no oceans and to be subject to violent dust storms. The thermal problem of the astronaut exploring Mars may be one of supplying heat rather than losing heat.

HEAT TRANSFER

The human body exchanges heat with the environment through four main channels, i.e., radiation, conduction, convection and vaporization, and in the micro-climate of the body surface these thermal exchange channels will continue to operate in space. The general equation of heat transfer can be written as the algebraic sum of the factors involved.[3]

$$H_L = H_R + H_C + H_D + H_V \tag{1}$$

in which

H_L = heat loss or gain
H_R = radiant heat loss
H_C = convective heat loss
H_D = conductive heat loss
H_V = evaporative heat loss

Depending upon the direction of heat flow, the quantities may be either positive or negative but are generally considered to be positive when the transfer of heat is from the body surface into the environment. As man must live in thermal equilibrium with his environment (except for small short-term transients which must be adjusted for) the heat balance equation can be stated as:

$$H_p - H_L = S \tag{2}$$

in which

H_p = heat production within the body
S = body heat storage (positive when body is gaining heat)

Heat balance requires that $S = 0$ over any extended period although under extreme physiological conditions body heat storage can fluctuate ± 300 kcal in a 70 kg man.

Heat production in man may be estimated most easily by measurement of the oyxgen consumption although CO_2 production is also sometimes used. The generalized equation for heat production can be written from a consideration of the food which man burns, as follows:

$$\left.\begin{array}{l}\text{Carbohydrate}\\\text{Protein}\\\text{Fat}\end{array}\right\} + O_2 \rightarrow CO_2 + H_2O + \text{Heat} + \text{Work} \tag{3}$$

At rest, the heat produced can be taken to be 40 ± 4 kgcal/m²/hr for normal man and 33 ± 3 kgcal/m²/hr for the normal woman. Thus, for the 70 kg man of 1.9 m² body surface area, the daily resting heat production will be 1824 kcal. The maximum heat production of which a man is capable depends on the degree of athletic training but is roughly twenty times the resting level for short periods of time (5–10 min); work at the rate of three to five times the resting metabolism can be performed for many hours without difficulty. The space environment may affect the amount of useful work which a man can do because of alterations in temperature, gravitational field, clothing restrictions, etc., but the associated heat loads must be eliminated from the body surface as they occur to prevent excessive body heat storage. The physiological factors which limit thermal exposure are discussed later in this chapter, the subject of body heat production being introduced at this point to indicate its importance in heat transfer problems.

RADIATION OF HEAT

By radiation in this sense is meant the exchange of thermal energy between objects in the form of electromagnetic energy and this process depends quantitatively only upon the temperature of the various exchanging objects and their abilities to absorb or radiate. The flow of heat by radiation does not require the presence of an intervening medium between the radiators and receivers and thus heat will pass by the process of radiation from a hot object to a cooler one through a vacuum. Two objects in equilibrium as regards the radiation transfer of heat can be said to be at the same temperature; in many respects temperature can be thought of as the property of matter which determines the direction of heat flow. Inasmuch as the radiant transfer of heat takes place through a vacuum, it is this mode of heat loss and heat gain which will be of greatest importance in the space environment and on the surfaces of the moon or other celestial objects having little or no atmosphere. The problem of maintaining a proper thermal environment for the astronaut in space will, to a great degree, revolve about the manipulation of the heat gains and losses by radiation.

Figure 1 shows the relative positions in the electromagnetic spectrum of the sun's radiation and the radiation from the hu-

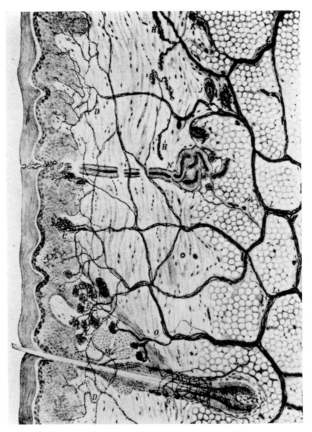

Fig. 3.   Cross-section of human epidermis.

man skin.   The sun's infrared radiation is almost entirely absorbed by the Earth's atmospheric CO_2 and water vapor before
it reaches sea level.   Ozone, water vapor and particulate matter
suspended in the atmosphere also contribute to the attenuation
of the sun's rays and greatly increase the scattering of solar radiation.   As solar radiation, including its infrared radiation, from
which we are normally screened, is so important throughout
the space environment in the solar system, the physiological
effects of this thermal radiation will be discussed in some detail.
    The capacity of solar radiation in producing changes in skin
temperature and in skin blood flow, as well as in evoking sensa-

tions of warmth and pain depend upon the optical and the thermal properties of human skin.

Figure 3 is a cross-section of the human epidermis, showing the general complexity of the structure. The skin has variable thickness over different parts of the body; the thickness shown in the illustration is roughly 1.5 mm. From the point of view of heat exchange, the skin is an extremely non-homogeneous substance and this is an important factor in the study of those optical and thermal properties of the skin which determine heating by radiation.

Optical Properties of the Skin: In a study of the effects of solar radiation on the skin, a first question concerns the reflectance and transmittance of the skin. Until these data are available, quantitative evaluations cannot be made of the heating and stimulating effects of sunlight.

Figure 4 shows the reflection curves for white and dark negro skin. The reflectivity of the skin has been studied from the ultraviolet clear through the far infrared.[4] From 3 to 20μ the

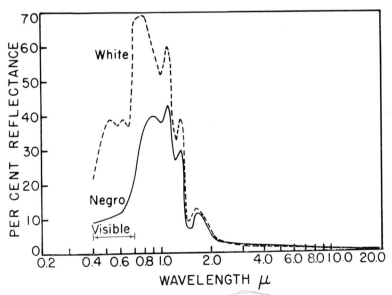

Fig. 4. Average values of spectral reflectance for white and dark negro skin.

reflectivity is low, approximately 1 per cent. Between 0.4 and
2μ the reflectivity is variable, depending to a great extent upon
pigmentation as well as skin blood flow. The maximum of reflectivity occurs at about $0.8–1.2\mu$. It is clear, from the reflection
curves, that the darkly pigmented individual will be heated more
by the direct radiation from the sun than the white individual
so far as his exposed skin surfaces are concerned. The difference between the white and dark individual is, of course, mini-

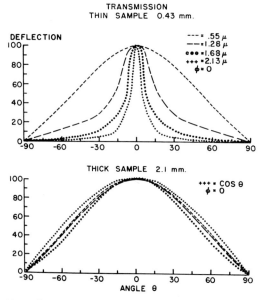

Fig. 5. Scattering of transmitted energy by
human skin. Normalized goniometric readings
in the zero altitude plane ($\phi = 0$) as a function
of azimuth angle θ measured from a line normal
through the sample.

mized by the effects of clothing. On the other hand, the stimulating effects of high intensity infrared rays may be significantly
less for the white than for the darkly pigmented individual.

A second important optical factor is the penetration of the
radiation into the skin surface. Because of its inhomogeneity,
the skin will scatter transmitted radiation. This effect is shown

in Figure 5, which is a study of the transmission of two samples of excised skin. The top of the figure shows the transmission through a thin sample for wavelengths 0.55 and 2.13μ as plotted on a goniometric spectrometer. If the skin were perfectly diffuse, such as a thick piece of paper, the transmitted radiation would follow the Cosine Law for all wavelengths. However, according to Rayleigh's Law, scattering is proportional to the inverse fourth power of the wavelength; thus, one would

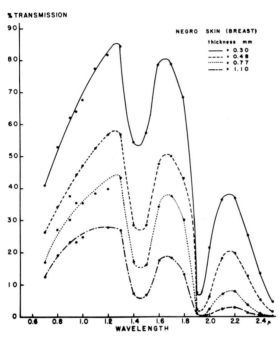

Fig. 6. Spectral distribution of total transmitted energy (as a percentage of the incident energy) as a function of skin thickness.

expect the shorter wavelengths to be scattered more than the longer wavelengths. This effect is shown at the top of Figure 5; the energy at 0.55μ is scattered diffusely, whereas the energy at 2μ penetrates almost directly through the thin specimen. As seen in the lower part of the figure, these differences due to wavelength largely disappear with greater thicknesses of skin.

The transmission spectrum of a specimen of white skin is shown in Figure 6 and indicates major absorption bands at 1.4, 1.9 and 2.4μ.

Absorption of light by the skin depends not only upon skin and blood pigments and other substances which absorb specific spectral bands, but also upon the degree of scattering action due to the microstructure of the skin. The absorption bands shown in Figure 6 are due to water, which is the principal absorber in biological tissues for infrared radiation. The skin is essentially opaque beyond 2.6μ. However, significant amounts of near infrared radiation penetrate considerable distances below the skin

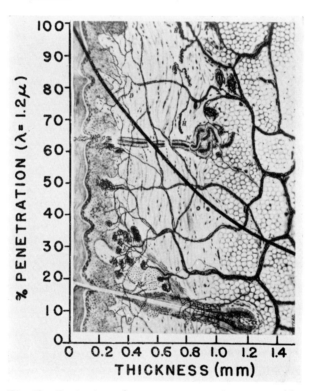

Fig. 7. Projection of average penetration curve (determined as per cent of energy in the incident beam which is not reflected) upon a schematic representation of skin tissues.

surface. The wavelength having the greatest penetrating power is 1.2μ. Figure 7 shows the average penetration of this energy below the skin surface for both negro and white skin. This illustration is schematic because the thickness of the layers varies greatly. However, at least 50 per cent of the radiation penetrates to a depth of 0.8 mm and thus interacts directly with nerve endings and small blood vessels. Partly as the result of scatter-

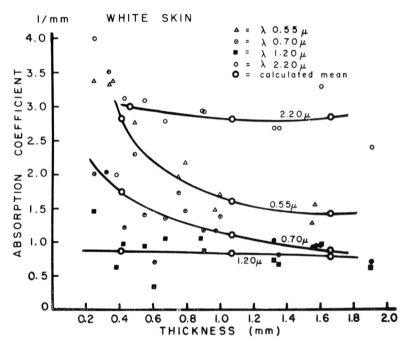

Fig. 8.   Absorption coefficients for white human skin.

ing action and partly because the several skin layers may absorb differently, the absorption coefficients for the skin are not constant as a function of skin thickness.

In Figure 8, the absorption coefficients are plotted as a function of skin thickness. For infrared radiation, the absorption coefficients are approximately constant. For visible radiation, the absorption coefficients increase the nearer one approaches the skin surface. The pigment layers lie near the surface. The accurate calculation of the penetration of radiation into the skin thus becomes difficult for sources emitting in the visible and near infrared. However, considering the complexity of the skin, it is perhaps not surprising that this complication exists. Also, for many purposes, an average absorption coefficient of about 2 reciprocal mm can be used.

Thermal Characteristics of the Skin: Changes in skin temperature caused by high intensity infrared radiation depend not only on the optical properties of the skin but also upon the thermal conductivity, density and specific heat of the living skin. With

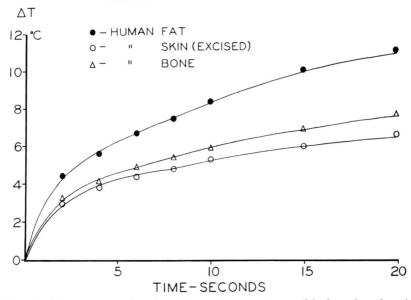

Fig. 9. Temperature elevation of some human tissues (blackened surfaces) during exposure to 0.04 gm-cal/cm² sec of thermal radiation.

the development of a dependable method for measuring skin temperature before and during exposure to known intensities of radiation, it became feasible to apply the theory of heat flow to the problem of skin heating. For non-penetrating radiation the relationship can be expressed as follows:

$$T_s - T_o = \Delta T = \frac{2Q\alpha\sqrt{t}}{\sqrt{\pi K \rho c}} \qquad (4)$$

and

$$K\rho c = \frac{1.13Q^2 t}{\Delta T^2} \tag{5}$$

In these equations,

T_s = final skin temperature
T_o = initial skin temperature
Q = radiation intensity
t = time in seconds
K = thermal conductivity
ρ = density
c = specific heat
α = absorptivity (0.94 for skin blackened with India ink)

The product $K\rho c$ will determine the temperature elevation of the skin or other tissue upon exposure to non-penetrating radiation. Figure 9 shows the surface temperature elevations caused by irradiating the blackened surface of specimens of human skin, fat and bone. The difference in heating rates is due to the differ-

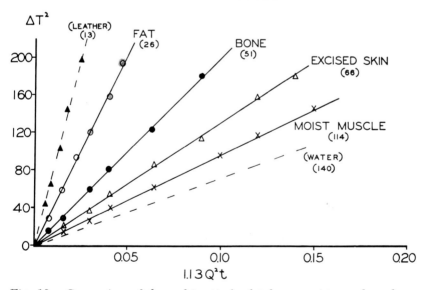

Fig. 10. Comparison of thermal inertia for fat, bone, moist muscle and excised skin, as compared with leather and water.

ence in the $K\rho c$ products for the different tissues. Fatty tissue, because of its relatively low specific heat, is heated considerably more rapidly than either moist skin or bone.

From this experiment, the $K\rho c$ values can be determined by plotting ΔT^2 against $1.13Q^2t$, as shown in Figure 10. In the brackets for each curve are the values for the $K\rho c$ product for the specific specimen ($\times 10^{-5}$). Comparing leather and water with body tissues suggests that the thermal inertia values depend to a large extent on the water content of the tissues.

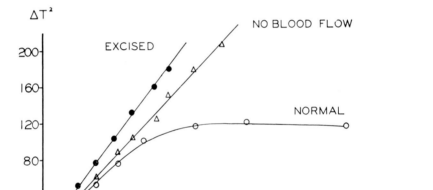

Fig. 11.   Thermal inertias of excised, bloodless and normal living skin.

Living tissues do not conform strictly to the simple mathematical formula outlined above. Figure 11 shows a comparison of excised skin with living skin with its normal blood flow and with the blood flow occluded. For short exposure times, the $K\rho c$ of normal skin is the same as that in which the blood flow has been stopped; excised skin heats more rapidly due to unavoidable dehydration which occurs post-mortem. However, for longer exposures to thermal radiation, skin blood flow increases through vasodilatation and serves to cool the skin. This important physiological response can be observed as early as 20 sec after the beginning of an exposure, but may be delayed for as long as several minutes, depending upon the initial state of the skin blood vessels. For the first 20 sec of irradiation, the skin with normally constricted blood vessels can be considered to have a $K\rho c$ value of 110–130 $\times$ 10^{-5} cal²/cm⁴/sec/C²; in hot environments $K\rho c$ values as large as 400×10^{-5} may be measured.

HEATING SKIN by SOLAR RADIATION

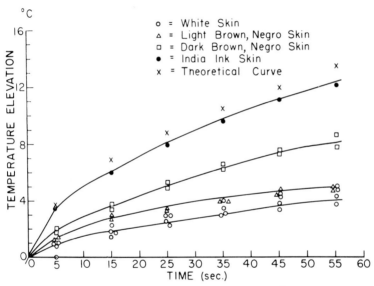

Fig. 12. Heating of the skin by solar radiation.

Heating of the skin by the sun involves all of the optical and thermal properties of the skin which have been discussed. For example, measurements were made of skin heating using sunlight which had passed through clear plate glass. The studies were made on clear days during the summer in Philadelphia, and it is seen (see Figure 12) that the white and light brown negro skin are heated least and to about the same extent. Some of the white subjects had sun-tanned skins and others did not. The dark negro skin is heated about twice as rapidly as the pale white skin, a result which is not unexpected, considering the high absorption of the negro skin for near infrared and visible radiation. The curve for skin blackened with India ink shows, however, that even dark negro skin is far from black. The rate of heating predicted from the equation is shown at the top by the x's using a value of $K\rho c$ of 100×10^{-5} cal^2/cm^4/sec/C^2. From this, it can be concluded that the heating of the skin by infra-red radiation is accounted for completely by simple heat flow theory and physiologic changes in skin blood flow.

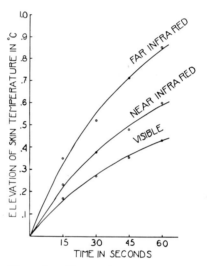

Fig. 13.   Skin surface temperature elevation produced by the same incident intensities of far infrared (λ = 3–20 μ); near infrared (λ = 0.8–3 μ) and visible (λ = 0.4–0.7 μ) radiation.

Inasmuch as pigment makes a significant difference in the heating of the skin, it is worthwhile studying the effects of the visible, near infrared, and far infrared separately. Figure 13 shows the skin temperature elevations produced by irradiating the white skin with the same intensity of visible, near infrared and far infrared radiation. Due to the differences in the spectral reflectivity and penetration, it is seen that the far infrared is much more effective in raising the skin temperature whereas visible radiation is least effective.

Effect of Infra-red Radiation in Evoking the Sensation of Warmth: If careful measurements are made of the skin temperature while the subject is sitting quietly in a darkened room at a comfortable and neutral temperature, and if the subject is asked to introspect and report upon his thermal sensations at specific intervals (say every 10 or 15 sec), it will be found, first, that the skin temperature is not constant but fluctuates spontaneously. These fluctuations are small (see top, Figure 14), usually less than 0.2 C, and are probably due to small changes in skin blood flow.

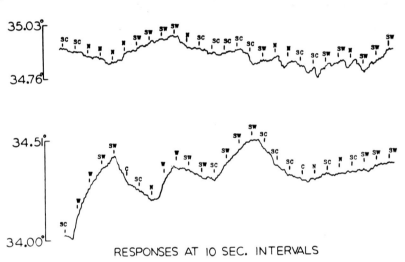

RESPONSES AT 10 SEC. INTERVALS

Fig. 14. Spontaneous fluctuations in skin temperature and the effect of weak thermal radiation in stimulating thermal sensation.

It will be found, secondly, that the subject continually reports thermal sensations other than neutral, such as slightly warm (SW) or slightly cool (SC). These sensory reports can be related to the skin temperature changes, since the subject will tend to report slightly cool with falling skin temperature and slightly warm with rising temperature. A generally neutral thermal environment is thus not one in which there is absence of temperature sensation, but a condition in which the subject will report slightly cool, slightly warm and neutral about one-third of the time each.

In such a situation, if a weak infrared radiation is projected on the skin, raising the skin temperature 0.4–0.5°C, definite sensations of warmth will be reported (see lower part of Figure 14) and the cycling frequency and amplitude of skin temperature are

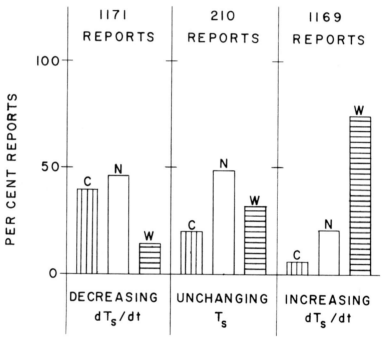

Fig. 15. Relation of skin temperature change to thermal sensation in the zone of thermal neutrality.

increased, being damped out after a few minutes. Thermal sensations become more distinct with reports of warm (W) alternating with cool (C). The warmth stimulus, i.e., infrared radiation, thus produces both warmth and coolness in the individual and these sensations will be in phase with skin temperature fluctuations. Not much is known about this stimulating action of infrared radiation. An analysis of these data is shown in Figure 15, in which the reports of sensation are categorized as to whether the skin temperature is decreasing, unchanging or increasing.

When there is little change in skin temperature, the subjects report with about equal frequency slight warmth, slight coolness and neutral. This result is not surprising since it is known that the temperature receptors in the skin are in continuous activity and change their activity with slight changes in skin temperature.

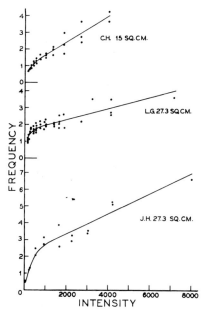

Fig. 16. Fusion frequency (flashes per sec of infra-red radiation) vs intensity of radiation in gram cal/sec/ $cm^2 \times 10^{-5}$.

From Figure 15 it can be seen that when the skin temperature falls slightly (0.001°C/sec) there is a marked diminution in the reports of warmth but an increase in the reports of cool and neutral. When the skin temperature is increased slightly, there is a marked increase in warmth reports, and a marked diminution in cold and neutral statements.

Rate of change of skin temperature is thus an important factor in the perception of warmth, or coolness; skin temperature level also has a stimulating effect, but to a lesser degree.   Factors which are important in the stimulation of sensation by infrared are: a) the size of skin area exposed, b) the intensity of the radiation, c) the color of the skin, d) the level of skin temperature and e) the time of exposure.

An additional factor with regard to temperature sensation should be pointed out.   The skin, due to its natural acuteness in the perception of temperature change, is extremely responsive to cycling of infrared radiation.   If a beam of infrared radiation is projected onto the face and cycled on and off, the subject will feel alternate pulses of warmth and cooling.   If the cycle frequency is increased, there will be a fusing of the sensation into a continuous feeling of warmth.   Figure 16 shows the fusion frequencies for warmth sensation for three subjects as a function of radiation intensity.   In general, the higher the radiation flux onto the face, the higher will be the fusion frequency and, as shown in Figure 16, a frequency of 4–7 cps may be perceived.   The phasic sensation of warmth, which results from perception of temperature change, dies away at between $1/2$ and $1/10$ cycle.

Heat transfer in the space environment will be due to the thermal radiation exchange between the surface of the astronaut's space suit or cabin and the sun, the low temperature space at $125°K$,[6] and the moon or planet surface.   The sun's radiation is "high temperature" and the other thermal radiation exchanges will be "low temperature" (see Figure 1).   Thus, the heat produced by the man in his suit will necessarily have to be balanced by the heat losses and gains from the outside, that is,

Heat production = heat loss to environment — heat gain from sun

If the astronaut's suit has a radiating surface area of two square meters, one can estimate the surface temperature of the suit with the astronaut operating outside of his space capsule, on the moon's surface while exposed to the sun and to the low temperature radiation of outer space.   Assuming moderate activity of 240 kgcal/hr, which is roughly equivalent to walking at 3 mph, the equations can be arranged as follows:

Heat loss to low temperature space $= S_o \epsilon_1 \epsilon_2 (T_{cl}{}^4 - T_\infty{}^4) \times A$ (6)

in which:

S_o = Stephan-Boltzman constant $= 4.93 \times 10^{-8}$ kgcal/m^2/hr/T^4
ϵ_1 = emissivity of the space suit for low temp. radiation
ϵ_2 = emissivity of the space environment $= 1$
T_{cl} = absolute surface temperature of the space suit
T_∞ = temperature of space in degrees absolute $= 125°K^6$
A = radiating surface area

Heat gain from sun $= H\epsilon_3 A' + H\epsilon_3 (1 - \epsilon_4)A$ (7)
$\qquad\qquad\qquad$ = Direct radiation + reflected radiation from moon's surface

in which: *or absorbtivity ?*

H = radiant flux from sun $= 1200$ kgcal/m^2/hr
ϵ_3 = emissivity of the space suit for sunlight
A' = area of suit exposed to sun $= A/4$, roughly, but has been experimentally determined for the clothed walking man as 0.62 m^{2,7}
ϵ_4 = absorptivity of lunar surface for solar radiation $= 0.9$

Also, the heat gain from or loss to the lunar landscape $= S_o\epsilon_1\epsilon_4 (T_{cl}{}^4 -T_L{}^4)A$ in which T_L = temperature of the lunar surface in degrees absolute $= 373°K$ in sunshine. If it be assumed that the astronaut is wearing a black suit which absorbs all the solar radiation falling on it and radiates as a perfect black body to outer space, then the thermal balance can be written as

Metabolic heat production $= Q_m = S_o\epsilon_1\epsilon_2(T_{cl}{}^4 - T_\infty{}^4)A$ (7a)
$\qquad - \epsilon_3 HA' - \epsilon_3 (1 - \epsilon_4)HA - S_o\epsilon_1\epsilon_4 (T_{cl}{}^4 - T_L{}^4)A$

and

$$\epsilon_1 = \epsilon_3 = 1$$

We can get an idea of the possible heat load on the man if we solve the above equation for T_{cl}, the temperature of the surface of the suit on the assumption that the astronaut is walking in the sunshine at a moderate pace over the lunar terrain. The results of this calculation are given in the first line of Table II which shows that the suit will heat up to 81°C (the temperature of piping hot coffee) which is not compatible with human life for any extended period. Should the man stop walking but remain in the sun, the situation would not be greatly improved as his suit temperature would decrease only 4°C. If the astronaut were to

TABLE II*

HEAT BALANCE AND AMBIENT (CLOTHING) TEMPERATURE OF MAN WALKING OR STANDING ON SURFACE OF THE MOON DURING A LUNAR DAY

Case	Exposure Condition	Heat Balance, kg-cal/m²/hr					Ambient Temp. °C
		Heat Gain by—				Heat Loss by Radiation to Space (Q_∞)	
		Metabolism (Q_M)	Direct Radiation from Sun (Q_H)	Reflected Radiation from Moon Surface (Q_P)	Re-emitted Radiation from Moon Surface (Q_L)		
A-1	Walking 3 mph; unshaded; dark suit ($\epsilon_1 = \alpha_3 = 1$)	240	738	238	309	1526	81
A-2	Same as A-1 except standing	80	738	238	385	1441	77
A-3	Same as A-2 except shaded	80	0	238	736	1054	51
B-1	Walking 3 mph; unshaded; reflective suit ($\epsilon_1 = \alpha_3 = 0.1$)	240	74	24	−73	265	134
B-2	Same as B-1 except standing	80	74	24	4	182	98
B-3	Same as B-2 except shaded	80	0	24	39	143	76
C-1	Walking 3 mph; unshaded; white suit ($\epsilon_1 = 0.8$, $\alpha_3 = 0.2$)	240	148	48	505	941	59
C-2	Same as C-1 except standing	80	148	48	578	854	52
C-3	Same as C-2 except shaded	80	0	48	647	775	45

* The Author wishes to express his appreciation to Mr. George Rapp for calculating these values.

shield himself from the direct rays of the sun (with a parasol!) a great improvement would be realized, but the sun's reflected radiation from the surrounding lunar landscape and the emitted radiation from the lunar surface would be so great as to heat the suit to 51°C. With sufficient sweat evaporation the astronaut could spend several hours at this temperature but the physiological stress would be extreme. The hot deserts of the Earth reach 50°C during the heat of the day on occasion. Situation B-1 indicates what might be expected if the astronaut's suit were highly polished so as to reflect 90 per cent of the sun's heat and the heat from the moon's surface. In spite of this great advantage, the astronaut would be even worse off than in the black suit because on the moon there would be no convection heat losses due to cooling breezes from the lunar oceans, and the man could not lose heat by radiation because of the low radiating power of his suit. Thus, his suit temperature would rise to 134° or 34°C above the boiling point of water! The best situation is provided by a pure white suit which is highly reflecting in the visible spectrum (sunlight) but is black and radiates well in the infrared. These conditions C-1, C-2 and C-3 are compatible with life for at least short periods of hours and by moving into a crater shadow could be tolerated for even longer periods. To explore the moon's surface during a lunar day will, in any case, be an exercise in heat tolerance. From Table II the following inferences may be drawn for the lunar day:

1. Man, standing or walking on the surface of the moon during a lunar day, will be exposed to ambient (clothing) temperatures ranging from 45° to 134°C—dependent on type of protective material worn, his specific work level (80–240 kgcal/m^2/hr) and whether or not he is shielded from the direct rays of the sun.

2. The type of clothing is the most important single factor; and highly reflective (polished metal) suits having low blackbody emissivity will produce temperatures (76–134°C) that are above the human tolerance ceiling for practicable working durations.

3. The most favorable (lowest) suit temperatures (45–59°C) will be obtained with *white* suits or materials having, similarly, high blackbody ($\lambda = 9$–10μ) emissivity and low solar absorptivity. These temperatures, approximately 50 per cent lower than those with reflective suits and about 10–30 per cent lower than black suits, are below the human tolerance ceiling for practicable working durations.
4. Shielding, or shading from direct rays of the sun, is second in effectiveness; and for a resting (standing) man, temperature reductions on the order of 13–34 per cent are indicated, the precise amount dependent on clothing type.
5. Body heat gain by absorption of solar radiation reflected from the lunar surface amounts to about one-third of the direct incident radiation from the sun.
6. The equivalent environmental or mean radiant temperature (*MRT*) of the moon during the lunar "day" for man (wearing white or dark clothing, walking or standing, shielded or unshielded from direct sun's rays) covers the approximate range 36–72°C (97–162°F).

In orbit about the Earth or on a space voyage between the Earth and the moon, the thermal exchanges can be calculated using equation 7a. For example, if the astronaut in a black suit were working outside of his space capsule making repairs or adjustments, requiring approximately the same effort as walking, and at the same time exposed to the sunlight, his heat balance would be (neglecting effects from the Earth and moon),

$$Q_m = Q_\infty - Q_H$$

or

$$240 = 4.93 \times 10^8 (T_{cl}^4 - \overline{125^4}) \times 2 - 738$$

From this, the suit temperature is $T_{cl} = 305°$K or 32°C. In this situation the suit temperature would be in the neutral range for the resting man. If the man stopped work for a while his suit temperature would tend to fall towards +16°C. If he moved into the shadow of his space craft, his suit surface temperature would tend towards −115°C, depending upon his activity level. On the other hand, in a highly polished suit ($\epsilon_1 = \epsilon_3 = 0.1$) the sun's rays would be reflected but the suit would not radiate to the space environment and thereby eliminate the astronaut's metabolic heat. Thus, with 240 kgcal/hr output from the man, the space suit would tend towards 467°C with the man in the sun, and even with a quiet man (80 kgcal/hr) the suit temperature would still heat up towards 340°C. A polished suit is not habitable in space for any length of time except in a shadow when the suit would tend towards +27°C for the quiet man. A white suit which reflects most of the sun's rays ($\epsilon_3 = 0.2$) and radiates well in the infrared low temperature region ($\epsilon_1 = 0.8$) would tend towards −12°C for an activity level of 240 kgcal/hr and would be much like a black suit otherwise.

The above examples are presented to illustrate the degree of temperature control that can be obtained by changing the emissivity values of the suit surface and the bodily activity of the man. By means of thermal radiation panels on his suit or cabin the man in space should be able to adjust his temperature rapidly. However, large and rapid changes in temperature will characterize the situation in which air convection and water masses are absent.

HEAT TRANSFER BY CONDUCTION

The flow of heat through a solid, liquid or gaseous medium without the physical transfer of material is called thermal conduction. Within the human body heat is conducted through the tissues to the skin surface and from the skin into any cooler objects with which the body may be in contact. The heat lost from the clothed body is largely conducted through the thin air layers between the skin and clothing, and through the fibers of the clothing layers. The nature of the contact of the skin with different objects is important when considering the amount of heat conducted into or out of the body. This is apparent to one who touches a cold smooth surface and compares this sensation to that from contact with a rough surface at the same temperature. In the same way, it is apparent that some objects conduct heat more readily than others, and further, that the greater the temperature difference, the greater the heat loss.

In a medium with uniform physical properties, the amount of

heat which flows from a warm area to a cool one is a function of
the length of the path, the nature of the medium, and the thermal
gradient. The equation for heat conduction in the steady state is

$$H_D = \frac{KA(T_2 - T_1)}{d} \times t, \text{ gm cal} \qquad (8)$$

where

H_D	= quantity of heat conducted
K	= thermal conductivity, a constant which depends upon the material
A	= area of the conducting surfaces
T_2 and T_1	= temperatures of the warm and cool surfaces
t	= time
d	= thickness of the conductor

This formula has been applied to the problem of the conduction
of heat from the interior of the body to the skin. On the basis of
computation Lefevre, Burton and others have arrived at the value
of $K = 0.0005$ gm/cm/sec/°C for the average thermal conductivity constant of human tissues. Experiments have yielded the
values 0.00097 and 0.00049 for the thermal conductivities of
muscle and fat tissue, respectively. Tables of thermal conductivities can be found for many substances in handbooks, and the following values are quoted only for comparative purposes:

Silver	0.99 gm cal/cm/sec/°C
Glass	0.0025 gm cal/cm/sec/°C
Soft wood	0.0003 gm cal/cm/sec/°C
Leather (tanned)	0.004 gm cal/cm/sec/°C
Cotton wool	0.00004 gm cal/cm/sec/°C
Air	0.000057 gm cal/cm/sec/°C
Water	0.001 gm cal/cm/sec/°C

It can be seen that muscle and fat tissue are among the substances
having low thermal conductivities, being a thousand times smaller
than silver and only ten times greater than cotton wool and dead
air. When the peripheral blood vessels of normal men are fully
constricted, between 9 and 10 kgcal/m²/hr/°C (rectal tempera-
ture-skin temperature) are conducted through the body tissues.
This insulation corresponds to a layer of tissue 18 to 22 mm in
thickness. For young women the thickness is even greater, being
about 24 mm.

If we consider three serial insulating layers of clothing through which body heat is flowing, the total thermal resistance or insulation will be

$$\frac{1}{K} = \frac{d_1}{k_1 A_1} + \frac{d_2}{k_2 A_2} + \frac{d_3}{k_3 A_3} \tag{9}$$

and the over-all thermal conductance, as the inverse of the insulation, is

$$K = \frac{1}{\dfrac{d_1}{k_1 A_1} + \dfrac{d_2}{k_2 A_2} + \dfrac{d_3}{k_3 A_3}} \text{ gm cal/sec/}^\circ\text{C} \tag{10}$$

Should the layers be in parallel,

$$K = \frac{k_1 A_1}{d_1} + \frac{k_2 A_2}{d_2} + \frac{k_3 A_3}{d_3} \text{ gm cal/sec/}^\circ\text{C} \tag{11}$$

The above type of calculation can be made to determine the effectiveness of the insulation afforded by clothing. The insulating value of clothing is often expressed in "*clo*" units[2] for practical purposes. The total insulation of a clothing assembly can be expressed as the sum of the individual insulative values from the skin out, as

$$I = I_a + I_{cl} \tag{12}$$

in which I_a is the insulation of the still air around the man, and I_{cl} is the clothing insulation. The ordinary business suit is assumed to have 1 *clo* insulation. Thus, if the heat loss by conduction be 38 kcal/m²/hr and the skin temperature 33°C at a comfortable room temperature of 21°C, then

$$\frac{H_D}{A} = 38 = \frac{K}{d}(T_2 - T_1) = \frac{1}{I}(T_s - T_1),$$

or $I_{cl} = 0.32 - I_a$

The best value for I_a as determined from experiment is 0.19°C/kcal/hr/m². Thus,

$$I_{cl} = \frac{I - I_a}{0.13} \text{ } clo \text{ units} \tag{13}$$

In the space environment insulation will be of the greatest importance in smoothing out the large changes in heat loss and heat gain that can occur with shifts of radiant heat loads. The time required for the development of a steady state after an abrupt disturbance is

$$t = \lambda I / (\rho c)$$

in which I is the insulation and ρc the volume heat capacity, and λ a constant. Thus, the larger the value of I, the longer the adjustment time for the same heat capacity. In space flight it is important to keep the mass down and this can be accomplished by increasing the insulation to provide a satisfactory time constant. Natural insulators such as fox fur (6–7 *clo*) provide the lightest and highest insulation values.

HEAT TRANSFER BY CONVECTION

Convection refers to the exchange of heat between hot and cold objects by the physical transfer of matter such as liquid or gas molecules with which the objects are in contact. This type of heat transfer depends upon the existence of a moving medium between the warm and cold objects and upon the actual streaming movement of warm molecules from the warm object to the cooler one. The transport of heat by such streams (convection) is to be distinguished from heat conduction through a gas or liquid, which is the type of heat transfer in which there is no streaming and in which the molecules of the medium remain essentially in their original locations, passing the heat energy from one to another by molecular vibration and collisions. The cooling of a surface with an electric fan is an example of *forced convection*, whereas the cooling by air rising about the warm skin surface is called "*natural*" convection. Natural and forced convection can contribute to heat transfer at the same time.

Natural Convection: In streamline flow the velocity of a fluid flowing across a surface or through a pipe varies from the side wall out, being highest away from the wall and approximately zero along the wall itself; that is, the gas molecules closest to the surface may be considered stuck or adsorbed to the wall, thus constituting a film of dead air. The importance of this film is seen in the transfer of heat across a thin metal plate separating a warm gas at temperature T_1, from a cold gas of temperature T_2. The two sides of the metal plate will be at nearly the same temperature, indicating a small flow of heat through the plate in spite of the plate's high thermal conductivity. The large temperature gradient T_1 − T_2, indicating a high insulation for the plate, is due mainly to the temperature drop across the stagnant air films (δ_0) in the immediate neighborhood of the plate, P. It is the low rate of conduction of heat through these films that forms the major portion of the heat barrier. The thickness of the air films will depend upon the temperature of the plate, velocity of the gas, the vis-

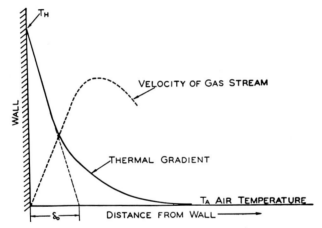

Fig. 17. A diagrammatic sketch of the convection loss from a hot wall, T_H, δ_0 marginal layer or *Grenzschicht*.

cosity of the gas and the gas density. The amount of heat carried through the film will depend upon the thermal conductivity of the gas and the thickness of the film and the temperature gradient. The transfer of heat from a solid to a liquid or gas can thus be visualized as being made up of two parts: 1) the conduction of heat through the surface layers of the gas, and 2) the transport of heat by the streams of molecules on the outside. This is illustrated in Figure 17 which shows a hot surface T_H in contact with a gas at a temperature T_A. The layer of gas next to the wall will be fixed to the surface so that it will not move, and the succeeding layers will partake increasingly of the convective streaming in an approximately linear fashion, the velocity increasing with distance from the wall until the maximum velocity is reached. The heat will therefore be transferred by pure conduction through the adsorbed layers of still air and will finally be transported away by streams of molecules which move faster and faster as they are removed from the surface.

Büttner[3] has called this surface layer the *Grenzschicht*, and the term *private climate* seems very appropriate. Büttner has made direct measurements of convection loss from spheres and cylinders as well as the human body. The formula for this case is

$$\frac{H_c}{A} = \frac{K(T_H - T_A)}{\delta_0} = K_c(T_H - T_A) \tag{14}$$

where

H_c = convection loss
K = thermal conductivity of air
A = *effective* surface area
T_H = average skin temperature
T_A = average air temperature
δ_0 = thickness of the surface layer
K_c = equivalent convective coefficient

All the quantities to the right of the equation are known except A and δ_0. To measure δ_0, the temperature gradient from the skin to the air is determined with a polished thermocouple mounted on a micrometer. Using this method, Büttner obtained values of δ_0 for different parts of the nude body while lying quietly on a hard surface which varied between 6 and 10 mm, depending on the temperature of the part. By proper weighting of the values for δ_0, he arrived at an average value for the thermal gradient,

$$\frac{T_H - T_A}{\delta_0} = 13.6°\text{C/cm}$$

Then

$H_c/A = 0.0035 \times 13.6 = 0.048 \text{ cal/cm}^2/\text{min} = 28.8 \text{ kgcal/m}^2/\text{hr}$
          or, an equivalent convective coefficient,
$K_c = 2.12 \text{ kgcal-cm/m}^2/\text{hr}/°\text{C}$

The methods for measuring A, the effective area for natural convection loss, have not been well worked out. Büttner assumed a value of about 80 per cent of the total area as the effective area for convection. Hardy and Soderstrom, by comparing the convection and radiation loss from nude men lying in the Russell Sage calorimeter with that from an elliptical cylinder, arrived at a value of about 75 per cent of the DuBois area for *A*. As *A* will depend upon the position of the man and his relation to his environment (for example, whether he is in bed or standing) its measurement is required for each circumstance.

Values for natural convection loss are quite variable as quoted in the literature, even for a nude subject sitting or lying motionless in almost still air. A few average values are given below:

Büttner........................2.12 kg cal-cm/m²/hr/°C
Winslow et al. (sitting subjects).....4.1–5.8 kg cal-cm/m²/hr/°C
Hardy and DuBois (men)..........0.85–1.40 kg cal-cm/m²/hr/°C
Hardy and Milhorat (women)......0.8–1.35 kg cal-cm/m²/hr/°C
Hardy (elliptical cylinder) ....0.6–0.8 kg cal-cm/m²/hr/°C

The slightest movement of the subject will increase the convection loss by stirring up air currents and by increasing the area effective in convection loss.

The variability of the convection constants and the difficulty of obtaining them makes it seem likely that convection will generally be measured not directly but by difference, as is the common practice.

Natural convection depends upon the movement of air of different densities under the action of gravity, cold air being heavier than warm air. In an acceleration-free space such as a space suit or capsule in orbit there will be no natural convection and thus the usual movement of air about the body will not take place. On the moon or in a rotating space station gravitational and acceleration fields will be weaker than on Earth and natural convection will be decreased correspondingly. Dependence for gaseous convection in space will be upon forced convection.

FORCED CONVECTION

By forced convection is meant all convection losses in excess of that natural minimum which is due to the rising of the gas or liquid

heated by the warm surface. Thus, the movement of the arms
and legs, whether the subject be walking or sitting, generates
forced convection. Generally speaking, for the quiet individual,
forced convection results from air or liquid streams generated by
outside forces. The relative velocity of the air stream with respect to the warm skin or clothing is the added variable which is
introduced when one considers forced convection as well as
natural convection in the total convective heat loss.

An analytical consideration of the basic concepts concerning
forced convection will lead to a statement of the factors upon
which this heat loss channel quantitatively depends. This dimen-
sional analysis considers the dependence of forced convection
upon the velocity of the air stream, the difference in temperature
between the gas and warm surface, air density, viscosity, etc.
That is,

$$H_c = f(K, V, \mu, \rho, \Delta T, D, C_p) \tag{15}$$

where

H_c = heat loss by convection, $cal/cm^2/min/°C$
f = the functional relationship which is not known a priori, but can
be determined from experiment
D = characteristic dimension of the object; for example, the diameter of a sphere or a cylinder
V = velocity of the gas
μ = viscosity
ρ = density
K = thermal conductivity
C_p = specific heat
ΔT = temperature difference between the warm surface and the air =
$T_s - T_a$

For convenience we can write $H_c = h_c \cdot A \cdot \Delta T$.

How these values can be combined to make the best formulation of h_c is a matter of experiment, and the final arrangement
which best fits both the experimental facts and theoretical considerations is

$$h_c = \frac{K}{D} [1 + a\frac{DV\rho^{1/2}}{\mu} + b\frac{DV\rho}{\mu}] \tag{16}$$

where *a* and *b* are constants depending upon the particular units
used. It is convenient to reduce irregularly shaped surfaces to

equivalent cylinders or spheres because most of the experimental work has been done on simple geometric forms. The convective heat losses from the nude man indicate that the adult human body loses heat like a cylinder 7 cm (3 in.) in diameter, or a sphere 15 cm in diameter, (a = 0.407; b = 0.00123).

h_cD/K is termed *Nusselt's Number* (*Nu*), and it can be seen that, neglecting free convection and the small last term, $b(DV\rho/\mu)$, one can write

$$Nu = a\,\frac{DV\rho^{1/2}}{\mu}$$

$DV\rho/\mu$ is called *Reynold's Number* (Re), so that

$$Nu = a\,Re^{1/2}$$

The usual method is now to plot Nusselt's number against Reynold's number and thus obtain the value of *a*. Büttner has done this for several velocity ranges and for spheres of several diameters, and finds a = 0.70, or

$$Nu = 0.70\,Re^{0.52}, \text{ if } V \text{ is greater than } 0.2 \text{ m/sec}$$

Applying the same methods to men lying on their backs on the floor, he arrived at

$$H_c = 0.021\ (V)^{1\ 2}\Delta T \text{ cal/cm}^2/\text{min} \tag{17}$$

for the human body.

The formula given above is valid only for a limited range of air velocities. Büttner extended his measurements to 10 m/sec and at about this velocity he found the relationship between Nusselt's and Reynold's numbers broke down, indicating turbulent flow.

EVAPORATION

The continual loss of weight from the body has been of interest to physiologists for about 300 years and the mass of experimental data that has been gathered by many workers under varied conditions has established the importance of this loss as a factor in the heat regulation of the body. F. G. Benedict[2] pointed out the usefulness of the fact observed by DuBois and Soderstrom;[2] namely, that about 25 per cent of the metabolic heat is carried away from the body by the water evaporated from the skin and lungs. The importance of the physiological control of the water evaporated from the skin has been repeatedly pointed out, and in the last twenty years the physical laws and physiological controls concerned with the loss of heat by evaporation from the body have been worked out.[2]

Although moisture is lost from both the skin and lungs, from a heat loss standpoint the former is the more important. Winslow et al measured the heat loss from the lungs of their subjects and obtained a value of 7 to 8 kgcal/hr, about 10 per cent of the total heat loss in the neutral temperature zone. This heat loss is dependent for the most part upon the respiration, and although it may vary considerably, it does not in general play so important a role in the heat loss regulation in man as it does in certain animals. Sweating from the skin is the important means of losing heat at elevated environmental temperature.

Büttner pointed out the importance of the amount of skin which can be considered wet and of the vapor pressure difference between saturated vapor at skin temperature and the vapor pressure of the environment. He proposed the following equation for the water loss from the skin:

$$W_V = A' \times C(E_s - E_a) \times f(VD) \; \text{gm/min} \qquad (18)$$

where

W_V = water loss by vaporization
A' = the wet area of the body (equals DuBois area for its maximum value)
C = 0.003 gm/min/cm Hg (proportionality factor)
E_s and E_a = vapor pressure of water vapor on the skin and in the air
$f(VD)$ = function of velocity V and the characteristic dimension of the body D; the function he proposed is $f(VD) = \sqrt{V/D}$

This formula is important mainly because of the introduction of the idea of a variable wet surface of the skin. Gagge's first exploited the physiological importance of the wetted area of the skin, and the work of the Pierce Laboratory contains the most complete information regarding the factors upon which the wetted area of the body depends.

Gagge's formula for the heat loss by vaporization is similar to Büttner's.

$$H_V = (W\mu) \, A \, (E_s - RH \, E_a) \text{ kg-cal/hr}$$

or

$$(W\mu) = \frac{H_V}{A(E_s - RH \, E_a)} \tag{19}$$

where

W = fraction of body area that is completely wet
μ = proportionality factor which contains the vaporization constant and the factors which depend on air velocity and direction
H_V = heat loss by vaporization
A = total body area
RH = relative humidity

It is seen from Gagge's equation that when the vapor pressure $(RH \times E_a)$ of the air equals that of the skin, no vaporization will take place, and if the air vapor pressure should be greater than that on the skin, moisture will condense on the skin and the body will gain heat.

Within the zone of evaporative regulation relative humidity does not change H_V, because the change in the vapor pressure factor $(E_s - RH \, E_a)$ is compensated for by an increase in the wet area of skin.

The effect of wind upon the wetted area and upon H_V will, of course, depend more upon the change in total heat loss than upon the immediate alteration in H_V caused by suddenly blowing air upon the body. That is, if the skin is sweating with a $(W\mu)$ of 50 per cent in quiet air, turning on an electric fan will cause a large initial fall in $(W\mu)$, with a subsequent readjustment to a new $(W\mu)$ which will just let H_V balance the heat equation. It is for this reason that the laws of vaporization relating air velocity, temperature, vapor pressure, and so forth, as determined from physical analogues of the skin, are valid only under conditions which are predetermined by observations made on the skin. The studies of wet cylinders and spheres are of value in elucidating the mechanism of moisture passage through clothing, but they are the strict analogue of the sweating skin only if they can be made to adjust wetted area as a man does, or in the limiting case where a man's skin is 100 per cent wetted.

In the space environment, with the astronaut clothed in highly insulated clothing, the control of the water vapor pressure in the air surrounding the man will be of greatest importance. In some of the first orbital space flights the vapor pressure in the astronaut's suit has built up to uncomfortably high values. Condensation of moisture by radiant heat exchangers exposed to the low temperature space environment should be able to take care of the problem, but the astronaut may have to pay some attention to his heat loss problems in order to keep his environment in the thermally neutral range. Training in a space chamber might be required.

SUMMARY

The over-all heat balance equations for the space environment can be written in two parts: the transfer from the man's skin to his suit or cabin, and the transfer from the suit to space. In the first case

$$\text{Metabolic rate} - \text{storage rate} = \frac{1}{I}(T_s - T_a)\,Af'\ \text{conduction term}$$
$$+\ 1.26\sqrt{V}(T_s - T_a)A\ \text{convection term} + 2.2\sqrt{V}(E_s - E_a)AW\cdot\mu \tag{20}$$
$$\text{evaporation term}$$

Storage rate may vary but the actual storage must be kept small enough to maintain body temperature within physiological limits. Thus, the heat loss from the astronaut's suit and cabin will have to keep pace with the metabolic rate of the man. An expression for this heat balance can be written in terms of the radiation gains and losses from the suit surface and the storage of heat in the cabin structures or space suit.

Advantage has been taken of the possibility of storing heat temporarily in cabin structures during re-entry of the Mercury capsule into the Earth's atmosphere. The large amount of frictional heat generated by the capsule during the slowing from orbital speed to a speed allowing parachute deployment caused a rise in the temperature of the cabin wall to several hundred degrees Centigrade for a short time. However, as the capsule

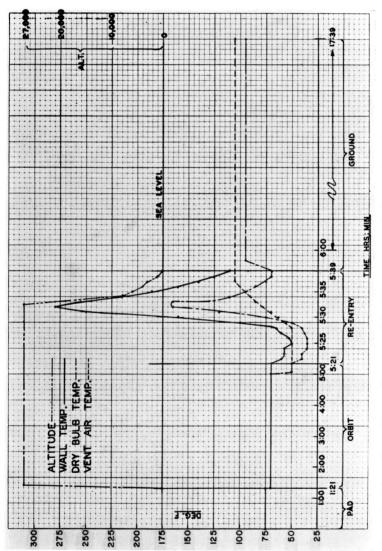

Fig. 18. The effect of heat of reentry of the Mercury capsule from 27,000 ft on the cabin wall and air temperatures and temperature of the ventilating air. (Courtesy of Dr. E. Hendler, U. S. Naval Air Crew Equipment Laboratory, Philadelphia, Pa.).

slowed down convective cooling by the air and radiative cooling brought the temperature of the cabin rapidly down to safe levels (Figure 18).

PHYSIOLOGICAL LIMITATIONS OF THERMAL EXPOSURE

Man's body temperature, both internal and external, is carefully regulated, under conditions of thermal stress, to remain within narrow limits.[3] Heat or cold stresses which are so great as to force a significant departure from normal tissue temperature will in time cause discomfort, pain, collapse and finally death. The magnitude

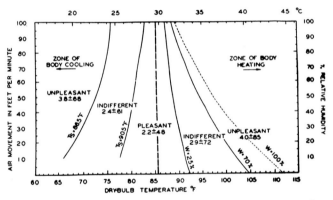

Fig. 19. The relation of air movement, relative humidity, and operative temperature, to thermal comfort experienced by unclothed subjects at rest. (After Winslow et al. Am. J. Hygiene *26*; 103, 1937)

of these departures has been determined for some special cases but the basic causes of the tissue injury and death from heat or cold are not understood in most instances. Two conitions, one of steady state and the other of temporary heat load, may be considered.

Steady State: Thermal comfort is achieved under those conditions which impose no thermal heat loads on the thermoregulatory system of the body. For a man at rest, an average skin temperature of $33° \pm 1°C$ and a rectal temperature of $37° \pm 0.5°C$ are measured under these conditions. There is a slight vasodilation of the skin blood vessels and no visible sweating. A departure of more than 0.5°C skin or rectal temperature above or below the range given above for comfort induces discomfort due to sweating on the hot side and shivering or other activity to maintain body heat on the other. The environmental conditions may, however, be well within the capacity of the thermoregulatory system. A description of the environment in terms of air movement, relative humidity and operative temperature[3] is shown in Figure 19. To the right of the dashed line on the right, man cannot lose sufficient heat even if at rest and an air movement of 100 ft/min (air movement above 35 ft/min is normally uncomfortable). Exposure of nude men to 5–10°C in still air for a period of about 10 days has

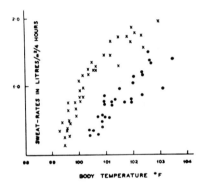

Fig. 20. Sweat-rates of raw (•) and acclimatized (x) laborers at average body temperature during 4 hr of work and heat-stress. (After Wyndham et al J. Appl. Physiol 6; 687, 1954)

caused peripheral tissue damage. For the health and safety of the astronaut his local private climate should not, as a steady state condition, exceed the limits of "pleasant" and "indifferent" indicated in Figure 19.

Temporary Heat Loads: Heat overloads may occur as the result of exercise which causes a rise in internal body temperature or changes in the heat losses to the environment. Exercise is self-limiting due to fatigue and although the internal body temperature is generally increased by exercise this is a physiological adjustment and poses no problem as long as the heat losses are able to dissipate the generated heat. During a severe bout of exercise, rectal temperatures as high as 39°–40°C are developed normally and without discomfort. During rest the body temperature falls rapidly, under continued sweating and vasodilation of the skin blood vessels. It is often necessary to work under hot conditions and the effort may exceed the physiological limitations even though the environment may be within acceptable limits for the quiet man. Heat acclimatization, water and salt replacement, and attention to the heart rate (160–180 beats/min maximum) can reduce the hazards of such a situation. The effects of heat acclimatization as found by Wyndham (see Figure 20) show that the heat acclimatized subjects sweat at a lower body temperature and increase sweat rate more rapidly as body temperature tends to rise than do unacclimatized subjects. Heat acclimatization also lowers the heart rate and induces greater comfort in the

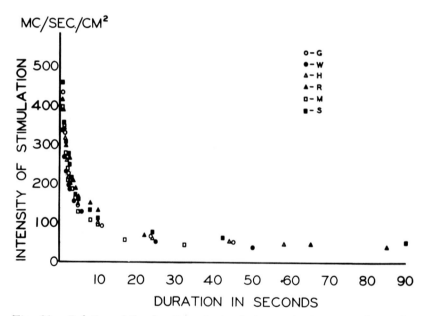

Fig. 21.   Relation of the duration of stimulation to the intensity of stimulus to produce pain.

individual. Methods for heat acclimatization during a two-week period are well worked out and as the effect lasts for several weeks after conditioning heat exposures, it would appear that such acclimatization should be a part of conditioning astronauts for lunar explorations and prolonged space journeys.

Heat overloads from thermal radiation may be troublesome during space exploration when the sun's radiation falls on the skin. The initial response to this radiation will be sensations of warmth, heat and pain. The intensity of the radiation which can be borne by the skin will depend upon the time of exposure and the initial skin temperature. In Figure 21 is shown the intensity duration curve of thermal radiation on blackened skin and the exposure time to produce pain. If the exposure be prolonged for half an hour or longer, it is observed that as little as 0.020 gm cal/sec/cm² will evoke pain in even a small area of blackened skin. As this is less than the intensity of the sun's rays outside the atmosphere of the Earth, pain could be produced by the sun shining on skin discolored by carbon or other black material. An appreciable amount of the sun's rays (25–35 per cent) will be reflected from

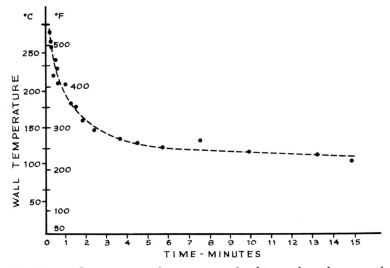

Fig. 22. Tolerance times for unprotected subjects abruptly exposed to high wall temperatures. (After Webb, P. in Chapt 3 Temperature. Its Measurement and Control in Science and Industry—Reinhold 1963.)

white skin or lightly tanned white or negro skin. Pain is stimulated when the skin temperature reaches 45° ± 2°C and at this
skin temperature burns are also produced.[5] Pain and skin burns
are the limiting factors for short high intensity heat overloads and
place the limits on physiological tolerance. In Figure 22 is shown
an intensity duration curve for pain limited radiant heat exposures on nude subjects sitting in a small chamber, the walls of
which could be suddenly raised to very high temperature with
quartz radiant heaters. Estimations of skin temperature indicated that "intolerable" pain, which was the limiting factor,
occurred at 45°C. A marked degree of protection is realized by
the wearing of an aluminized suit. However, the danger of such
a suit for a steady-state condition in space has been noted above.

In summary, it appears that with care thermal loads in space
near the Earth and moon will be manageable by control of radiation exchanges. Heat acclimatization and training of the astronaut in a space chamber with the thermal characteristics of the
space environment appear warranted.

REFERENCES

1. BERKNER, L. V., and H. ODISHAW: *Science in Space.* McGraw-Hill
   Co., Inc., New York. 1961.
1a. WYSOCKI, J. J.: Photon Spectrum Outside the Earth's Atmosphere.
   Solar Energy, 6:(3), 104–105. 1962.
2. HARDY, J. D.: Physiology of Temperature Regulation. *Physiological
   Reviews, 41:*521. 1961.
3. NEWBURGH, L. H., ed.: *Physiology of Heat Regulation and Science of
   Clothing.* W. B. Saunders Co., Philadelphia. 1949.
4. LICHT, S. ed.: *Therapeutic Heat and Cold,* 2nd ed. Licht Publishing
   Co., New Haven. 1958.
5. HARDY, J. D. H. G. WOLFF, and H. GOODELL: *Pain Sensations and Reactions.* Williams & Wilkins, Baltimore. 1952.
6. SPITZER, JR., L., and M. P. SAVEDOFF: Measured Temperature of Interstellar Matter. *Astrophysical J., 111.*(3)(593–608. 1950.
7. Quartermasters Research & Engineering Center: *Tech. Rep. EP-157,*
   1961.

2

HIGH ENERGY RADIATIONS

Carl Clark, Ph.D.

I. INTRODUCTION

The space traveller may encounter high energy radiations due to

1) Galactic and solar cosmic rays,
2) Interactions with particles "trapped" in planetary magnetic fields,
3) Interactions with the radiation fields such as aurorae produced by the energy degradation of such particles,
4) Emissions from auxiliary power supplies or main thrust engines utilizing nuclear reactions,
5) Emissions from materials made radioactive by cosmic rays or by nuclear power sources,
6) Emissions from high voltage electronic equipment,
7) Emission from nuclear explosions whether of origin by accident or by anger, and
8) Collisions at high speed with interplanetary gases not in themselves possessing such "high energy."

"High energy radiations" include both electromagnetic radiations and particulate or corpuscular radiations. The high energy electromagnetic radiations include x-rays, Bremsstrahlung, and gamma rays, with wavelengths shorter than 100 Angstroms, but are here taken to exclude ultraviolet, visible, infrared, microwave and radio quanta, of longer wavelength.

These high energy radiations produce very generally harmful biological effects, from slight to fatal depending on the nature of the radiations, the location, duration, and intensity of the exposure and many other factors. With special and generally localized use, beneficial biological effects may be produced such as the arresting of a cancerous growth. The benefit of improved medical diagnosis using high energy radiations may also offset any hazard due to such use.

This chapter will review: 1) problems of measurement and terminology, 2) the physical characteristics of the various types of high energy radiations, 3) the energy spectra, component radiation and time variations of the natural and man-made radiation sources of concern to a space traveller, 4) the biological effects due to these radiations, and 5) means of protection. The material here presented is but a brief introduction to large fields of study which are developing rapidly, with still limited human experience. Radioactivity was discovered by Becquerel in 1896, x-rays were first identified by Roentgen in 1895, the first induced radioactivity was discovered by Joliot and Joliot-Curie in 1934, the first self sustaining nuclear reaction under human control occurred in 1942, and the "trapped particle" radiation belt about the earth was not measured until 1958. With only eighteen days of total human experience above an altitude of 30 km (as of September, 1963), most of our views of space radiation problems are estimates from preliminary space physical measurements and from ground biological exposure experiments. Cosmic particle energies to 10^{19} ev have been measured. The most powerful terrestrial particle accelerators still attain only 10^{10} ev.

But the preliminary data does establish that high energy radiations are of major significance to manned space exploration. Solar cosmic "storms" pose a threat of possible catastrophy similar to although of less probability than ocean storms for the early terrestrial explorers.

II. TECHNIQUES OF MEASUREMENT

Mankind's information about space radiations is growing at a rapid rate; we can expect present concepts to be further evolved and perhaps even new means of energy transport and new particle

TABLE I

HIGH ENERGY RADIATIONS

Radiation	Symbol	Relative Rest Mass	Charge	Range for 1 Mev energy			
				Lead	Aluminum	Water	Air (STP)
Electromagnetic: x-ray or Brems-strahlung or γ ray	x or γ	0	0	8.8 cm	41 cm	97 cm	86,000 cm
Corpuscular:							
Neutrino	ν or z	0	0				
Electron or beta particle	e or β⁻	1/1840	−1	0.035	0.15	0.40	310
Positron	β⁺	1/1840	+1				
μ Meson	μ	210/1840	±1	0.0032	0.0066	0.011	10
π Meson	π	276/1840	±1	0.0025	0.0050	0.0087	8.0
Proton	p or H⁺	1	+1	0.000016	0.0013	0.0022	2.3
Neutron	n	1	0			23	
Alpha Particle	α	2	+2	0.00016	0.0003		0.5
Heavier Particles	Li, Be, B, C, etc.	3, 4, 5, 6, etc.	+3, 4, 5, 6, etc.				
For example:	Fe	26	+26				

Note: "Cosmic rays" include p, α, and heavier particles. Energies of the heavier particles to 10^{19} ev have been observed.

* The "range" for the electromagnetic and neutron radiation is given in terms of the distance penetrated which reduces the intensity to 1/1000, i.e., ten half value layers or 3 tenth value layers. For the other corpuscular radiation, the "range" is the forward distance traversed before the particles loose their identity and are absorbed. In this process, the secondary radiation produced, particularly Bremsstrahlung, may be considerably more penetrating than the primary radiation.

types to be identified. The early balloon flights of ionization chambers by Gockel, Hess and Kohörster (1910–1914) which led to the naming of "cosmic radiation" were in the same tradition of the radiation measurements of Sputnik II (November, 1957), Explorer III (March, 1958) and many other rocket experiments down to the present Orbiting Solar Observatory (March, 1962). We can expect further changes of our view of space radiation as refinements of measurements are added, just as the 1958 picture of inner and outer "Van Allen radiation belts" about the earth is now being replaced by the 1963 picture of a "magnetosphere" of trapped particles of differing characteristics at different positions and different times.

Table I summarizes the principal types of high energy radiations. Note the major subdivisions into electromagnetic radiation and corpuscular radiation. Table II lists the principal high energy

TABLE II

High Energy Radiation Measurement Devices on Techniques

1. Electroscope
2. Vibrating reed electrometer
3. Ionization chamber
4. Proportional counter
5. Flow counter
6. Geiger-Müller counter
7. Crystal counter
8. Scintillation counter
9. Čerenkov counter ($E_p > 20$ Mev)
10. Cloud chamber (with photography)
11. Film: track microscopy and radio-autography
12. Film: densitometry
13. Chemical dosimetry (color change, fluorescence change, pH change)
14. Foil activation dosimetry
15. Gas activation counters (BF_3 for counting neutrons for example)
16. Mass spectrometry
17. Time of flight spectrometry (especially for neutrons)
18. X, γ, β, and neutron diffraction and spectrometry
19. Biological effects dosimetry (erythema, epilation, lethal dose, etc.)
20. Radio noise: riometer
21. Thermal detectors (Temperature change following absorption)
22. Shielding (filter) effects
23. Magnetic field effects
24. Coincidence and anti-coincidence circuits

radiation measurement techniques. Many of the radiations will produce some effects with several of the detection techniques, severely complicating the analysis of particularly mixed radiation beams. Complete analysis involves identification of the particular electromagnetic quanta or particles present and the numbers of each at each energy interval, and the changes of these spectra as the radiations penetrate and deliver energy through ionizations in the materials of interest.

When high energy radiation passes through a gas, ionizations are produced as the radiation is absorbed. These ions may be attracted to charged poles or plates, causing a current flow or charge dissipation which can provide a measure of the amount of incident radiation (Table II, 1–6). With the electroscope or simple ionization chamber, an initial potential difference between the electrodes of perhaps 100 volts is dissipated, providing a count of the number of ions formed by the incident radiation but no specific information as to whether these are produced by interactions with many low energy particles or quanta or with a few high energy particles or quanta. The common "pencil dosimeter" is such a low voltage ionization chamber.

If the voltage between the plates of a gas chamber is increased to perhaps 600 volts, ions once formed are accelerated sufficiently to produce a "cascade" or "avalanche" of additional ions before they reach the plates. A "gas amplification" of numbers of ions of up to 10^7 is produced, and a pulse of current due to a single particle or quantum interaction with the chamber gas can now be detected. In the proportional counter, the electrode voltage is such that the current pulse amplitude is proportional to the number of initial ions formed as energy is absorbed by the gas from the incident particle or quantum. If the electrode voltage is further increased, to perhaps 1000 volts, any ionization produced within the chamber will now "cascade" to fill the entire chamber with ions, and the current pulse amplitude will now be independent of the energy of the incident quantum or particle; the chamber is operating in the "Geiger-Müller counting region." With further increase of electrode voltage, the chamber gas will remain ionized, in the "discharge region," without incident radiation.

Radiation detectors can only respond to energy absorbed in the sensitive volume of the detector, a principle which in another context is called the first law of photochemistry. Hence detectors will have different "sensitivity factors" for radiation differently absorbed. For example when an alpha emitter is placed between the plates of a chamber, perhaps by flow of a gas containing the emitter through the chamber, the range of the alpha particle is so short that essentially all ions formed by it will be collected and the efficiency or *sensitivity factor* given by the energy detected divided by the energy incident on the detector can be almost 1. On the other hand, a gamma ray beam traversing the gas chamber will be only slightly absorbed; the sensitivity factor may be less than 0.01. Moreover, the detector may receive only a part of the energy emitted by a source, due to its size and position with respect to the source; the *geometry factor* is usually less than 1. It is common practice to use a combined *geometry-sensitivity factor* for a particular source measured in a defined way by a particular detector.

The disadvantage of the low efficiency of the gas chambers for gamma rays can be avoided by having a solid crystal, of silver chloride, cadmium sulfide, or diamond for example, between the electrode plates of the chamber. Ionizations produced in the crystal counter by the radiation, now more effectively stopped within the sensitive volume, produce through a cascade effect a detectible pulse in a counting circuit. A serious disadvantage however is that most crystals must be used at liquid air temperature to reduce conductance without radiation to a sufficiently low value.

In certain materials, the ionizations produced by absorption of high energy radiations will include outer orbit electron transitions. When the atom very shortly thereafter recaptures an electron, a quantum of visible light is emitted. Indeed, Rutherford in 1911 observed the high angle scattering of alpha particles by thin metal foils by observing with a microscope the scintillation of a zinc sulfide screen when the alpha particles hit it. From this experiment he concluded that the atomic nucleus must be concentrated, and he named the electron.

Modern scintillation counters use a photocell or photomultiplier to detect the flash, and electronic counters to determine the number of flashes in a given time. In traversing the scintillation crystal, the incident high energy quantum or particle will produce a track of flashing ions; if the radiation is completely absorbed, the brightness of the track which is proportional to the number of ions formed will be a measure of the quantum or particle energy of the incident radiation. Just as with the proportional gas chamber counter, a "pulse height analyzer" may be used to determine the incident radiation energy. Whereas the gas chambers are suitable for short range alpha or beta particles but have low efficiencies for high energy quanta, the scintillation counter, with its solid or liquid sensitive volume (of sodium iodide-telluride, anthracene, a solution of terphenyl in xylene, etc.) is particularly suitable for gamma radiation.

When particulate radiation velocities exceed the velocity of electromagnetic radiation in a medium, given by the velocity of light in a vacuum divided by the refractive index, the resulting relativistic electron motions produce electromagnetic radiation, partially in the visible spectrum, at specific angles of incidence from the particle path, as described by Cerenkov. Photoelectric observation of this Cerenkov radiation can be used to count these very high energy particles.

The cloud chamber is a device for visualizing ionization tracks. When a piston is withdrawn, expanding the vapor in a transparent cylinder, the gas temperature drops, and the vapor becomes supersaturated. Radiation passing through the chamber forms ions which act as condensation nuclei for the vapor. These condensation tracks can then be photographed in intense light, to indicate the paths of the radiation (if the radiation produces a sufficiently dense track of ions), the formation of secondary radiations, the deflection in electrical or magnetic fields, and so on. Positrons and mesons were first identified by cloud chamber studies.

Permanent tracks may also be directly formed in film. A thick photographic emulsion or a stack of emulsions with a high concentration of silver halide is used. Development reveals the ionization tracks, particularly for radiations giving high ion densities, such as alpha particles, protons, fission fragments and cosmic radiations. Absorbers may be used between the layers of emulsion, and magnetic fields, to aid in identifying the particles and their energies. Overexposure of the films must be prevented to allow recognition of tracks, and microscopy is commonly used in their measurement. Radio-autography is a technique in which high energy radiations emitted by a sample (a bone section for example) expose a film closely applied to the sample.

With continued exposure of film, a general blackening develops, which may be related to the source exposure by the film densitometry, previously calibrated by known source exposures. The technique is most accurate in the linear range of the film density (or absorbance) vs exposure curve; a series of absorbers over parts of the film may be used to extend the useful range. Careful control of development is necessary to maintain calibration. By careful shielding from light the film can be used to integrate exposures over long periods. "Film badges" are widely used in radiation protection monitoring. Film blackening cannot indicate the type of radiation exposure. Separate calibration (and badges) must be used when the source spectrum is changed. Neutron film badges may be provided by using a beryllium absorber over the film. The film is exposed primarily by the Bremsstrahlung secondary radiation emitted from the beryllium when it is exposed to neutrons.

Chemical dosimetry involves the measurement of radiation in terms of a chemical change produced by the radiation in a sensitive organic or inorganic chemical system. Color, fluorescence and pH changes are notably used. A glass disc radiation dosimeter has been developed for civil defense applications. Changes of the fluorescence of the glass measure the integrated exposure of the individual.

Foil activation dosimetry involves the use of thin metal foils in the radiation. The extent of nuclear transmutation, as measured by more easily identified radiation from the daughter products, is proportioned to the flux of the radiation (particles or quanta/ cm^2/sec) times the cross-section (or effective opacity or stopping power, in cm^2/atom) of the particular metal for the radiation of particular type and energy. The activities of a series of foils of different metals (gold, indium, etc.) in an unknown radiation beam can therefore provide a rough indication of the presence and energy range of the transmuting radiation, particularly neutrons. With gas activation counters, a transmutation product may be measured directly. Thus boron trifluoride gas, in an ionization chamber, may be used to count neutrons. (Or boron may line the walls of the chamber.) A portable neutron chamber of this type is called "Rudolph," because its chamber "nose" is painted red to distinguish it from an ordinary ionization chamber. Because of the nuclear reaction $_{10}^{5}B$ (n, α) $_{3}^{7}$ Li, the ionization chamber responds to the alpha transmutation products, to which it is far more sensitive than to the incident slow neutrons. It is emphasized however that these devices measure a transmutation amount; a high flux of a radiation for which the material has a low cross-section may give the same reading as a low flux of a radiation for which the material has a high cross-section. To adequately identify a broad spectrum radiation will require the use of several materials.

The mass spectrometer, by providing a measure of the current carried by a stream of ions deflected specified amounts (determined by slits) by known electrical and magnetic fields, can indicate, by varying the field strengths, the particle velocities and charge to mass ratios of the incident ions. Hence this technique has great potential for identifying particulate radiation components. The time-of-flight spectrometer, used particularly with neutron beams, by measuring the velocities of the detected particles, can indicate particle energies if the masses are known. The source is pulsed, by mechanical shutter or other means, and the detector sensitivity is pulsed shortly thereafter, so that only those particles travelling at the certain velocity are detected.

X-rays, gamma rays, beta particles, and neutrons all interact with crystalline materials to produce diffraction patterns, with pattern spacings depending on crystal lattice spacings, the quantum or particle energies, and the diffraction angles and order. Hence knowing the crystal lattice spacings, and measuring the diffraction angles by rotating a suitable detector about the crystal, the incident energies may be determined. Analyses of mixed radiations would require different detectors, collimation procedures and perhaps crystals.

An amount and quality of radiation may be approximately identified by its biological effects. The skin "erythemal dose," to just produce reddening, was a typical end point in early x-radiation therapy work. The tissue depth of the effects provides indication of the radiation penetrating power. Other secondary effects of the radiation may be noted: solar storms may be detected by the resulting changes in radio noise. The "riometer" (radio ionospheric opacity meter) for example measures "cosmic" radio noise changes at 28 and 50 megacycles/sec. The changes are produced by effects of radiation incident on the ionosphere.

The energy absorbed from a radiation beam, after a series of specific interactions, finally is "degraded" as target heat, which may be measurable as a temperature change. Within the radiation beam, atomic collisions may produce high local or individual target atom velocities, called "point heat" which are not directly measurable thermally.

A major preliminary means to distinguish different types of radiation is by determining shielding or filtering effects. Table I above includes the ranges of certain radiations in lead, aluminum, water, and air. See also section IV and Table III below. By careful measurement of radiation transmission through filters of varying thickness, simple mixtures of radiations of differing penetrating power or quality may indeed be distinguished, but the method is tedious and not accurate if the mixed radiation is complex. The use of magnetic or electrical fields can provide additional means to separate the radiations, and electronic "gating" circuits can turn on and off a series of aligned detectors, in "coincidence" or "anti-coincidence" circuits, to assure that the observed events are happening in proper temporal relationship or spatial direction.

It can be seen from this brief discussion of high energy radiation measurement that most techniques are affected to some extent by most radiations. It is small wonder that our knowledge of the complicated mixed radiations of space is still developing, as additional measurement techniques are brought to bear.

TABLE III

RANGE IN GM/CM^2* FOR VARIOUS ENERGY RADIATIONS INCIDENT ON SEVERAL MATERIALS

Radiation	Lead	Aluminum	Tissue	Air (STP)	Energy
γ**	98	112	109	108	1 Mev
	137	300	332	344	10 Mev
	73	274	386	426	100 Mev
e†	0.39	0.41	0.40	0.40	1 Mev
		5.3	4.7	4.7	10 Mev
p	0.008	0.0035	0.002	0.003	1 Mev
	0.34	0.17	0.12	0.14	10 Mev
	16.6	9.85	7.59	8.70	100 Mev
	629	406	322	636	1 Bev
n**	691	124	18.7	115	1 Mev
	854	308	77.4	451	10 Mev
α	0.002	8×10^{-4}	5×10^{-4}	0.05	1 Mev
	0.04	0.016	0.010	0.010	10 Mev
	1.6	0.86	0.6	0.6	100 Mev
	78	48	38	35	1 Bev
(Density	11.3 gm/cm^3	2.70	1.03	0.00122)	

* The range in cm may be determined by dividing the range in gm/cm^2 by the density in gm/cm.^{3}

** The "range" of γ and n radiations are here represented in terms of the thickness in cm of material which will pass only 1/1000 of the incident radiations (i.e., three tenth value layers) times the density of the material in gm/cm^3. Note that the higher atomic number (higher Z) materials are better x-ray absorbers even when the shield thickness is expressed in these mass per unit area units.

† Attention is called to the fact that the higher the shield atomic number Z the more Bremstrahlung x-radiation is produced as the high energy electrons are absorbed. Since this x-radiation is often more penetrating than the initial electron beam the dose rate behind the shield may be reduced by having the initial electron absorption in a low Z material.

III.   TERMINOLOGY

Atoms may be designated in this manner:

Mass number		valence or charge
	symbol	
Atomic number		number of atoms in a compound

The mass number, A, is the sum of the number of protons and neutrons in the nucleus. The atomic number, Z, is the number of protons in the nucleus, and hence for a neutral atom, the number of orbital electrons. Isotopes are atoms with the same number of nuclear protons (and hence essentially the same orbital electrons and chemical properties) but different numbers of nuclear neutrons. Thus a rare isotope nitrogen gas would be designated $^{15}N_2$, and a cosmic ray potassium atom, fully ionized, might be $^{39}_{19}K^{+19}$. For convenience, isotopes with their mass numbers are sometimes designated in the form carbon-14, or Cs-137, for example.

Particle or quantum energies are generally given in electron volts, or multiples of the kinetic energy acquired by an electron in accelerating across a potential difference of one volt. Thousand (Kev), million (Mev) and billion (Bev) electron volt symbols are also used. This is a small unit of energy: 1 Bev = 10^9 ev = 3.83×10^{-11} cal = 1.60×10^{-3} ergs. Because of the different significance of the word "billion" in Europe, more recent usage is that 10^9 ev be called the giga electron volt, or Gev.

A quantity of radiation may be specified by a graph called an energy spectrum showing number of quanta or particles of specified type with energies within the range E and $E + dE$ (specified) vs the energy E. More commonly, since these are often highly penetrating radiations and effects depend only on the absorption processes, the quantity of radiation is expressed in terms of the energy absorbed by a suitable test sample. Thus the roentgen (r) is essentially that amount of x-radiation absorbed by dry air at $0°C$ and 1 atmosphere pressure, to produce 1 electrostatic unit of charge of either sign (or 2.08×10^9 ion pairs) per cubic centimeter or air, and the statement that the astronaut received a 25 r exposure means that he was in a beam which could produce 25 e.s.u. of charge per cc of air if this were measured by a suitable ionization chamber.

Because the absorption processes are different for different forms of radiation (see below), other radiations will produce different relations of charge density in an ionization chamber per amount of energy absorbed. Here the roentgen unit should only be used for x-radiation. Other radiations should be compared in terms of this energy absorption. Thus the rad unit, representing the absorption of 100 ergs of energy per gram of absorbing material, is recommended for general dose comparisons. Since 1 r of x-radiation on biological tissue (or water) gives an absorption of about 93 ergs/gm, these units for x-radiation are similar.

Different radiations have different ranges in materials, and hence their *linear energy transfers* (*LET*) in ergs per centimeter of penetration are different. This difference may produce significant differences in the biological effects. Thus alpha particles may produce short dense ionization tracks, locally killing cells, whereas gamma rays may produce fewer ionizations per cell but over a far greater length. The different radiations will then expectly have different *relative biological effectiveness* (*RBE*), defined as the absorbed energy in rads of x-radiation to produce a given biological effect divided by the absorbed energy in rads of the radiation of concern to produce the same biological effect. (This *RBE* concept is further discussed in section V). If the rad dose to produce a specified biological effect is multiplied by the *RBE* for that radiation, the resulting number may be called the *dose in rem units* (roentgen equivalent-man, or roentgen equivalent-mammal). Thus the same effects will be produced by the same rem doses, whatever the radiation used, although the rad doses may differ by an order of magnitude.

The difficulty with the *RBE* and rem concepts is that the biological effects must be carefully circumscribed to be considered "the same," and the responses may be quite non-linear and must be treated statistically because of biological variation. When not otherwise specified, the most commonly used relative biological effectiveness values concern the lethal dose for half of an exposed population, with death in thirty days (abbreviated as the LD$_{50}$-30. Some biological effects may be delayed for years.

A radioactive isotope, or radio-nuclide, will spontaneously disintegrate into daughter products, specified by its "decay scheme," with the release of energy. This decay occurs in an exponential fashion, $A = A_o e^{-\lambda t} = A_o e^{-0.693/T_{1/2}}$, in which A_o is the initial amount of radionuclide, A is the amount after t, λ is the decay constant, and $T_{1/2}$ the "physical half life," or the time for half the radioactive material to decay. If a nuclide, radioactive or not, is put into the body by a specified route in a specified chemical form, the time for half of these atoms to leave the body is called the "biological half life." This elimination process may be quite non-exponential. If a radionuclide is put into the body, the time for half of it to leave the body or decay is called the "effective half life." The total amount of a nuclide in the body, is called its "body burden." If it is selectively assimilated by a particular organ (as strontium is by bone, or iodine by the thyroid), this is called the critical or "target organ."

The amount of a radionuclide may be measured in terms of the number of atoms disintegrating per second. If the decay scheme for example involves the release of one gamma per disintegration, one can count the number of gamma quanta released from the material per second. If there are 3.7×10^{10} disintegrations per second, there is "one curie" of radionuclide present. This is approximately the disintegration rate of 1 gm of refined radium. Defining the "specific activity" of a sample as the number of millicuries of activity present per gram of total sample, one can see that a pure radionuclide decaying more rapidly than radium ($T_{1/2}$ of 19.9 years for R-226) would have a higher specific activity. Isotopes are typically used with such an amount of carrier material that the specific activities are generally far below 1000 mc/gm. Indeed with some radionuclides, pathological effects will occur with total body burdens of just a few microcuries.

IV. RADIATION ABSORPTION PROCESSES

When high energy *electromagnetic* radiation passes into material, three processes occur, with importance depending on the quantum energy. 1) At quantum energies below about 1 Mev, the x- or gamma ray may give up all of its energy to an electron, which then has the quantum energy as its kinetic energy, or about 30 ev less if the electron is stripped from an atom. The electron does not necessarily travel along the previous path and is subsequently slowed as discussed below. This is called the photoelectric effect. 2) At energies up to about 15 Mev, especially above 1 Mev, the gamma ray may give only part of its energy to an electron, and proceed on a new path with the remaining energy. This is called the Compton effect. 3) At energies above 1.02 Mev and especially at higher energies the gamma ray may disappear near a nucleus and an electron and a positron appear travelling along different directions with about but not necessarily equal kinetic energies. This is called pair production. The positron is subsequently slowed, then combines with an electron and both disappear in an annihilation process, giving rise to two gamma rays, each of 0.51 Mev, travelling in opposite directions.

For an incident beam dose rate I_o of many quanta per second, the absorption of electromagnetic radiation is essentially exponential, that is $I_x = I_o e^{-\mu x}$, where I_x is the dose rate at depth x in the material and μ is the linear absorption coefficient, with units of cm^{-1}. At each wavelength or quantum energy, the linear absorption coefficient of a specified material has components due to photoelectric effects, Compton effects, and pair production. Absorption may also be represented in terms of the mass absorption coefficient $\mu_M = \mu/\rho$, in units of cm^2/gm, where ρ is the density of the absorber. In general, x-ray absorption increases with increasing atomic number of the absorber and decreases with increasing quantum energy of the source. Note that the photoelectric and Compton effects depend on interaction of the x-ray quantum with electrons. Since electron density increases as Z increases, absorption due to these effects increases as Z increases.

A thickness of material which absorbs half of the incident dose rate is called the "half value layer"; HVL $= 0.693/\mu$. Similarly a thickness of material which absorbs all but one tenth of the incident radiation is called a tenth value layer; TVL $= 2.30/\mu$. For a monoenergetic incident beam, successive tenth value layers will reduce the transmission by successive multiples of 1/10; three layers reduce the transmission dose rate 1/1000 of the incident dose.

For a broad spectrum incident beam, the less energetic ("softer") radiation is more strongly absorbed than the more energetic ("harder") radiation, so that the spectrum is shifted to higher and hence more penetrating quantum energies (although lesser numbers of quanta) as material is traversed. Hence successive shielding layers will absorb decreasing proportions of the incident beams.

As *electrons* penetrate material, they collide with other electrons, giving up significant proportions of their kinetic energies and hence causing scattering as well as ionization, and they interact with nuclei and are slowed, giving up portions of their kinetic energies which appear as electromagnetic x-radiations called Bremsstrahlung or "braking radiation." Both of these processes rapidly redirect the energy transport, and so electrons take very erratic courses on successive collisions, that is, the radiation is highly scattered. Because of its low mass and its charge, a given electron has a negligible probability of traversing an absorber beyond a certain distance. For each given energy of electrons incident on a specified material, a maximum range or distance of electron transport may be specified (see Table III). Empirical relations have been established relating the number of electrons penetrating to the depth of penetration. It must be recognized that the majority of those electrons which do traverse an absorber are slowed, that is, they have less kinetic energy than the incident electrons.

Neutrons are particles released in nuclear reactions, rarely with kinetic energies above 15 Mev and generally below 1 Mev. They spontaneously disintegrate into a proton and an electron, with a half life of about twelve min. Hence, essentially no stellar or solar neutrons reach the earth, although some neutrons are found in space due to man-made nuclear reactions, or reactions produced by cosmic particles in the upper atmosphere.

Neutrons are absorbed by elastic collisions, in which the total momentum of the recoil particles equals the momentum of the incident particles, or by inelastic collisions, in which momentum is not conserved due to ionization, gamma emission, or other energy exchange than kinetic recoil, or by nuclear absorption or "capture" in which the neutron disappears, and a transmuted daughter nucleus is produced which is generally artificially radioactive. In the capture process some radiation may be given off ("capture gamma" emission) before the daughter nucleus disintegrates. Neutron energies are described broadly by saying that the neutron is "thermal" when its kinetic energy matches that of the thermal motion of the other particles (about 0.025 ev at 20°C), that the neutron is "slow" when its kinetic energy is up to about 1 Kev, and that the neutron is "fast" when its kinetic energy is greater than 0.5 Mev. Neutron capture is most probable with slow or thermal neutrons, hence fast neutrons must be slowed or "moderated" by collisions, which are generally inelastic, prior to their absorption. Due to the lack of charge of the neutron, fast neutrons will penetrate several centimeters in solids between collisions; that is, they have a mean free path of several centimeters. The radiation is thus very penetrating.

Since a neutron has a mass close to that of a hydrogen atom, the neutron can deliver up to its entire kinetic energy to a hydrogen atom in an elastic collision; elastic collisions with heavier atoms are not as effective in slowing the neutron. Hence hydrogenous or organic materials or water make good neutron moderators. Moreover, when the slow or thermal neutron is captured, for shielding, it is desirable that the excited nucleus not give a strong gamma ray. Lithium and particularly boron, both with high thermal neutron "cross-sections," that is, high thermal neutron capture probabilities, yield no or low energy gamma rays after excitation, and the daughter products are non-radioactive. Lithium hydride for example is therefore a good neutron shield. A high atomic number material would then be used on the inside of the shield to stop these gamma rays.

It can be seen that neutron penetrations into material involve a complicated series of interactions. Although the reduction in numbers of neutrons of a specific energy is essentially exponential with absorber thickness, the net energy transport into each successive layer, including all effects of secondary radiations produced, is not so simple a relation.

A few materials on capturing neutrons undergo nuclear reactions releasing sufficiently more neutrons such that if sufficient material (the "critical mass") is provided to reduce effects of neutron loss at the edges of the material a continuing or "chain reaction" is initiated. The materials "fissioned" by thermal neutrons include U-233, U-235 and Pu-239. The materials fissioned by fast neutrons include U-238, Th-232 and Pa-231. Energy is released at about 1 megawatt-day per gram of fissioned material, as compared to 1 megawatt-day per 3 tons of carbon chain chemical combustion (requiring in addition 6 tons of oxygen). Although nuclear powered rocket motors have not yet flown, their development is progressing.

Because of their charge and low weight, *protons,* like electrons, penetrate only a certain distance into material. This range varies with proton energy approximately to the 1.8 power for energies between 10 and 200 Mev. A proton can deliver essentially all of its kinetic energy to another hydrogen atom in one collision, producing a secondary proton with essentially the same direction. Less direct collisions with hydrogen or collisions with heavier atoms will produce more scattering and less slowing of the primary proton. Hence higher atomic weight materials are less effective proton absorbers. Lead for example is only about 40 per cent as effective in stopping high energy protons as water. (See Table III). These collisions are typically inelastic, so that moderately dense ionization tracks are left by a proton.

At energies above about 0.5 Mev, protons may be absorbed by target nuclei, to produce nuclear transmutations, commonly with the emission of gamma or particulate radiation. For example, protons falling on aluminum produce the nuclear reaction $^{27}_{13}\text{Al}$

(p, γ) $^{28}_{14}$Si, and shielding must be provided for the secondary gamma radiation released. At higher proton energies (up to 10^{19} ev observed in cosmic radiation) very complex nuclear reactions may occur. Multiple radial track "stars" are formed when a light target nucleus breaks into its component nuclei after such a collision. Alternately, a heavy target atom may undergo a "spallation reaction," emitting a series of nuclei but leaving a principal daughter nucleus residue.

Alpha particles produce very dense usually straight ionization tracks in penetrating matter, with specific ranges depending on energy. At particle energies below 5 Mev most of the energy is delivered to electrons. Since an average of about 32 ev is required to strip an electron from a tissue molecule, a 5 Mev alpha particle (and its secondaries) will produce about 150,000 ion pairs before stopping within its range of 0.0045 cm (45 microns) in tissue. Some of these electrons leave the alpha track with significant energies and are slowed by further ionizations and the release of Bremsstrahlung.

For alpha particle energies above about 5 Mev, nuclear reactions become increasingly important. Since the secondary radiations (for example, gamma rays or neutrons) may penetrate far greater distances than the primary radiation, these must be considered in shielding analyses.

V. PROPERTIES OF SPACE RADIATIONS

A. Galactic Cosmic Rays

Indications that the atmosphere shielded terrestrial man from intense space radiations data from the first balloon radiation measurements in 1910. This passive shielding indeed amounts to about 1000 gm/cm² at the surface, sufficient to stop most of the primary particles and transmitting mainly the penetrating secondary mesons formed by nuclear reactions in the atmosphere. In the 1920's it was established that the earth's magnetic field provides an additional shielding effect, deflecting all but the more energetic cosmic particles (i.e., the 5 per cent with energies above 15 Bev) from approaching the earth on the equator but having far less influence on particles approaching along the magnetic poles.

Satellite measurements since 1957 have clarified the description. Primary galactic radiation is now viewed to consist of high energy fully ionized nuclei (i.e., no orbital electrons), with about 85 per cent protons, about 14 per cent alpha particles, and about 1 per cent heavier particles, in their sequence of prevalence in the universe. These nuclei are apparently boiled off distant stars and accelerated in galactic space by magnetic fields (Fermi theory) to approach the earth presumably isotropically with a flux of about 5 particles/cm² sec, an average energy of about 4×10^9 ev/nucleon, and a total energy density near the earth about equal to that of visible starlight, 0.6 ev/cm³ (Winkler, 1960). The proton spectrum in the energy range of 5×10^8 to 2×10^{10} ev is well represented by $N(E) = 0.3/(1 + E)^{1.5}$ particles/cm² sec ster. (Winkler, 1960). During periods of minimum solar activity (see below) these approach the earth to interact with its magnetic field, to contribute to the "magnetosphere" radiation belt, and with the atmosphere. During periods nearer maximum solar activity, the lower energy half of these particles are deflected in interplanetary space by the magnetic fields of the "solar wind," which are in the range of 10^{-4} to 10^{-5} gauss.

Because of the high energy and low number of the light (low Z) galactic cosmic particles, they penetrate materials to give a low linear energy transfer or ionization density and hence a low rem dose. However, particular concern has been expressed for effects of the heavy primary cosmic particles, for each one of these produces a very dense ionization track within the body, with secondary particle ranges of the order of 5 microns, commensurate with the radii of biological cells, and "ionization column" doses of the order of 10^4 rem, sufficient to severely damage or kill these cells. If one heavy primary cosmic particle can indeed kill cells in its path, damage might not be adequately represented by the average rem dose of the body, particularly when critical non-regenerating localized tissues such as the retina or hypothalamus might be hit. With estimates of six (solar maximum) to forty (solar minimum) heavy primary cosmic particles passing through each cubic centimeter of a lightly shielded person in space (or on the lunar surface) per day, uncertainties remain as to how long it would be before detectible biological effects would occur. Estimates are that David Simons, in the Man High II balloon flight of August, 1957, with 15 hr above 90,000 ft, experienced about two hits by particles of atomic weight above 6 per cm^3, or about 150,000 hits in the entire body, without apparent biological effect.

Without material or geomagnetic shielding, the galactic cosmic radiation gives a dose rate of about 25 rem/year during a solar maximum period, and about 50 rem/year during a solar minimum period. (Including secondary radiation effects, these values may be doubled to 50 and 100 rem/year.) Shielding by 40 gm/cm^2 of water or low atomic number material (equivalent to the atmosphere above 70,000 ft) is sufficient to stop essentially all of the heavy primary cosmic particles. Because of secondary radiation buildup, the total rem dose inside a shield actually increases until the shield exceeds about 80 gm/cm^2 of low atomic weight material.

B. Solar Cosmic Rays

The sun, as our small moderate temperature local star, boils off ions and electrons with a far greater variation in particle energies and with time than we see for galactic cosmic radiation. Much of this variation is correlated with visible changes.

The average numbers of sunspots observable on one day vary approximately on an eleven year cycle with the last minimum (about 5 sunspots) in 1954 and the next minimum "year of the quiet sun" to receive international study in 1964–1965. The maximum typically occurs $4^1/_2$ years after the minimum. A maximum number (about 200 sunspots seen in one day on the average) occurred in 1958, and a new maximum expectedly will occur again in 1968–1969, unfortunately in an expected critical period of space and lunar exploration before boosters are able to carry the very heavy shields for complete radiation safety.

Different maxima may differ in numbers of sunspots by a factor of 4, in a manner not yet reliably predicted until the cycle is at least $1^1/_2$ years beyond its minimum (Anderson, 1961), although with an increasing trend over a ninety year cycle, then an abrupt decrease, which should occur in the next one or two cycles. X-radiation intensity in the 2–8 Angstrom range may increase several hundred times in the maximum vs the minimum emission. Particulate radiation (principally protons and electrons) may increase in spasmotic flare periods as much as a million times, with greater probabilities of occurrence of these "solar storms" when there are many sunspots.

The sunspots generally appear in latitude bands between 5° and 40°, north and south of the equator. The latitude of greatest probability of sunspot appearance shifts from about 24° (north and south) shortly after a sunspot cycle minimum, to about 8° (north and south) at the next minimum, indicating basic solar vortices, not yet understood. Particular spots are visible from one day to several months and are seen to rotate with the sun, which surprisingly has a shorter rotation period at the equator, 25 days, than towards the poles, for example 31 days at 60° north or south. The sunspots (through a very dark filter or in a projected sun image) are seen as a dark umbra surrounded by a less dark penumbra, against the bright photosphere.

The solar surface experiences continuous turbulence, with vast amounts of material irregularly boiled off. The solar corona, irregularly extending beyond the photosphere, generally circles the sun at solar maxima but at the poles shrinks to "small tufts of light" (*Encyclopedia Britanica*) during the minima. The sunspots, which generally appear in pairs, are interpreted from the motions of ejected material as north and south poles of intense (up to 4000 gauss) magnetic fields maintained by ion transport. Near the sun the average magnetic field is about 50 gauss; near the earth it is 0.5 gauss. Large streams of high speed ions completely ejected from the sun carry significant magnetic fields as well. The north pole sunspot may lead in the direction of solar rotation in the northern hemisphere and the south pole may lead in the southern hemisphere, with a reversal of this condition on successive solar cycles, again indicating underlying solar mechanisms not yet understood with a cycle of 22 years rather than 11.

Solar prominances, visible in photographs of the corona or by special techniques across the photosphere, (such as the use of narrow band filters transmitting the hydrogen Hα line at 6565A) are masses of material, spectrographically principally hydrogen, ejected from the photosphere, most of which fall back to the sun. They are of two types: associated with sunspots or not, the former characteristically having a close loop path imposed by the sunspot magnetic field and the latter with much longer curving projections seen at the Hα line as dark furrows or hedge-rows or "filaments" across the photosphere. These prominences seem suspended in the network of sunspot magnetic fields, and may ascend or descend with the abrupt changes of these fields. As the material progresses outwards it expands and increases temperature or speed, from the 6000° K of the sun's surface or 4000° K of the sunspots, up to the 150,000° K of the outer promi-nences to the perhaps two million degrees of the outer corona. Local interactions of the magnetic and electrical fields ("pinch effects" and cyclotron effects) with rising "bubbles of gas" are thought to cause some of this material to escape from the sun as the solar plasma or "solar wind," the more energetic components of which we detect as solar cosmic radiation.

These instabilities of the solar surface are particularly frequent in regions (or at times) with many sunspots. The abrupt bright-ening (particularly visible at the Hα wavelength) of up to one per cent of the solar disc in such regions is called a "solar flare," an event occurring simultaneously with a detectible increase at the earth in radio noise and x-ray emission and usually but not necessarily correlated with an eventual increase in ejected solar plasma, which, because of its slower velocity, reaches the earth 30 min to several hours after the x-ray changes. The appearance of the flare, and surrounding sun, changes abruptly, with the luminous flare border appearing to expand at up to a thousand kilometers a second and other features of the sun as much as 10^5 km away (such as a dark filament) briefly disappearing within minutes. These changes may reflect a transmission of instability within the solar atmosphere as well as different aspects of a common subsurface solar instability. The flares last on average 30 min; the resulting increase in solar cosmic radiation, called a solar storm, as detected at the earth, may last several days, due to the transmission delays of the different particulate radiations.

Attempts are being made to predict the occurrence of the large flares, which are usually associated with solar storms. Anderson (1961) states, "The large flares that produce fluxes of protons occur predominantly in sunspot groups having lifetimes of at least one week, and particularly in those that have reached a fair degree of complexity." Solar cosmic ray events were found to occur particularly when sunspot groups had large unbroken penumbral areas, but since these cannot be predicted prior to their observed development, or appearance ready formed on the sun's eastern limb as the sun rotates, this criteron cannot be used in scheduling space flights with low shielding lasting more than about four days. We must await improvements in solar structure theory to provide longer term solar storm prediction criteria. Preliminary indications from 1957–1958 data are that the ratio of number of solar proton events to large flares is greatest in the July–September quarter of the year (Anderson, 1961). Likewise, intense geomagnetic events, associated with the arrival of solar cosmic rays, appear most probably (1943–1960 data) in the periods from August 6 to October 6, and February 6 to April 6, as the earth in the ecliptic plane moves above or below the solar magnetic equatorial plane (Adamson and Davidson, 1962).

During the 1957–1958 solar maximum, about ten large solar flares occurred per month; one to two of these per month produced notably elevated solar cosmic radiation. All of the 1957–1958 storms were of the type with few protons with energies above 1 Bev, which may be called a "low particle energy solar cosmic radiation storm," or simply a low energy proton event. Near the solar minima, a year may go by with no solar cosmic storms. Storms tend to occur in multiples, several possibly arising from the same sunspot group.

About every four years, generally not at a sunspot cycle maximum but still from solar areas of complex sunspot activity, a "high particle energy solar cosmic radiation storm" occurs; the high energy event of February 23, 1956 was the most notable of these since 1932. Counting rates of over 1000 protons/cm² sec with energies above 1 Bev have been estimated for the early period of this storm, able to penetrate over 300 gm/cm² (or 3 m) of water. A few protons had energies above 10 Bev. It is these high energy solar cosmic radiation storms which are of particular concern for space flights beyond the protection of the earth's

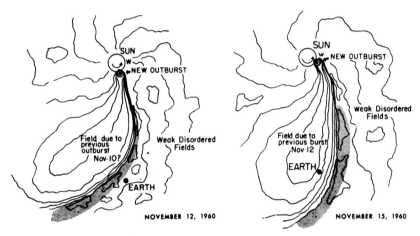

Fig. 1. Magnetic field effects on solar cosmic storms. (From Steljes *et al.*, 1961, by permission.)

magnetic field. Such "giant" high energy storms occurred on 2/28/42, 3/7/42, 7/25/46, 11/19/49, 2/23/56, 7/14/59 and 5/4/60. Moderate energy solar cosmic radiation storms also occur, with higher frequency than the high energy proton events but a lower frequency than the low energy proton events.

The mechanisms of transfer of particulate matter from the sun through interplanetary space are now under intensive study with the aid of satellites and international cooperative programs of observation of solar flares, aurorae, magnetic field effects, secondary cosmic neutrons and mesons, etc. Motion away from the sun of these particles, non-uniformly emitted, expectedly distorts the solar magnetic field, to create disordered field regions and "magnetic bottles" of closed magnetic field loops more strongly localized in solid angle than the hypothetical undistorted solar magnetic field loop. These "magnetic bottles" created by one localized solar outburst and maintained for several days by the slower motions of the lower energy particles can expectedly trap the faster moving particles of a subsequent outburst as well as "store" particles as a consequent of their distorted spiral paths, to subsequently release these particles over a longer time course and wider angular dispersion than would be the case for travel of single particles in the hypothetical undistorted solar magnetic field. Figure 1, from Steljes, Carmichael and McCracken, 1961, shows a hypothetical view of the solar magnetic field effects of the low energy solar cosmic radiation events of November 12 and November 15, 1960.

A charged particle, moving at right angles to a magnetic field is deflected in a circular path, in a plane perpendicular to the magnetic field. If the velocity has a component parallel to the magnetic field, this component is unaffected, and the particle travels with a helical path. A large number of charged particles moving together create a significant moving magnetic field with complicating interaction effects. Ions entering regions of increasing magnetic field will turn in tighter helices and may be reflected at a "mirror point" characterized for ions of particular energy by specific changing magnetic field conditions. Moreover, ions travelling in helices about magnetic lines of force may reverse direction as the lines of force bend sharply and reverse direction. In moving magnetic fields, ions may gain or lose energy.

It may be seen that a cloud of particles of varying kinetic energies starting together from a solar eruption will rapidly separate into more and less rapidly travelling components, with differing helical paths in the disturbed solar magnetic field. Whereas the electromagnetic radiations, such as the visual optical flare and elevated radio noise and x-radiations, take 8 min to traverse the 93 million miles from the sun to the earth, the solar cosmic protons due to magnetic field effects continue to arrive for several days as they are released from magnetic trapping.

The high energy proton events yield protons which travel faster than the low energy events. These protons are less affected by magnetic effects, and hence have less spread in direction and time of arrival at the earth than is the case for low energy protons. Hence at the earth the high energy solar storm may be over in a day or so, whereas the low energy storm may continue for ten or twelve days.

For reasons not yet understood, the high energy proton events involve fewer numbers of protons, i.e., have a lower intensity, than the moderate energy events. Hence with the slight shielding of present spacecraft (under 10 gm/cm²), the biological dose of the moderate energy high intensity storm of May 10, 1959 would have been greater than the dose from the high energy moderate intensity storm of February 23, 1956, as shown in Figure 2.

It is emphasized that our information on the spectra of solar cosmic storms, and their time changes, is still sparse. Most analyses have relied on temporal and altitude extrapolations from sub-orbital rocket and balloon measurements, and the few interplanetary orbital measurements. Hence the doses indicated in Figure 2, calculated using such extrapolations, may be in error. Improved data may be expected, for example from the Orbiting Solar Observatory series of experiments of the United States National Aeronautics and Space Administration. However the point can be made that solar storms can increase the unshielded dose rate from the 0.02 rad/day of the galactic cosmic radiation to perhaps several thousand rad/hr at the peak of the most severe storm, requiring shields of perhaps 25 to 100 gm/cm² to reduce the integrated dose below 25 rem.

Although emphasis for solar cosmic radiation has been placed on the protons, and heavier particles have not yet been identified in this radiation, in order for the sun to maintain charge neutrality and continue to emit charged particles, solar particulate radiation (and indeed also galactic cosmic radiation) must also include electrons. These will take different paths than the protons

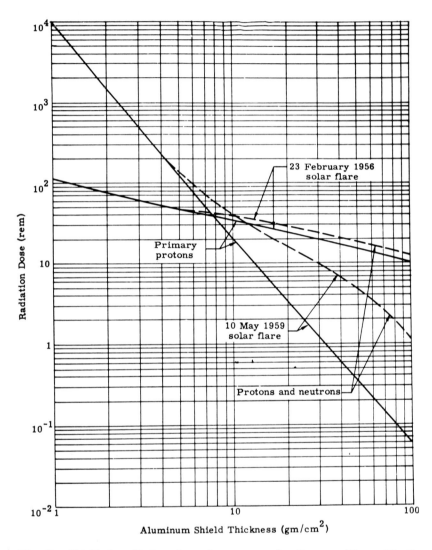

Fig. 2. Shielded radiation dose from two solar flares. (From Martin Company analysis by S. Russak *et al.*)

through the swirling magnetic fields, and localized charge differences may occur, which may be of significance to the space traveller. Slowing of these electrons involves Bremsstrahlung production, not usually considered in analyzing solar cosmic radiation effects.

Because of the magnetic spiralling and trapping effects, charged particles take very devious paths away from the sun, and may arrive in the vicinity of the earth from any direction, not just that towards the sun. Indeed preliminary indications are that at an interplanetary point the particulate radiation arrives essentially isotropically in direction. Hence "shadow shielding," by orienting the bulky unmanned part of a space vehicle towards the sun, would not be effective. We look forward to obtaining measurements to show whether indeed a solar storm is just as severe on the dark side of the moon as on the side towards the sun. Although the delayed solar cosmic radiation is approximately isotropic in direction at a point beyond the earth's magnetic field, it is re-emphasized that points several million miles apart could experience quite different solar cosmic radiation intensities.

C. The "Magnetosphere" Radiation Belts

The trapping of changed particulate radiation by the earth's magnetic field has been well reviewed by Singer, 1960, Vernov and Chudakov, 1960, and Van Allen, 1959. Laboratory experiments by Birkeland over sixty years ago with a magnetized sphere, simulating the earth, in a discharge tube, led to theoretical predictions by Störmer of the limited "allowed" regions for the motions of charged particles in the earth's magnetic field. Further analyses and simulation experiments were made by Alfvén and coworkers; the paths of charged particles moving in a dipole magnetic field, shown in Figure 3, may called "Störmer-Alfvén trajectories." Because of the convergence of the magnetic lines of force toward the magnetic poles, i.e., an increasing field strength, the helix angles of the particles as they spiral about these lines of force will increase, until the particle reverses direction, at a "magnetic mirror," and this is repeated towards the

opposite pole. The "Störmer-allowed" region is a "magnetic
bottle," trapping the charged particles within the magnetic field
lamellae appropriate to their energies and headings. The trajectories precess in azimuth, with protons drifting to the west and
electrons to the east, producing a "ring current" effect.

Prior to satellite measurements, attempts were made to interpret
ground based and sub-orbital rocket measurements to explain
cosmic ray intensities, aurorae and magnetic storms. A contribution to cosmic ray intensities as measured by rockets was sug-

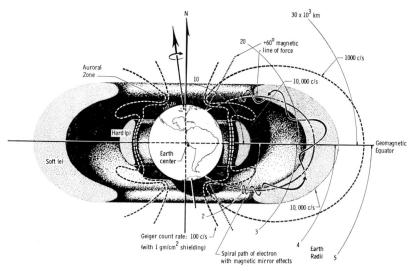

Fig. 3.   Diagrammatic representation of interactions between earth magnetic fields and charged particles forming inner and outer Van Allen belts.

gested to come from "albedo neutrons" produced as daughter
products of nuclear interactions of primary cosmic particles with
the upper atmosphere. These neutrons could penetrate the
regions of the magnetic field "forbidden" for charged particles,
and on spontaneous decay to a proton and an electron could
deliver these charged particles to an allowed region, where they
could be trapped. Some fifty years ago, Störmer had suggested
that a "ring current" at about the distance of the moon, of
unspecified origin, could deflect solar particles into the auroral

zones, some 20° from the geomagnetic poles. Chapman and Ferraro in 1931 interpreted magnetic storms in terms of a modified ring current hypothesis. Singer, in 1957, suggested that the azimuth drift of trajectories of trapped charged particles could comprise this ring current, with the particles arriving in sufficiently large groups from the sun to penetrate through the regions "forbidden" by a simple dipole magnetic field. Hence before the satellite measurements, the elements of the present view were presented, but there was no expectation of the great intensity of the radiation belts.

Sputnik II (November, 1957) provided the first satellite radiation measurements. Over the USSR at heights up to 700 km when satellite latitude exceeded 60°, gas discharge tube count rates increased 50 per cent over rates at the same altitude at lower latitude. It was later recognized that the lower border, at high latitudes, of the outer radiation belt had been traversed. It is the "dumping" of primarily electrons, with energies generally below 100 Kev, from the outer radiation belt through these high latitude borders (north and south) which produce aurorae.

Explorer 1 (January, 1958) provided Geiger counts of radiation in latitudes within ±33°. Quite unexpectedly, the counter was blocked near peak altitudes by an excessive count rate exposure; the lower border of the inner radiation belt had been contacted. Explorer-3 (March, 1958) provided additional data, interpreted by Van Allen and co-workers in May, 1958, in terms of particulate radiation trapped in what came to be called the inner Van Allen radiation belt, then thought to be of solar origin. The "Argus" experiments of August, 1958, involving high altitude nuclear explosions, showed the possibility of artificially filling a laminar magnetic force zone, strongly supporting the trapped radiation interpretation. Sputnik-3 (May, 1958), with an inclination of 65°, showed that the inner belt was limited within the magnetic lines of force which intersect the earth within the geomagnetic latitudes of ±50—55°. Sputnik-3 also measured the lower energy electron flux at higher latitudes, providing the first indication that there were different inner and outer regions of the space radiation. The Russians call this "terrestrial corpus cular radiation" of the "earth's corona," or simply the "radiation belt." Singer (1958) made a theoretical interpretation of the inner belt arising from cosmic ray albedo neutron decay (an hypothesis independently developed by Vernov and co-workers) and hence consisting notably of energetic protons (100 Mev), and predicted an outer belt of less energetic particles trapped from solar particulate radiation.

Separate belts were indeed identified by the U. S. Pioneer-1 and Pioneer-3 probes (October and December, 1958) and by the Space Rockets I (Lunik-1, January, 1959) and II (Lunik-2, September, 1959). Lunik-2 also established the absence of a radiation belt around the moon, related to the absence of a significant lunar magnetic field. Subsequent probes, with varying detectors and filters have clarified the structure of the radiation belt. Present emphasis is on the intergradation of solar and cosmic albedo effects within the "magnetosphere." At the time of this writing the United States probe to Venus indicated no magnetic field for this planet. The Soviets had a probe en route to Mars to find whether magnetic fields and radiation belts exist about this planet; apparently communication failure prevented getting such data.

The earth's dipole magnetic axis is offset from the axis of rotation, being tipped 11.5° towards Canada, with the north magnetic pole (eccentric dipole approximation) presently near 80°N, 83°W. Present interpretation (Vestine) is that the dipole center is located some 350 km from the earth's center along a geographic heading towards 16°N, 149°E. The radiation belt is approximately symmetrical with respect to the dipole axis. Hence the inner belt is closest to the earth (600 km altitude) off Brazil and furthest from the earth (1600 km altitude) above the western Pacific.

In more detail, the geomagnetic field has other anomalies. A particularly strong depression of the field over Cape Town, South Africa, may allow the charged particles to spiral deeper into the atmosphere, where they give up their charge to lower energy neutral particles or are scattered out of their Störmer trajectories, thereby depleting the particles in this magnetic shell.

Indeed, this may be one mechanism explaining the reduced population "slot" within the radiation belt, at about 2.6 earth radii at the geomagnetic equator.

Figure 3 shows some of the Geiger count rate contours estimated by Van Allen (1959), for counters shielded with 1 gm/cm² of aluminum equivalent. More extensive measurements, with ion chambers, scintillators, use of various shields over counters, and including nuclear emulsion analysis (Naugle and Kniffen, 1961), have extended this description. Because of a charged particle trapping time in the inner belt judged to be tens of years, present indications are that the natural inner belt intensity would vary less than an order of magnitude over the years, although human contamination, and indeed possible decontamination of this region is changing this condition. Trapping time in the outer belt region on the other hand may be a matter of days, for even moderate solar storm fluxes penetrate into and distort the magnetosphere even down to two earth radii, causing a loss of the "magnetic mirror" effects and a rapid "dumping" of particles, particularly into the auroral zones.

Figure 3 shows a Geiger count rate for a broad inner magnetosphere region of above 10,000 counts/sec with the center located at an altitude of about 3500 km above the geomagnetic equator. In the core this count, corrected for the 20 cm² surface of the counter, is estimated to be produced primarily by 2×10^4 protons/cm² sec with energies above 70 Mev, with 10 per cent of these protons in the energy range 300–700 Mev and 1 per cent with energies above 700 Mev (Wallner and Kaufman, 1961). In addition, the inner zone core is estimated to contain some 10^7 electrons/cm² sec with energies above 600 Kev (Van Allen, 1961). With 1 gm/cm² shielding, the equivalent inner zone dose rate is of the order of 10 rad/hr, and very much higher for the 0.2 gm/cm² shielding of the present design pressure suit alone. Because of the high energy protons, extensive shielding would be required to remain safely in this region. A 700 Mev proton has a range of 250 gm/cm² (9 ft H_2O). Rapid traversals or the use of the polar escape route can keep exposures below 2 rem (Schaeffer, 1959). Because of the spiralling particle trajectories, the radiation is not omni-directional. Some shadow shielding benefits would be obtained by traversing both belt regions with the longer vehicle axis perpendicular to the local magnetic field.

The outer zone has a maximum count rate at an altitude of about 18,000 km above the geomagnetic equator, produced during a solar maximum period by some 10^7 electrons/cm² sec with energies above 200 Kev. The proton count, for energies above 75 Mev, is less than 1 proton/cm² sec (Van Allen, 1961). For a shielding of 1 gm/cm² this would produce about 10 rad/hr, with a reasonable traversal time of 15 min for a lunar flight. These electrons are far more easily slowed, and their Bremsstrahlung stopped, than the high energy protons of the inner zone. Dose rates of 0.01 rad/hr (10 counts/sec) behind 1 gm/cm² shielding extended out to an altitude of 55,000 km (Pioneer-4, March, 1959), then retracted to 38,000 km. (Explorer VI, August, 1959) with a reduced solar activity. (Arnoldy, Hoffman, and Winckler, 1961). Although intensity variations of the outer region of the magnetosphere are attributed to the solar cosmic radiation whose energetic components are protons, the high energy component in the outer zone is apparently mainly electrons, with the solar cosmic protons being dumped into the atmosphere. Apparently an unknown mechanism exists for accelerating the trapped electrons in the outer zone, a problem emphasized by S. N. Vernov.

Earth magnetic field effects are indistinguishable from "quiet" interplanetary field effects at about 13.5 earth radii (86,000 km), with a magnetic field intensity of about 10^{-5} gauss or 1 gamma. During solar storms, the solar wind fields extend much further into the earth's magnetosphere, with apparently extensive interface instabilities. Explorer VI showed that the earth magnetic field has a large scale anomaly in the region of five to eight earth radii attributed to the "ring current" effect of the spiralling trapped protons and electrons. This also apparently changes position with solar storm action.

On July 9, 1962, the United States exploded a 1.4 megaton equivalent nuclear device at an altitude of 400 km over Johnson Island, in the Pacific. Expectation was that the nuclear particles would distort the lower magnetosphere and ionosphere, seriously but temporarily affecting radio communication and perhaps moderately depleting or increasing the lower zone of the radiation belt. Instead, communication was little affected, and the lower belt was not depleted, but was apparently augmented near its core with additional high energy electrons with energies up to 8 Mev, to perhaps 10^9/cm^2 sec with energies above 200 Kev, with perhaps half with energies above 1 Mev, at an altitude of 3200 km, now expectedly to remain near the core for one to many years (Hess and Nakada, 1962). A week after the explosion, intensities of 2×10^6 electrons/cm^2 sec were still detectable at an altitude of 320 km over Brazil, where the inner belt dips most closely to the earth, posing a possible radiation hazard to manned orbital flights which were safely below the natural radiation belt. This lower altitude contamination is moderately rapidly being attenuated; the orbital flights of Nicholayev (August 10–14, 1962), Popovich (August 11–14), and Schirra (October 3) were not jeopardized. However five unmanned satellites (Injun: 1961 omicron 2; Transit 4B: 1961 Alpha eta 1; Traac: 1961 alpha eta 2; Ariel: 1962 omicron 1; and Telstar I: 1962 alpha epsilon 1) were apparently damaged by this major extension of man's "cosmic garbage" capability.

D. Nuclear Power

Nuclear power has been used in space for military explosions and for radioactive decay thermoelectric power generation, the SNAP-3 2.7 watt nuclear generators of the Transit satellites (Morse, 1963). Developments are progressing well for higher power SNAP (Space Nuclear Auxiliary Power) sources, including the SNAP-8, 30 electrical kilowatt fission reactor, weighing 60 lb/kw (hopefully to be reduced to 10 lb/kw in later reactor electrical systems). Reactor designs (SNAP 50) of up to one megawatt to operate for one year for nuclear powered thrust engines are also under development (Finger, 1961, 1962.) The "Kiwi" reactor thrust engine prototypes have already operated, using a "direct pass" of hydrogen heated in the reactor as the thrust medium. The NERVA ("nuclear engine for rocket vehicle application") engine is under development from the Kiwi work with thrust in the 100,000 lb range, and the RIFT (reactor in flight test) third stage 85 ft long and 33 ft in diameter for C-5 Saturn flights with the operating reactor engine in 1966–1967 is under development. In addition nuclear reactors can be used to generate electrical power to drive "ion rocket" engines thus far of less than 1 lb thrust by accelerating mercury vapor or cesium ions by electrostatic or electromagnetic fields. Ion rockets of 40 megawatts (supplied by a nuclear reactor) are under consideration (Langmuir, 1962.) With thrusts of less than 10 lb/megawatt, these engines must operate for perhaps half of the flight time during an interplanetary voyage.

The advantages of nuclear propulsion are seen by comparing energy release per gram of chemical reactants or U-235 nuclear fuel burned, and specific impulse (pounds of thrust acting for a time in seconds per pound of chemical reactants or thrust medium ejected, hence with a reduced unit of "seconds") of chemical and nuclear engines.

Engine	Specific Impulse	Energy Release
Solid chemicals	250 sec	1 kcal/gm
Liquid hydrocarbon-oxygen chemicals	300 sec	1 kcal/gm
(TNT + O_2)		1 kcal/gm TNT ($+ O_2$)
(Bituminous coal + O_2)		4 kcal/gm C($+ O_2$)
Nuclear reactor + H_2	1000 sec	2×10^7 kcal/gm U-235
Nuclear reactor + electrostatic mercury vapor rocket	4000 sec (Possible developments to 10,000 sec)	2×10^7 kcal/gm U-235

It is estimated that the Mars mission nuclear rocket, with a 10,000 megawatt first stage assembled in earth orbit, would weigh one tenth as much as a comparable mission chemical rocket (Finger, 1961), and indeed more severe missions may not be possible until the higher energy efficiency of nuclear propulsion is available.

A fission reaction may be approximately represented by

$$^{235}U + 2n \rightleftharpoons A + B + 5\gamma + 2.5n + 195 \text{ Mev/atom}$$

Of the 195 Mev released per atom of U-235 fissioned, about 160 Mev is carried as kinetic energy of the primary fission fragments A and B, about 20 Mev is released with the subsequent radioactive decay of the primary fission fragments to produce further fragments and about 5γ and 10β in addition, and the rest of the energy is carried by the gamma rays and neutrons. In approximation, the β, γ, and n radiations of fission originate with about 1 Mev energy each. The fissioning of one gram of U-235 or $6 \times 10^{23}/238 = 2.5 \times 10^{21}$ atoms, releases one megawatt-day of energy, equivalent to the explosion of 20 tons (18 million grams) of chemical explosive, and the order of 10^{22} gamma rays and neutrons. Hence a one megawatt reactor releases 10^{22} gamma rays and neutrons per day, and a one megaton equivalent explosion, involving the fissioning of 50 kg of U-235, releases on the order of 10^{26} each of gamma rays and neutrons. It is this radiation which must be shielded against when there is use of nuclear power in space.

Fortunately, this radiation is far less energetic than the galactic cosmic radiation. Local shield thicknesses adequate for long duration flights (more than one year) in galactic and solar cosmic radiation may also be adequate for protection against the radiation of these early nuclear reactors, which leak less than 1% of their radiation through their moderator and containment vessel, particularly when the reactor is positioned at some distance (more than 100 ft) from the crew and shielded by remaining fuel and some "shadow shield" required for equipment operation.

As we attempt larger space missions, with larger reactors, fleets of space vehicles may be utilized for safety reliability. The Mars mission for example might be attempted with three vehicles, with all three crews able to return in any one ship. Moreover, rendezvous with nuclear powered vehicles such as a nuclear earth-lunar shuttle stage may also expose crews to radiations from adjacent vehicles if rendezvous is not affected within the umbra of the shadow shield. Hence we may find it necessary to use more direct crew compartment shielding, with less dependence on shadow shielding. Clearly, as local shielding requirements due to expected radiation levels grow beyond 100 gm/cm^2 (a meter of water), the increased storage of supplies which can make up this shield places a decreasing requirement for the reutilization (as closed food cycles for example) of these supplies, and allows greater safety margins of available supplies. Instead of a lead shield, we can store extra cans of water, steaks, books, etc.

E. Induced Radioactivity, Residual Radioactivity, Radionuclides and Electronics as High Energy Radiation Sources

As incident quantum or particle energies exceed 1 Mev, or particularly 10 Mev, or as neutrons are absorbed, nuclear reactions become possible, and artificial radioactivity may be induced. The extent of this radioactivity may be said to depend on the "capture cross-sections" of the material involved in these nuclear reactions. Materials with large capture cross-sections become rapidly radioactive, if the nuclear reaction products are radioactive, but these radioactive products in turn have short half lives, and more rapidly loose their radioactivity. As compound materials continue to be exposed, equilibria will be approached for each of the possible radionuclides, in which the rate of production and rate of decay of the radionuclide just balance for the particular incident dose rate. Analysis of the radiations from these induced radionuclides may be used to quantify the concentrations of parent elements, the basis of the chemistry technique of "activation analysis." Alternately, knowing the sample chemistry (often in the form of metal foils), the nature of the induced activity in a certain time can indicate the dose and quality of the radiation, the basis for "foil dosimetry."

In the space environment, the astronaut must be prepared for such induced activity outside of his shielded areas, particularly following intense solar storms or the recent use of his reactors. Design of the space vehicle should utilize materials having low capture cross-sections, such as aluminum in preference to iron, or materials with high capture cross-sections such as hydrogen or boron, as desired for shielding purposes, whose nuclear reaction products are not radioactive. Likewise on the surface of the moon and other bodies without atmospheric shielding, with long exposure to cosmic radiations, an induced radioactivity will be present, although an analysis by Barton (1960) indicates that this would give an unshielded human a dose of the order of 30 millirem/year, commensurate with the dose from the "natural" radio-activity of K-40, U-235, U-238, Th and their daughter products.

Following the shutdown of a nuclear reactor, its radioactivity does not drop off instantaneously; the residual gamma radiation a day after shutdown may still be one third of its operational gamma activity. One does not conceive of our spaceman retro-firing to a landing on nuclear power, shutting down the reactor, then hopping out of his shielded cabin to be about his business. Moreover, the space logistics and population hazards of having gigawatt reactors land on earth bespeaks our using chemically powered planetary or lunar landing vehicles which rendezvous with planetary or lunar nuclear power shuttle stages which are maintained in space, perhaps even to the extent of doing fuel reprocessing there.

The use of reactors can increase the contamination by radionuclides of the astronaut's environment, although the "closing" of this environment provides a considerable isolation. To the extent that atoms from outside the cabin can enter the life support cycles, contamination can occur. Thus on the Mars mission, a nuclear fuel element failure may coat the vehicle with fission products. If an emergency requires an astronaut to work on the outside of the vehicle, even months later, he may bring some of these products back into the cabin. Clearly, radionuclide radiation monitoring and decontamination procedures will be desirable when extra-vehicular operations are planned on nuclear vehicles. The symposium edited by Dougherty *et al.,* 1962, provides a recent review of this "internal irradiation" problem.

As high energy radiation sources, one should not forget the high voltage electronic equipment utilized in spacecraft for radar ranging, telemetry, scientific measurement, etc. The high voltage vacuum tubes in such devices produce significant x-radiation, which through propinquity to the astronaut (for he may indeed be almost straddling a TV tube for large portions of the flight) may without careful and retained shielding give significant proportions of the total trip radiation dose. In addition, microwave beams may produce injury.

VI. BIOLOGICAL EFFECTS

No attempt can be made here to describe the breadth of radiation biology; the reader is referred to the excellent brief works by Browning, and Loutit, the more extensive books edited by Hollaender, and Campbell, an introduction to the Soviet work edited by Kiselev, Gusterin, and Strashinin, and the authoritative works under United Nations sponsorship, such as *The Use of Vital and Health Statistics for Genetic and Radiation Studies 1962*, and particularly the *Report of the United Nations Scientific Committee on the Effects of Atomic Radiation, 1962*. This section will note a few of the high energy radiation effects of consequence to manned space flight.

To understand the radiation sensitivity of man, who is killed by a radiation dose of a few hundred rad, in comparison to the sensitivity of inanimate objects for changes of properties, requiring doses of 10^8 rad or more, the dynamic molecular characteristics of the living state must be emphasized. We eat, drink and breath our body weight of new substance about every three weeks. The living state is a fabric of organization through which washes the temporary realization which is today's set of atoms. Whereas for the transitor for example a significant proportion of fixed molecular constituents must be altered by radiation interaction before its properties are changed, with man changes of structure of a few molecules which affect organization leads to an altered reproduced organization from then on, with a "biological amplification" from an effect of the few changed organization molecules to an effect of the many molecules altered by that changed organization in subsequent biochemical "turnover" processes. Doses of radiation which may change only one molecule in one cell, producing a dominant lethal mutation, may kill an organism, as an extreme case. More typically, doses of radiation which change only one molecule in perhaps 10^7 will kill mammals.

Biological amplification is most clearly seen in looking at the dividing cell; a reproduced change in a stem cell will lead to a similar change in every daughter cell. Moreover, the dividing cell may be viewed as having the reproductive abilities of all of its organization tested, whereas the specialized cell no longer dividing may be utilizing only part of its organization capabilities. Thus, by 1906, Bergonié and Tribondeau were able to say, "X-rays are more effective in cells which have greater reproductive activity; the effectiveness is greater on those cells which have a longer dividing future ahead, on those cells the morphology and function of which are least fixed." Thus radiation induced morphology changes are seen at lower doses for the rapidly dividing tissues of the blood, germinal epithelium, intestinal mucosa, ectodermal epithelium and the embryo than for the undividing cells of mature muscle and nerve, for example. Changes of other aspects of cell function following radiation may show a different order.

But "biological amplification" also occurs in this continuous biochemical turnover of the functioning but not dividing cell. A primary organization is maintained, in spite of the vast flux of changing individual atoms. Mechanisms of this functional control are just beginning to be determined, with a primary importance being given to the nuclear deoxyribonucleic acids (or "DNA," which may turnover only on cell division), which control "messenger" ribonucleic acids, and in turn these control or determine the structure of proteins, including enzymes. The mechanisms of most of this control are still far from clear; we have no idea how DNA codes, or other cytoplasmic codes, can control aggregates of molecules to make one species' mitochondria typically of different form than those of another species—or indeed one man's nose longer than another's. But a basic organization with a consequent biological amplification of the consequences of changing just a few of the molecules of this organization appears to be involved.

Apparently some of this organization involves resultant action by groups of molecules. Thus a change of one molecule is not effective in changing this resultant action, and a "threshold dose" or level of molecular change is required before the net action is changed. Moreover, there is expectedly a time span required to affect a complex biochemical turnover process; it is not surprising that radiation effects can be altered by other changes introduced during this critical time span, brought about by different doses or dose rates for example, or apparently even changes of environment, such as oxygen tension, temperature stress or hormone level.

Whereas the genetic effects of radiation appear generally to be proportional to dose, without a threshold or dependence on dose rate, somatic effects do vary with dose rate, and may have thresholds of dose below which no effect can be identified. The statistical problems of identifying these thresholds are formidable (see the United Nations statistical report, 1962). The reports that exposed populations do not differ significantly in incidence of an effect from control populations too often must be interpreted in terms of excessive variability of the control populations or inadequate size of the populations, rather than a certain lack of an effect.

The variability of individual responses must also be considered. For lethality of apparently equivalently healthy individual animals of the same species, a factor of more than two may separate the acute dose required to kill the first and last within a certain time span (usually 30 days). Means are not yet at hand to predict tolerance, and select astronauts for radiation resistance. For mice, an inherited effect on resistance has been identified. With the lower dose rates of chronic exposure, a considerable recovery effect occurs for lethality, so that doses acquired over years may exceed the acute dose lethal in thirty days for 50 per cent of a population, the LD_{50}-30 dose, by even a factor of 10.

Long duration space flight exposes the astronaut to both categories of exposure: the chronic dose of weeks' duration from galactic cosmic radiation, radioisotope contamination, and long term nuclear power use as well as the acute dose of a day's duration or less from flights through the magnetosphere radiation belts, solar storms and the use of short duration high thrust nuclear engines. In this early period of short duration flight, emphasis is on reducing the acute dose, particularly that due to solar storms. Early thrust limitations may preclude completely adequate spacecraft shielding, so that to the extent that solar storm prediction capabilities are inadequate, exposures to astronauts may occur which are significantly beyond the "maximum permissible dose" of 5 rem/year or 25 rem in any single emergency exposure for terrestrial workers with radiation (Morgan, 1963). A synopsis of expected effects is presented, drawing particularly on nuclear reactor and weapon radiation experience (Glasstone, 1957; United Nations, 1962).

For exposures of 25–100 rem, just detectible blood changes may be seen microscopically, but the astronaut may not be subjectively aware of the exposure. Animal studies show detectible changes of conditioned reflexes at this exposure level, emphasizing that functional nervous system effects may be more sensitive than morphological nerve cell effects (see Haley and Snider, 1962, and Kiselev *et al.*, 1962). The genetic "doubling dose" for germ cells is in this range, with a doubling of probabilities of occurrence of mutations. Since most of these mutations are not fully dominant, the increased probability of the astronaut's child showing visible damage because the astronaut received a doubling dose is perhaps 0.1 per cent, where some 6 per cent of the general population's offspring before age five, including stillbirths, show some visible damage (United Nations report, 1962). Most of the damage appears in later generations, hidden in the damage the rest of society and nature effect on our gene pool. Somatic cells also mutate, with an increased probability of leukemia for example suggested to be 2×10^{-6}/rem year (Lewis, 1957), although Taylor (1962) hopes that one can set a "practical threshold" before one considers an increased probability of leukemia of 50 r.

In this moderate dose level, chromosomal abnormalities might be looked for by astronauts on long duration flights, using arrested leucocyte metaphase smear or other techniques. These should also be used following a flight; Bender and Gooch (1962) report up to 23 per cent of the chromosome counts of men exposed to accidental whole body irradiation 2.5 yr earlier were abnormal, with rings, dicentrics, minutes, pericentric inversions, translocations and deletions being seen.

For exposures of 100 to 250 rem, nausea and vomiting may develop within a few hours. If the astronaut has instruments which detect the onset of the solar storm, the sooner nausea develops thereafter, the more severe the warning of radiation injury.

Since the prompt x-radiation of the storm gives a warning of the approach and perhaps even an indication of the quantity of the consequent particulate radiation, the astronaut has time to take chemical protection and movable shield protection measures. Following nausea, finger prick blood smear microscopic examinations should be made to estimate prognosis of the radiation sickness. If the leucocyte count goes below $500/mm^3$ in three to six days, survival is not expected, unless extensive supportive therapy is provided. Following a few hours of nausea, a "latent period" of feeling well insues, a favorable time to make an emergency termination of the flight, if possible. This may be followed in about two weeks by loss of appetite and a general malaise, and at the higher doses, loss of hair (epillation) which will grow back in about two months, sterility lasting one or two years, diarrhea, and small skin hemorrhages (petechiae), with a gradual recovery in the next month or two. The delayed effects, such as leukemia and other cancers, and life shortening of perhaps 1–15 days/rem, with perhaps a dependence on dose and dose rate (Browning, 1959; Jones, 1956) appear much later. The leukemia incidence after Hiroshima peaked in about 6 yr. In this exposure range, the skin epidermis thickness may be reduced; finger print ridge height might be measured before and after flights.

For exposures of 250 to 750 rem, the onset of nausea and vomiting will occur sooner, perhaps in 1 hr after a 750 rem dose given in seconds, and a state of shock develops. In the space environment, the dose rate will be lower than for a nuclear explosion, with the solar storm passing in 2 hr to two days rather than 1 to 10 min. However, early nausea during a solar storm is a severe warning of trouble. It is emphasized that a motivated and well trained astronaut can continue many of his control tasks during nausea, and indeed even during moderate shock if he is conscious, as evidenced by stress simulation experience. However, some training on maintaining task performance during induced nausea may be appropriate. The falling blood pressure accompanying nausea would probably reduce acceleration tolerance; the astronaut should have drugs available to counteract this effect if a re-entry is necessary.

Space helmet design should consider vomiting problems. Clearly, the "face seal" design is less adequate than the "free head" design, but face plate splattering and aspiration of vomitus remain problems made even more severe in the weightless state. Possibly astronauts flying in groups should be trained in the tracheotomy procedure in case one is gaging. If the cabin has pressure, the astronaut can open the face plate and use a throw-up bag. Diarrhea is an even more severe problem in a pressure suit. Hence in a translunar flight if a severe solar storm is experienced in this early period of marginal shielding, it may be the necessary course as diarrhea commences to get out of the pressure suit and trust that cabin pressure will not fail before the flight can be terminated.

For this possibly lethal range of exposure, the latent period of apparent recovery after perhaps a day of nausea and vomiting is shortened from two weeks (for 250 rem) to perhaps two to four days (for 750 rem) before nausea, vomiting and diarrhea return. The lymphocyte and leucocyte blood counts fall to minima in perhaps six days, then hopefully rise, although their protection against infection is drastically reduced in this period, requiring antibiotic support of the astronaut. (The granulocytes may triple in number on the first day, before falling.) The blood platelets reach a minimum in about eight days, with increasing small hemorrhages, nose bleeds and bloody diarrhea. At the higher dose levels, the lips and gums ulcerate, the mouth and throat are inflamed, and fever and rapid emaciation develop. At about two weeks, the red blood cell count reaches a minimum, perhaps as low as 10 percent of the normal value. Without supportive therapy, death for half of those exposed to 400 rem will occur within 30 days (i.e., LD_{50}–30 for man is about 400 rem). In this dose range, this is called a "blood death." Supportive therapy of antibiotics, venous fluid infusion providing foods and maintaining water and mineral balance, blood transfusions, and possibly bone marrow injections (ideally from a marrow "bank" established by the particular astronaut before his flight) can save most of these people, although the self administration and automatic monitoring of these means while in space flight will take some preparation effort. With survival the long term effects of increased probabilities of cancers, cataracts of the eye lens, life shortening, and at the higher dose level, permanent sterility remain.

Additional stress applied during this period, such as cold stress, hypoxia, etc., may reduce the survival (see Kewsom and Kimeldorf, 1963). Just as shock therapy in any of its forms (such as

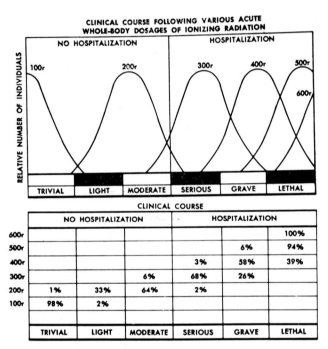

Fig. 4. Summary of expected clinical effects of whole-body ionizing radiation. (From Gerstner.)

attenuated tetanus fever therapy) may mobilize the body's defenses and lead to an improved recovery, it is not unreasonable that we will find physiological or biochemical procedures to counteract radiation effects. Perhaps the astronauts should increase exercise regimes when there is a chance of receiving a nominal lethal dose. A summary of the clinical effects to be anticipated following whole body radiation is shown in Figure 4 from a study by Gerstner based on data from Hiroshima and Nagasaki victims, nuclear accidents and effects on patients. It appears reasonable that short term exposures should be kept below a maximum of 200 r to avoid serious clinical consequences.

For exposures from 750 to perhaps 2000 rem, heroic supportive therapy measures as listed above are indeed required for any survival. Nausea and vomiting develop within less than an hour after accumulating this acute dose, and a state of shock develops, and perhaps unconsciousness. A return to alertness may occur in a few hours to a day, with perhaps one day of possible additional minimal activity during the latent period. Then nausea, vomiting, diarrhea and fever return, with death expected even if fluid and mineral balance are maintained in less than a week at the higher dose. The intestinal mucosa is extensively sloughed, oozing fluid and blood, to produce a "gut death" even before the maximum blood effect has time to develop.

For exposures above 2000 rem, disorientation and virtual unconsciousness may occur within minutes. Nausea and vomiting develop, with a minimum recovery, to be followed by death. A number of the human cases occurring from reactor accidents are well documented in the United Nations report (1962). These may be called "nerve deaths." Pickering mentions a human exposure of 10,000 r, with death in 38 hr (Jacobs, 1960).

It must be re-emphasized that only during a very intense solar storm with the astronaut inside the spacecraft of 10 gm/cm² shielding equivalent, or during a moderate solar storm with the astronaut outside the spacecraft in a pressure suit of less than 0.2 gm/cm² shielding, and only when beyond the earth's magnetosphere, or when within the radiation belts, would these extreme radiation doses be received. Extreme solar storms may have unshielded dose rates as high as 5000 rad/hr. Nicholeyev's exposure in a four day flight (August 11–15, 1962) was only 43 millirads (Space Log, Vol. 2, No. 4, Space Technology Laboratories, Redondo Beach, California, December, 1962). It must also be emphasized that the chronic exposure dose can be considerably above these values for a comparable effect. Thus Schaefer (1961), using Blair's (1952) "non-recoverable fraction" estimate of about 10 per cent and a recovery half time for man of 25–35 days, concludes that if a 50 rem acute dose is acceptable for equivalent short term somatic effects, 86 rem spread over thirty days, or 336 rem spread over a year, or 478 rem spread over three years should also be acceptable. Others are more conservative, although an emergency dose of 100 rem on a flight, with a probability of a lower dose of 95 per cent, seems more comparable to the other hazards than to jeopardize these other aspects of the flight by attempting to get even the emergency dose below 5 rem/flight.

A final note must be made concerning the preliminary nature of our space radiation measurements, estimations of the effects of complex beams of mixed radiations of vastly different penetration powers, and biological studies with very high energy particulate radiation. To paraphrase John Stapp's comment concerning acceleration, the best measure of the effect of space radiation on man is man.

VII.   MEANS OF PROTECTION

The quite adequate protection from space radiations is the 1000 gm/cm² shielding by the earth's atmosphere or the deflection shielding provided near the equator by the earth's magnetic field. Alternate but far less successful protection may be provided by certain chemical effects.

To attain 1000 gm/cm² requires a water layer of 10 m or a lead layer of 0.9 m, not feasible for passive shielding in this early era of costs to attain orbit of perhaps \$2000/kg. On the other hand, present (Apollo type) spacecraft walls and equipment provide a shielding of less than 10 gm/cm², giving doses approaching 100 rem if more than one large solar storm occurred during a flight (see Figure 2 above). For the Mars type flights of more than one year's duration, particularly with nuclear power sources (Konecci and Trapp, 1959), shielding approaching 100 gm/cm² appears necessary (Wallner and Kaufman, 1961). Means should be developed to have this shielding assembled from otherwise needed materials during solar storms or reactor use. Of particular interest is the use of rubber bags which can be inflated with air about the astronaut to provide vibration and impact isolation during exit and re-entry, inflated with fuels, water or wastes drawn in from the service module during radiation periods, then deflated out of the way during other periods (Cooper, Blechschmidt and Clark, 1963).

Analyses are progressing of means to provide magnetic shielding of space vehicles (Kash and Tooper, 1963). This approaches feasibility utilizing nuclear generated electrical power in the coils, made of super-conducting materials. However more needs to be learned about the biological effects of the magnetic fields required (Davis *et al.*, 1962).

Chemical protection is not as successful as one might hope (see Hollaender, Campbell and Doull *et al.* for examples). Protective agents, notably the thiols cysteine, cysteamine and "AET," must generally be given just before the radiation at a concentration level approaching toxic, in order to less than double the LD_{50} dose or double the survival time for an LD_{75} dose. However, the astronaut facing such doses would welcome such drugs, although he may have to be pre-conditioned to their toxic effects in advance. Hypoxia provides a similar magnitude of protection, so that it may be safer for the astronaut to use this means, automatically controlled under anesthesia. Indeed, the hypoxic action of ethanol may make this approach the most pleasant, albeit not the most effective. Post-radiation injections of stored bone marrow from the same astronaut can improve chances of survival up to doses of perhaps 750 rem, when "gut death" effects predominate.

Hence thus far it is material shielding which provides the best protection against space radiations. A typical engineer's response is to say that if man and his support equipment leave too little weight for the payload, then he would just take man out of the system and send his chunks of metal by themselves. Indeed, he should do this for the first flights. But the chunks of metal are there for the man, not man for just the tending of the chunks of metal. Indeed, man and his support equipment are the payload in this remarkable adventure, as man takes his fledgling steps from being "citizen-terra" to becoming "citizen-comos."

As far as we now know, for all of his evolution up to April 12, 1961, man has lived within a narrow shell of atmosphere on one of the smaller planets of one of the smaller stars of one of the smaller galaxies. In this first three years, of space flight up to 188 miles, he has acquired 18 days of experience above 100 miles. Man is about to leave his hereditary cradle; it is probable that space radiations will not stop him.

BIBLIOGRAPHY

1. ADAMSON, DAVID, and DAVIDSON, ROBERT E.: Statistics of solar cosmic rays as inferred from correlation with intense geomagnetic storms. *Technical Note D-1010, National Aeronautics and Space Administration.* Washington 25, D. C., February, 1962.
2. ANDERSON, KINSEY A.: Preliminary study of prediction aspects of solar cosmic ray events. *Technical Report D-700, National Aeronautics and Space Administration.* Washington 25, D. C., April, 1961.
3. BARTON, JOHN A.: An estimation of the nuclear radiation at the lunar surface. Preprint No. 60–54, American Astronautical Society, Boeing Airplane Company, Seattle, Washington, 1960.
4. BENDER, M. A., and GOOCH, P. C.: Persistent chromosome aberrations in irradiated humans. *Radiation Res., 16:*44–53, 1962.
5. BERGONIÉ, J., and TRIBONDEAU, L.: Interpretation de quelques résultats de la radiothérapie et essai de fixation d'une technique rationnelle. *C. R. Acad. Sci. (Paris), 143:*983–985, 1906. See translation, *Radiation Res. 11:*587, 1959.
6. BLAIR, H. A.: A formulation of the injury, life span, dose relations for ionizing radiations. *AEC Report UR-206.* University of Rochester, Rochester, New York, 1952.
7. BROWNING, ETHEL: *Harmful Effects of Ionizing Radiations.* Elsevier Publishing Company, New York, 1959.
8. CAMPBELL, PAUL, editor: *Medical and Biological Aspects of the Energies of Space.* Columbia University Press, New York, 1961.
9. COOPER, BRUCE, BLECHSCHMIDT, CARL, and CLARK, CARL: Human vibration and impact isolation with a full length airbag restraint system. *Engineering Report 12799,* Martin Company, Baltimore, 1963.
10. DAVIS, LEROY D., PAPPAJOHN, KRISTALLO, and PLAVNIEKS, ILGA: Bibliography on the biological effects of magnetic fields. *Federation Proc. 21,* Suppl. 12, September, 1962.
11. DOUGHERTY, THOMAS F., LEE, WEBSTER, S. S., MAYS, CHARLES W., and STOVER, BETSY J., editors: *Some Aspects of Internal Irradiation.* Pergamon Press, New York, 1962.

12. DOULL, JOHN, PLZAK, VIVIAN, and BROIS, STANLEY J.: A survey of compounds for radiation protection (USAF Radiation Laboratory, University of Chicago). *Report 62-29, School of Aerospace Medicine.* Brooks Air Force Base, Texas, April, 1962.

13. FINGER, HAROLD: Nuclear rockets and the space challenge. *Astronautics,* 6:24–26, 94–96, July, 1961.

14. FINGER, HAROLD: Nuclear energy, the space exploration energy source. In *Proceedings of the Second National Conference on the Peaceful Uses of Space.* Report SP-8, NASA, May, 1962.

15. FOELSCHE, TRUTZ: Current estimates of radiation doses in space. *Technical Note D-1267, NASA.* Washington 25, D. C., July, 1962.

16. GLASSTONE, S., editor: *The Effects of Nuclear Weapons.* U. S. Department of Defense, Washington, D. C., 1957.

17. HALEY, THOMAS J., and SNIDER, RAY S.: *Response of the Nervous System to Ionizing Radiation.* Academic Press, New York, 1962.

18. HESS, W. N., and NAKADA, PAUL: Artificial radiation belt discussed in symposium at Goddard Space Center. *Science, 138*:53–54, 1962.

19. HINE, GERALD, and BROWNELL, GORDON L.: *Radiation Dosimetry.* Academic Press, Inc., New York, 1956.

20. HOLLAENDER, A., editor: *Radiation Biology.* McGraw-Hill Book Company, Inc., New York, 1954.

21. JONES, H. B.: A special consideration of the aging process, disease, and life expectancy. *Advances of Biol. and Med. Phys.,* 4:281, 1956.

22. KASH, S. W., and TOOPER, R. F.: Correction on active shielding for manned spacecraft. *Astronautics,* 8:43, 1963.

23. KEWSOM, BERNARD D., and KIMELDORF, DONALD J.: Alterations in physiological accommodation to stress induced by irradiation. *Aerospace Med., 34*:226–230, 1963.

24. KISELEV, P. N., GUSTERIN, G. A., and STRASKININ, A. I., editors: *Problems of Radiobiology (Voprosy radiobiologii).* Volume 3: Collection of papers in honor of the 60th anniversary of Professor M. N. Pobedinskii. Translated by Y. S. Halpern and S. Shoshan, Israel Program for Scientific Translations. Sivan Press, Jerusalem, 1962. Available from the Office of Technical Services, U. S. Department of Commerce, Washington 25, D. C., as OTS 61-31017.

25. KONECCI, E. B., and TRAPP, R.: Calculations of the radiobiological risk factors in future nuclear powered space vehicles. *Aerospace Medicine, 30*:487–505, 1959.

26. LANGMUIR, DAVID: Electric spacecraft—progress 1962. *Astronautics,* 7:20–25, June, 1962. See also other papers of this "Electric spacecraft design" issue.

27. LEWIS, E. B.: *Science, 125*:965, 1957.

28. LOUTIT, JOHN F.: *Irradiation of Mice and Men.* The University of Chicago Press, Chicago, Illinois, 1962.

29. Menzel, D. H., Moreton, G. E., von Kenschitzki, C. H., Malville, J. M., *et al.:* Solar phenomena. *Proceedings of the Lunar and Planetary Exploration Colloquim,* Vol. 3, No. 1, May, 1962. (Office of Lunar and Planetary Exploration Colloquia, Space and Information Systems Division, North American Aviation, Inc., Downey, California.)

30. Morgan, Karl Z.: Permissible exposure to ionizing radiation. *Science, 139:*565–571, 1963.

31. Morse, J. G.: Energy for remote areas. *Science, 139:*1175–1180, 1963.

32. Nangle, John E., and Kniffen, Donald A.: The flux and energy spectra of the protons in the inner Van Allen belt. *Technical Note D-412, NASA.* Washington 25, D. C., August, 1961.

33. Price, William J.: *Nuclear Radiation Detection.* McGraw-Hill, New York, 1958.

34. Schaefer, Hermann J.: Radiation dosage in flight through the Van Allen belt. *Aerospace Med., 30:*631–639, 1959.

35. Schaefer, Hermann J.: The role of the time factor in the dosimetry of ionizing radiation in space. *Aerospace Med., 32:*909–914, 1961.

36. Schaefer, Herman J.: Permissible dose and emergency dose from ionizing radiation in space operations. *American Rocket Society Report 2137-61,* Space Flight Report to the Nation, October, 1961.

37. Shapiro, Maurice M.: Supernovae as cosmic ray sources. *Science, 135:*175–193, 1962.

38. Sharpe, J.: *Nuclear Radiation Detectors.* Methuen and Company, London, 1955.

39. Shcherban, E. I.: Effect of moderate physical strain during x-ray irradiation on the course of acute radiation sickness. In Kiselev *et al.* (*Ibid.*), p. 329–336, 1962.

40. Siegbahn, Kai: *Beta and Gamma-Ray Spectroscopy.* Interscience Publishers, Inc., New York, 1955.

41. Simons, David G., and Hewitt, John E.: Review of biological effects of galactic cosmic radiation. *Aerospace Med., 32:*932–941, 1961.

42. Steljes, F. F., Carmichael, H., and McCracken, K. G.: Characteristics and fine structure of the large cosmic ray fluctuations in November 1960. *J. Geophys. Res., 66:*1363–1377, 1961.

43. Singer, S. F.: On the nature and origin of the earth's radiation belts. In Bijl, J. K., editor: *Space Research, Proceedings of the First International Space Science Symposium.* North Holland Publishing Company, Amsterdam, 1960.

44. Taylor, L. S.: Radiation hazards in realistic perspective. *Physics Today, 15:*32–40, 1962.

45. Thomson, John F.: *Radiation Protection in Mammals.* Reinhold Book Division, New York, 1962.

46. TOBIAS, CORNELIUS A., and WALLACE, ROGER: Particulate radiation: electrons and protons up to carbon. In Campbell, P. (*Ibid.*), p. 421–442, 1962.

47. UNITED NATIONS: *The Use of Vital and Health Statistics for Genetic and Radiation Studies.* Proceedings of the Seminar Sponsored by the United Nations and the World Health Organization, held in Geneva, September, 1960. United Nations, New York, 1962.

48. UNITED NATIONS: Report of the United Nations Scientific Committee on the Effects of Atomic Radiation. General Assembly Official Records, Seventeenth Session, Supplement No. 16 (A/5216), United Nations Sales Section, New York, 1962.

49. VAN ALLEN, J. A.: The earth and near space. *Bull. Atomic Sci., 18*:218–222, 1961.

50. VERNOV, S. N., and CHUDAKOV, A. E.: Terrestrial corpuscular radiation and cosmic rays. In Bijl, H. K., editor. *Space Research, Proceedings of the First International Space Science Symposium.* North Holland Publishing Company, Amsterdam, and Interscience Publishers, New York, 1960.

51. WALLNER, LEWIS E., and KAUFMAN, HAROLD R.: Radiation shielding for manned space flight. *NASA TN-D-681, NASA.* Washington, D. C., July, 1961.

52. WINKLER, J. P.: Primary cosmic rays. In George Jacobs, editor, Proceeding on Conference on Radiation Problems in Manned Space Flight. *Technical Note D-588, NASA.* Washington, D. C., December, 1960.

53. YAGODA, HERMAN: *Radioactivity Measurements with Nuclear Emulsions.* John Wiley and Sons, Inc., New York, 1949.

54. YAGODA, HERMAN: Bioastronautics measurements of ionizing radiations in space: nuclear emulsion monitoring report. *Report AFCRL 62-244, GRD Research Notes No. 76.* Geophysics Research Directorate, U. S. Air Force Cambridge Research Laboratories, Bedford, Massachusetts, February, 1962.

55. ZELLMER, ROBERT W., and ALLEN, RALPH G.: Cosmic radiation laboratory observations. *Aerospace Med., 32*:942–946, 1961.

3

THE GASEOUS REQUIREMENTS
(RESPIRATION)

EDWIN HENDLER, PH.D.

When penetrating the unknown, hostile reaches of space, man must provide himself with the minimum of those elements from his earthly environment which will assure his unimpaired performance over prolonged intervals of time. Chief among these necessities are the gaseous constituents which he must breathe. Limitations of available vehicular space and propulsive power make it necessary to eliminate as many as possible of the superfluous items composing the equipment and materials of the life support system. Consequently, man's inherent physiological flexibility and adaptability must be fully exploited to reduce penalties of equipment weight and complexity. However, exploitation of this kind involves risks. Achievement of the optimum compromise so as to minimize these risks is the goal being sought. In order to realize this goal, knowledge of man's capabilities and limitations is essential.

GASES IN THE ATMOSPHERE

Oxygen

To support the complex physico-chemical reactions occurring in the cell of living organisms, the continual release and use of free energy is essential. Even in the resting state, the cell's continued existence as a living entity depends upon the extraction and use of energy to carry out those functions which distinguish it from inanimate material. The energy source used by the cell is the nutrient material made available to it. By combining with O_2, this nutrient material provides some of its chemical energy to sustain a variety of functions characteristic of life. The cell as the smallest living entity, the tissues formed by aggregations of cells, and the organism arising as a discrete unit made up of a variety of tissues, all depend upon the utilization of O_2 for their individual and collective existence. For this reason, of all the gases in the environment, O_2, by far, is the most critical.

Unfortunately, in spite of the continual need for O_2 by the tis-sues, only about 1 l of this gas is stored within the human body.[1] Consequently, when the usual external O_2 supply to the cells is reduced or cut off entirely, the vital metabolic processes quickly slow down and then stop. An over-all view of human tolerance to various concentrations and pressures of O_2 is provided in Figure 1.

TABLE 1

ALTITUDE AND BAROMETRIC PRESSURE

Altitude, ft	Pressure, mm Hg	Pressure, psi
0	760	14.7
5,000	632	12.2
10,000	523	10.1
50,000	87.5	1.69
100,000	8.29	1.60×10^{-1}
500,000	3.72×10^{-6}	7.20×10^{-8}
1,000,000	1.78×10^{-7}	3.44×10^{-9}

In general, the lower the concentration of O_2, the higher the pressure which can be safely breathed. When the inspired pO_2 is reduced because its concentration in the atmosphere is low, or because the total barometric pressure is low, the major danger is from anoxia. Conversely, when the pO_2 is high, and the total barometric pressure is also high, the major danger is from oxygen toxicity. Because it is not likely that barometric pressures greater than 1 atm will be met with in space flight operations, our attention will be concentrated on the pressure region between sea level and altitude. Table 1 shows some relationships between altitude and barometric pressure.

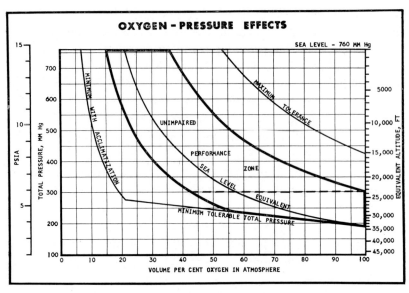

Fig. 1. Physiological effects of oxygen percentage as related to total pressure of the atmosphere for continuous, long-term (one week or more) human occupancy. Acclimatization involves continuous exposure to conditions of successively lower pressure. Dashed line shows bends level in non-denitrogenated subjects. (From *Physiological Performance Charts*, The Garrett Corp., AiResearch Mfg. Div., Los Angeles 45, Calif.)

The atmospheric gases which enter the lungs during respiration are carried to the pulmonary alveoli before being transferred to the circulating blood. The volume of gases filling the respiratory passages, across the walls of which occurs no gaseous exchange with the blood, comprises the dead air space. The gases in the alveoli are saturated with water vapor which, at body temperature, exerts a partial pressure of 47 mm Hg. Inspired gases are diluted with the gases already present in the alveoli, so that the pO_2 in the alveoli drops to about 100 mm Hg at sea level, when breathing room air. It is the difference in the pO_2 in the alveolar air and its tension in the blood entering the pulmonary capillaries which provides the driving pressure necessary to almost completely saturate arterial blood leaving the lungs, under normal conditions. The hemoglobin of the red blood cells enables each

100 ml. of oxygenated blood to transport about 20 ml of O_2, in addition to the 0.3 ml of O_2 dissolved in the water of the blood. It is interesting to note that in order to increase the normal saturation of arterial blood from 97.5 to 100 per cent, the pO_2 to which the blood is exposed must be increased from 100 mm Hg to well over 300 mm Hg.[2] On the other hand, blood saturation is almost linearly related to pO_2's up to 40 mm Hg, ranging from 0 to 70 per cent. The O_2 dissociation curve for human blood relating saturation to pO_2 is shown in Figure 2.

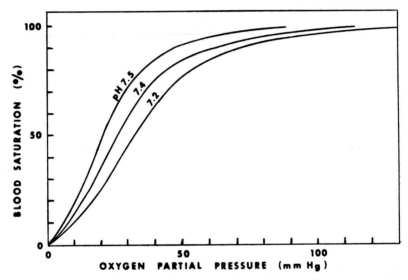

Fig. 2.   Oxygen dissociation curves for human blood. (From Scarpelli, E. M.: *Physiological Training*, Gunter Branch, Sch. of Av. Med., USAF, Air Univ., May, 1955.)

Since the pO_2 within the tissues is below 60 mm Hg, arterial blood bathing these tissues loses about 5 ml of $O_2/100$ ml of blood. In exercise, consumption of O_2 by the tissues increases, so that over 12 ml of O_2 /100 ml of blood can be extracted. Thus, the utilization of O_2 can be increased from about 25 per cent during rest to 60 per cent during exercise. By breathing 100 per cent O_2 instead of room air, the amount of physically dissolved O_2 in the blood is noticeably increased, and is capable of supplying tissue needs while sparing a portion of the O_2 combined with hemoglobin. If pure O_2 is breathed at a pressure of about 3 atm, sufficient O_2 becomes dissolved in the blood to satisfy resting tissue requirements without necessitating the dissociation of O_2 combined with hemoglobin. However, the toxic effects of breathing high pressure, pure O_2 for appreciable durations are well established, and make such a practice extremely dangerous.[3]

Deficiency in O_2 supply to the tissues, or anoxia, can be produced in a number of ways, depending upon which portion of the O_2 transportation system is affected. In otherwise healthy individuals exposed to environmental conditions of reduced O_2, a condition of anoxic anoxia (or, as it has more recently been classified, hypotonic anoxemia[4]) may be produced. In this condition, both the amount and tension of O_2 in arterial blood are below normal. Clinical signs of hypotonic anoxemia include breathlessness, cyanosis, tachycardia, and, in extreme cases, convulsions. When the supply of O_2 being breathed is suddenly reduced, the ensuing behavior is very similar to that seen in alcoholic intoxication. A limited decrease in ambient O_2 occurring over a prolonged period produces symptoms of fatigue. Some of the clinical conditions produced in the unacclimatized, healthy individual upon exposure to various altitudes breathing ambient air is shown in Table 2.

TABLE 2

SIGNS AND SYMPTOMS OF ALTITUDE HYPOXIA IN A NORMAL PERSON*

Altitude, ft	Art. O_2 Sat., %	Clinical Condition
Sea level	95–98	Normal, fatigue on long exposure
10,000	88–90	Headache
14,000	80–81	Sleepiness, headache, dizziness, impaired vision, personality changes (euphoric or quarrelsome), impaired judgment, loss of muscular coordination, pulse increase, respiration increase, cyanosis
18,000	74–75	Same as above, only more marked
22,000	67–68	Convulsions, collapse and coma
25,000	55–60	Collapse and coma in about 5 min

* From Scarpelli, E. M.: *Physiological Training*, Gunter Branch, School of Aviation Med., USAF, Air Univ., May, 1955.

Anoxia has its earliest and most profound effects on the most susceptible tissues of the body, namely those of the central nervous system and the heart. Phylogenetically more primitive parts of the central nervous system appear to be more resistant to anoxia, with the result that cortical activity is quickly affected, while lower vegetative centers continue to function. In a recent study, nerve cells of hamster cerebral cortex were examined with the electron microscope following acute anoxia. Submicroscopic changes were regularly seen involving the perikaryon and mitochondria, suggesting a rise of intracellular osmotic pressure following O_2 deficiency in the tissue or suppression of the activity of the respiratory enzymes.[5]

TABLE 3

TIME OF USEFUL CONSCIOUSNESS AT ALTITUDE*

Altitude, ft	Time, min
22,000	10
25,000	5
28,000	2.5–3
30,000	1.5
35,000	0.5–1
40,000	0.25
65,000	0.15

* From Scarpelli, E. M.: *Physiological Training*, Gunter Branch, School of Aviation Med., USAF, Air Univ., May, 1955.

Abrupt withdrawal of O_2, such as could occur in high-altitude vehicles with failure of the structural integrity of the inhabited compartments, causes an almost immediate loss of consciousness. The time of useful consciousness is the period following interruption of an individual's O_2 supply, at an O_2-breathing altitude, during which he is capable of taking effective and purposive action. Average useful consciousness times are shown in Table 3 for various altitudes. Greater O_2 utilization during exercise would be expected to shorten the times shown in Table 3. Continued lack of O_2 produces collapse followed by coma, as shown for various altitudes in Figure 3.

The minimum pO_2 in the lungs capable of preventing symptoms of hypoxia is 61 mm Hg. Such a situation is produced when the ambient air is breathed at an altitude of 10,000 ft, or when 100 per cent O_2 is breathed at about 39,500 ft. In order to ascend to higher altitudes, the pure O_2 breathed must be supplied at greater than ambient pressures. Continuous positive pressure equal to 10 in. of water enables military flying personnel to perform their duties at an altitude of 43,000 ft. However, under these circumstances, blood saturation drops to about 85 per cent, a marginal

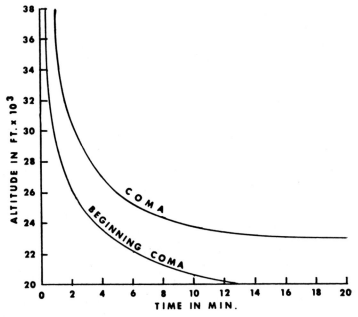

Fig. 3. Effects of oxygen deprivation at various altitudes. (From Scarpelli, E. M.: *Physiological Training*, Gunter Branch, Sch. of Av. Med., USAF, Air Univ., May, 1955.)

level which involves a definite risk from progressive anoxia. In addition, respiratory and circulatory embarrassment due to positive pressure breathing result in fatigue and discomfort which cannot be tolerated indefinitely. Pressurized or sealed compartments, or pressure suits, obviate the need for pressure breathing. For extended flights, an inspired pO_2 of 122 mm Hg is considered the minimum necessary to prevent the fatiguing effects of anoxia.[6]

The seriousness of an anoxic, or hypoxic state cannot be over-emphasized. Impaired judgment and reduced performance may be the first external signs of anoxia, but other important changes also occur. Pulse rate and respiratory rate increase, and at an ambient pO_2 of 65 mm Hg (equivalent to 22,000 ft altitude breathing air), circulatory collapse is imminent.[7] In spite of peripheral vasodilatation, systolic blood pressure increases while diastolic pressure falls.[8] The heart increases its output, which, together with the other circulatory changes, places it under considerable strain.[9] Hyperventilation accompanying the anoxia may lead to alkalosis and cerebral vasoconstriction.[10] Finally, since the effects of anoxia are cumulative, repeated or prolonged exposures to low pO_2 may lead to irreversible brain damage in susceptible individuals.[11] The emotional disturbances, nausea and rapid fatigue following muscular exertion which commonly result from anoxia could prove particularly disturbing to astronauts exposed to the additional rigors of space flight.

The consumption of O_2 by an individual depends upon such a wide variety of internal and external factors, that estimates deduced from values given in the general literature can be in serious error when applied to a specific situation. A few of the more important of these factors are: body type, posture, age, sex, training, diet, elapsed time, clothing, task, emotion and environment. The resting consumption of O_2 for the "average" man can be assumed to be 350 ml, obtained by ventilating the lungs with 8 l of air/min. At maximum exertion, about 5.4 l of O_2 may be used each minute, and the volume of air breathed may reach 120 l/min. Naturally, this rate of breathing cannot be sustained for periods longer than a few minutes, at most.[12] The ventilation coefficient, or amount of air breathed for each liter of O_2 consumed, is lower during rest and heavy work than it is during light, or moderate work. Animal experiments have shown that ambient temperatures above and below 20–24°C increase O_2 consumption, rectal temperature and heart rate, while respiration rate remains relatively constant over a wide range of ambient temperatures below 24°C. Good correlation was found between O_2 consumption and the difference between ambient and skin temperatures.[13]

Other animal experiments have shown that over a temperature range from 6° to 30°C, no difference in O_2 consumption was observed whether pure O_2 or air was breathed.[14]   In performing the same total amount of work using various rest and work intervals, shorter intervals (0.5 and 1 min) produced less of a physiological strain in a trained subject than longer intervals (2 and 3 min).[15] Mechanical efficiency was shown to be practically the same when a given quantity of work was done continuously at a relatively low load or periodically with higher loads.[16]   Rodents, and certain other "warm-blooded" animals, have the capability of reducing metabolic rate, and therefore O_2 consumption, by lowering body temperature when the pO_2 is reduced.   Thus, rats were shown to be able to tolerate an altitude of about 28,000 ft for 35 min when the air temperature was kept at 24°C, but raising the air temperature to 33°C (and thus impeding heat loss from the body) decreased this time at altitude to only 10 min.[17]   Along these lines, Hock has considered the advantages of reduced O_2 and food consumption and waste production to be gained during space travel by hibernation.[18]

The inherent capability of man to adapt to hostile environmental conditions is shown nowhere so impressively as in his acclimatization to high altitudes.   The principal physiological changes characteristic of this acclimatization include increases in pulmonary ventilation, cardiac output, capacity to carry O_2 in arterial blood and ability of the tissue cells to function at very low levels of pO_2.   Balke and his associates in an extensive series of field experiments showed that physical training not only increases altitude tolerance, but when performed during the acclimatization period (six weeks spent at altitudes between 10,000 and 14,000 ft) provides faster and more effective adaptation to altitude.[19, 20] Acclimatization raised the critical altitude (highest level of simulated altitude at which subjects become unconscious) from 24,000 to 30,000 ft.   During the fifth week of acclimatization, subjects suddenly exposed to the O_2 pressure equivalent of 25,000 ft remained alert for 30 min, with little decrement in neuro-muscular coordination.   Of two acclimatized subjects suddenly exposed to a 30,000 ft level, one remained conscious for 5 min, the other for

30 min, although unconsciousness in unacclamitized subjects at this altitude usually occurs within 2–3 min. In trained and acclimatized subjects, bends resistance at altitudes between 42,000 and 56,000 ft increased, pressure breathing was maintained at an average level of 55,000 ft for as long as 30 min, sensitivity to CO_2 was increased 10–30 per cent, and resistance to fatigue increased. From these experiences, the benefits to be gained by using properly trained and conditioned men for the initial space probes are obvious.

Prolonged exposure to pure O_2 may remove most of the N_2 normally present in various body cavities. If these cavities are poorly ventilated, the O_2 trapped within them may be absorbed by the circulating blood. The relatively low pressure thus produced within the cavities can either cause their collapse (pulmonary atelectasis) or pain (middle ear and paranasal sinuses). In relatively rare instances, subjects who have become severely anoxic show a brief respiratory arrest upon first being given pure O_2 to breathe ("oxygen apnea").[21] In addition to these undesirable effects produced by inhalation of O_2, the important question of O_2 toxicity will be briefly considered in what follows.

When high concentrations of O_2 are breathed for prolonged periods, toxic symptoms related to the respiratory system (when the pO_2 exceeds about 456 mm Hg) and the nervous system (when the pO_2 exceeds about 1500 mm Hg) have been observed. Partial pressures of O_2 greater than 1 atm result primarily from underwater operations, such as diving, and the toxicity of O_2 under these circumstances will not be considered here. The work of three groups of investigators showed that when 70–100 per cent O_2 is breathed for 24 hr or longer at sea level, normal subjects experience substernal distress, coughing and irritation of the respiratory tract. In many subjects, vital capacity was also reduced. Occasionally, other symptoms, including fatigue, pain in the joints, peculiar sensations in the hands and feet, loss of appetite, nausea and vomiting were reported. In some subjects, one or more of these symptoms persisted for several days after the experiment.[22-24] In order to investigate the factor of exposure duration more thoroughly, six men spent seven days in a closed chamber breathing from an atmosphere containing a pO_2 of 418 mm Hg. Although no acute symptoms were noted, some signs of pulmonary irritation occurred which may have indicated that the limits of tolerance were being approached.[25] No completely satisfactory explanation has yet been offered to explain the toxic effects produced by prolonged respiration of air containing a high pO_2.

Carbon Dioxide

The normal sea level CO_2 content of air is about 0.04 per cent. In contrast to atmospheric O_2, when the CO_2 content of the air is reduced, that within the body remains almost unchanged. Since the tissues continuously produce CO_2 as an end product of metabolism, one of the chief objects of respiration is to expel excess quantities of this gas which have been transported to the lungs. Again in contrast to the 1 l of O_2 stored in the average man's body, almost 130 l of CO_2 are stored there.[1] Most of this CO_2 (about 110 l) which is stored in the bones, is largely independent of changes in the ambient CO_2, while the remaining 20 l stored primarily in the muscles and blood, is more responsive to external pCO_2. Apparently even among the soft tissues, the extent and speed with which CO_2 is gained or lost depends largely upon the local rate of blood flow. Because tissues have the capability of absorbing CO_2 when man is confined to a relatively small space from which he must rebreathe, he himself acts as a storage depot for this gas as its tension in the atmosphere increases. Thus under certain arbitrary conditions, it has been estimated that for every 3 additional liters of rebreathing space, time of consciousness would be extended by 1 min; a 1 cu m rebreathing volume (assuming, of course, that sufficient O_2 were present) would provide an estimated consciousness time of 5.5 hr.

The stimulant effects upon respiration produced by CO_2 are physiological in nature and much greater and more consistent than the pathological stimulatory nature of either anoxia or acidemia.[4] Table 4 summarizes the effects of various CO_2 contents of air when breathed for sufficient periods of time. Subjects who become adapted to altitude show an increase in sensitivity to CO_2, but no change in the sensitivity of the respiratory system to O_2

TABLE 4

EFFECTS OF INSPIRING AIR CONTAINING VARIOUS LEVELS OF CO_2

CO_2 level, %	Effect
<1	None noticeable
4	Pulmonary ventilation doubled
7	Headache, dizziness, nausea, uneasiness, pulmonary ventilation increased 5 times over normal
10	Above symptoms exaggerated, brain dysfunction, pulmonary ventilation increased 10 times over normal
15	Unconsciousness, muscular rigidity, tremors, generalized convulsions, maximum increase in pulmonary ventilation
25–30	Surgical level of anesthesia

seems to occur.[26] Lower concentrations of CO_2 directly stimulate the respiratory center located in the gray reticular formation of the pons and medulla. Concentrations of CO_2 in inspired air above about 15 per cent do not produce further consistent increases in respiratory minute volume, and the values shown for the higher inspired CO_2 concentrations represent peaks between convulsive seizures.

In order to reduce the work load on equipment which may be used to remove CO_2 from a sealed space vehicle, with consequent gains in efficiency and reliability, Bartlett and Phillips suggested that an elevated CO_2 concentration in the enclosed atmosphere be permitted. The rapid physiological response of increased respiratory minute volume to the higher than normal levels of inspired CO_2 would maintain internal bodily homeostasis without producing respiratory fatigue.[27] Under carefully controlled conditions, ten monkeys were exposed to an atmosphere containing 21 per cent O_2 and 3 per cent CO_2 for a period of 93 days. No significant consistent variations in activity, body weight, blood glucose, nonprotein nitrogen, serum chloride, hematocrit, hemoglobin, serum calcium, serum phosphorus, total leucocyte count, erythrocyte sedimentation rate, serum bilirubin, serum cholesterol, cephalin flocculation, arterial and venous CO_2 and adrenal function were observed.[28] Lambertsen suggested a gas mixture containing low pO_2 and relatively high pCO_2 to produce acute acclimatization to low inspired pO_2. The presence of high pCO_2 would prevent hypocapnia and resulting respiratory alkalosis and cerebral vasoconstriction. By thus utilizing the CO_2 metabolically produced in a space capsule environment, equipment requirements for removing CO_2 could be eased, the fire hazard from high O_2 atmospheres could be reduced, and photosynthetic processes for O_2 production could be enhanced.[28a] Schaefer, on the other hand, emphasized the physiological and histopathological changes which may occur following chronic exposure to even slightly elevated

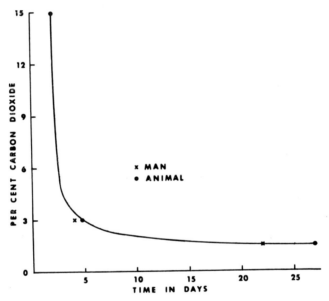

Fig. 4.   Concentration time relationship in adaptation to CO_2. Adaptation is the time to reach compensation of CO_2-induced respiratory acidosis. (Redrawn from Schaefer.[29])

pCO_2. His "strength-duration" curve for adaptation to CO_2 is shown in Figure 4. Three levels of activity are used to express tolerance limits, the first at 3 per cent CO_2 and above, the second at 1.5 per cent CO_2 and the third at 0.5–0.8 per cent CO_2. No adaptive processes occur at this last level, although the physiological and histopathological changes already mentioned may presumably occur.[29] The effects of acute exposure to CO_2 are shown in Figure 5.

The effects upon the respiratory center of pCO_2 and pO_2 in the blood are mediated by cerebral vasomotor activity. Cerebral vasoconstriction is produced by increased pO_2 and decreased pCO_2, while cerebral vasodilatation is produced by decreased pO_2 and increased pCO_2.[30] By this mechanism, compensation is provided, so that although marked changes of the arterial pCO_2 occur, consequent changes in the pCO_2 of the tissues comprising

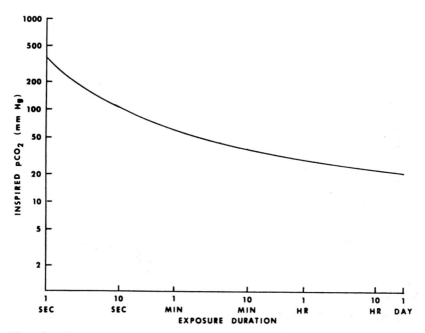

Fig. 5. Human tolerance to inspired pCO_2 for various exposure durations. Region below the curve represents safe conditions. Region above the curve represents conditions producing CO_2 narcosis. (Redrawn from Thompson.[6])

the respiratory center are minimal. Either breathing air containing higher than usual amounts of CO_2 or hyperventilating to remove CO_2 from the body causes marked changes in arterial pCO_2, but relatively small changes in the pCO_2 of the cerebral tissues.

Increased respiratory activity such as that induced by O_2 lack or anxiety, results in a "washout" of CO_2 contained in the lungs. The resulting hypocapnia is accompanied by alkalosis, and the latter has its chief effect on the neuromuscular system. Cerebral vasoconstriction, following reduction in blood CO_2, traps blood in the brain until its O_2 content is reduced to a low level. Symptoms of tetany and deterioration of cerebral functioning eventually lead to unconsciousness. An alveolar pCO_2 below about 20 mm Hg results in a decrement in performance,[10] so that acapnia and anoxia are each capable of adversely affecting normal cerebral function. Voluntary hyperventilation at sea level which causes alveolar pCO_2 to drop by only 0.2 per cent is sufficient to produce apnea. If air containing 4.7 per cent or more CO_2 is breathed during voluntary hyperventilation, apnea cannot be produced.[31]

Nitrogen

Nitrogen comprises about 79 per cent of the gas mixture making up the earth's atmosphere. If pure O_2 is continuously breathed and the amount of exhaled N_2 measured, after approximately 10 hr, about 1 l of N_2 is collected. The curve relating N_2 elimination to time of O_2 breathing (or denitrogenation) is shown in Figure 6. About 61 per cent of the N_2 exhaled during O_2 breathing is given off within the first 105 min.[32] In an average man, almost 70 per cent of the N_2 contained in his body is dissolved in the 20 per cent of his mass composed of fat. The brain and most of the visceral organs have a plentiful blood supply, and rapidly lose N_2 when pure O_2 is breathed. Although the skeletal muscles and body fat have approximately the same blood perfusion rates, the latter tissue contains much more N_2, and consequently requires an appreciably longer time to become desaturated during denitrogenation. In addition to fatty tissues, such poorly perfused tissues as tendon cartilage may lose N_2 only after a long period of denitrogenation.

The importance of N_2 retained in body tissues, as related to space flight, concerns its role in decompression sickness or aero-embolism. The incidence, manifestations, history and recurrence of decompression sickness depends upon such personal factors as age, individual susceptibility, activity, physical condition and past injuries, and upon such environmental factors as temperature, gaseous composition of the atmosphere, rate of decompression, pressure change and duration of exposure to reduced pressure. The accumulated evidence gives strong support to the theory that decompression sickness results when N_2 dissolved in the body fluids and tissues comes out of solution and forms bubbles under conditions of reduced atmospheric pressure. At altitudes above 35,000 ft, even though all N_2 has previously been removed from the body, bubbles may still form in the tissues due to CO_2, O_2 and

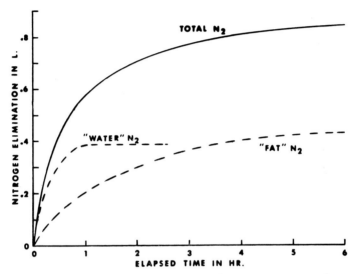

Fig. 6. Nitrogen elimination by breathing 100 per cent O_2 at sea level. "Water" and "fat" N_2 elimination curves are hypothetical, and approximate the total N_2 elimination curve when summed. (From *Submarine Medicine Practice* (NAVMED-P 5054). Washington, U. S. Government Printing Office, 1956.)

water vapor. Decompression sickness is characterized by some or all of the following symptoms: joint pains, paresthesias, skin changes, paralysis, convulsions, ineffective coughing, visual disturbances and coma. Treatment of this condition consists primarily of recompression, by means of which the gaseous constituents of the bubbles are forced once again into solution. Prevention of decompression sickness can be achieved by denitrogenation before exposure to altitudes of about 25,000 ft and above. Experience has shown that preoxygenation at any altitude up to 20,000 ft is as effective as at sea level, while at altitudes between 20,000 and 30,000 ft, it is only about one-third as effective as at sea level.

Decompression sickness is a constant threat to the well-being of astronauts traveling in space. Under normal cruise conditions, it is anticipated that certain astronauts will be wearing unpressurized full-pressure suits, in order to enjoy maximum mobility and comfort. Should the space vehicle cabin lose pressurization, however, the pressure suit will automatically inflate and maintain a pressure of 180 mm Hg around the wearer at ambient altitudes of 35,000 ft and above. The pressurizing gas consists of 100 per cent O_2. One of the atmospheres considered for space vehicle living compartments is 50 per cent O_2–50 per cent N_2 at 380 mm Hg pressure. If a decompression should occur in such an atmosphere, the astronaut would be transferred rapidly from the mixed gas atmosphere at 380 mm Hg pressure to a 100 per cent O_2 atmosphere at 180 mm Hg. Would this change in pressure and gas composition be expected to result in decompression sickness? Let us assume that the astronaut has spent sufficient time in his mixed gas environment to allow his tissue pN_2 to equilibrate with the 190 mm Hg pN_2 of the respired gas. The gaseous pressure in his veins can be estimated as $pN_2 = 190$, $pO_2 = 40$, $pCO_2 = 47$ and $pH_2O = 47$ for a total pressure of 324 mm Hg. Behnke assumed that the total venous gaseous pressure could be double the atmospheric pressure without causing decompression sickness.[32] Therefore, in his pressure suit–100 per cent O_2 atmosphere at 180 mm Hg following decompression, the astronaut could safely tolerate a total venous gas pressure of 360 mm Hg. Since this total tolerable pressure is larger than that present before decompression, no decompression sickness would be expected. Results of a study to validate this conclusion showed that about 18 hr were necessary for subjects to equilibrate with the mixed gas environment, so that subsequent decompression could be accomplished without producing aeroembolism. This equilibration time could be shortened considerably by having the subjects preoxygenate. Using the same criterion to predict occurrence of decompression sickness, it can be calculated that the above mixed gas composition can be safely used at a pressure as high as 452 mm Hg, or about 14,000 ft. On the other hand, if the gas mixture were changed to resemble the proportions found in air (80 per cent N_2, 20 per cent O_2), the maximum safe pressure for equilibration before decompression is 282 mm Hg, or about 25,000 ft. From this calculation, it can readily be appreciated that decompression from sea level breathing air directly to 35,000 ft breathing 100 per cent O_2 would result in severe decompression sickness.

In order to decrease the complexity of equipment required to store, meter and monitor the gases enclosed within the living compartments of a space vehicle, and to decrease probability of bends in case of explosive decompression, it has been proposed that a N_2-free atmosphere be maintained.[27] Data relating to prolonged exposure to altitude while breathing 100 per cent O_2 at non-toxic pressures are limited. Recently, one subject breathed 100 per cent O_2 at an altitude equivalent of 35,000 ft for a period of 72 hr. This subject exhibited no other untoward effects than reddening of the pharangeal and nasal mucosa and irritation of the eyes, which were attributed to the dryness of the O_2 breathed.[33] Atelectasis produced by absorption of O_2 from poorly ventilated, or blocked alveoli has been suggested as a possible cause of the decreased vital capacity measured in subjects who have breathed pure O_2 for prolonged intervals.[21] Schaefer has also pointed out the danger of pulmonary atelectasis in the absence of an inert gas in the breathing mixture.[34] Depending upon its severity and extent, pulmonary atelectasis may decrease arterial pO_2, stiffen the lung, and reduce the effective alveolar surface for diffusion of gases. Several studies carried out in three different U. S. laboratories in 1962 were designed to evaluate the probability of atelectasis induced by fourteen-day, continuous exposures of over twenty-five persons to pure O_2 atmospheres at reduced pressures. In one of these studies, a simulated launch acceleration pattern preceded, and a simulated re-entry acceleration pattern followed each exposure to the O_2 atmosphere. Oxygen electrodes were used to measure directly arterial pO_2, and a variety of pulmonary function tests were also conducted. For the exposure duration tested, atelectasis proved to be no problem, but there were indications of rapidly reversible changes in peripheral vision and delayed changes in morphology of the formed elements of the blood. In view of the limited data presently available, the complete elimination of N_2 in the gas mixture breathed over a prolonged period, at altitudes where pure O_2 is non-toxic, has yet to be proved entirely safe.* The use of $He-O_2$ mixtures in space vehicles has been considered, but experience breathing this inert gas has been limited to diving operations. In animal experiments, a $He-O_2$ mixture was found to result in increased body heat loss, thereby evoking an increased metabolic response with decrease in liver glycogen, increase in O_2 consumption and body weight loss.[35]

Another reason for including N_2 or another inert gas as part of the space vehicle atmosphere is to reduce the fire and explosion hazard of O_2. Thus, although the same pO_2 may be supplied at altitude as exists at sea level, combustion at altitude will be supported better because of the limited interference resulting from reduction in the amount of N_2 (or other inert gas used in place of N_2). That this is of more than academic interest is emphasized by two separate experiments conducted in 1962, in which prolonged habitation by human volunteers in practically pure O_2 atmospheres were suddenly terminated by the outbreak of fires. Each of these experiments was carefully planned, and attempts were made to incorporate every reasonable precaution to prevent fire. However, its occurrence demonstrated most dramatically the real difficulties involved in preventing and fighting fires in pure O_2 atmospheres.

Toxic Substances

The sealed atmosphere of the space vehicle designed for extremely long habitation presents unusual problems with regard to the presence of toxic substances. The toxic substances referred to here are those which contaminate the atmosphere,

---

* For further discussion of these and related matters see: Physiology Symposium—Respiratory Physiology in Manned Spacecraft. *Fed. Proc.*, 22:1022, 1963.

usually in relatively low concentrations. Much of the present knowledge regarding the toxic concentration and effects of these substances has been based upon relatively acute experiments, where exposure time has been limited to hours or days. Most toxic agents of industrial importance have had their maximum allowable concentrations determined on the basis of daily exposure for the usual number of working hours. In space flight, the duration of exposure may be months or years. In addition, the unknown interactions of cosmic rays, or other substances found in space, with the materials comprising the space craft and its contents may produce toxic substances whose nature and action are entirely unanticipated.

The sources of known toxic substances are many. From the intestinal tract of man, with its bacterial flora, come many substances which are not only malodorous, but poisonous and explosive as well. On the basis of 100 cu ft of volume per occupant, it has been estimated that after 14 mo, the concentration of intestinally arising hydrogen sulfide would cause lacrimation and nausea, while hydrogen and methane, from the same source, would reach explosive concentrations in about 4 and 5.5 mo, respectively.[36] Ammonia could arise from the decomposition of urea incidental to the operation of waste disposal or water recovery processes. Non-metalic oxidation of ammonia could produce contaminating oxides of nitrogen. In addition to human sources, atmospheric contaminants could also arise from construction materials, adhesives, fuels, refrigerants, lubricants, foods, solvents, paints, electronic components, etc. Some compounds which have been identified in submarine atmospheres include: acetylene, ammonia, carbon monoxide, chlorine, freon, "hydrocarbons," hydrogen fluoride, hydrogen, methane, methyl alcohol, monoethanolamine, nitrogen dioxide, stibine, arsine, benzene, ethylene, hydrogen chloride, mesitylene, propane, pseudocumene, sulfur dioxide, toluene and xylene. Cigarette smoke contains at least twenty-three hydrocarbons in gaseous and vapor form, many of which become toxic when sufficiently concentrated. Some substances, like skatol and mercaptan, are smelled in concentrations as low as 3.3×10^{-7} and 3.3×10^{-5} ppm, respectively, which are considerably lower levels than are detectable by any other means now known. Because of their objectionable nature in even minute quantities, they must be removed from any sealed enclosure which is to be inhabited for even relatively short periods of time.

Incomplete combustion of carbon leads to the formation of the colorless and odorless gas, CO. Carbon monoxide has over 200 times the affinity for hemoglobin as does O_2; it not only prevents the hemoglobin with which it combines from carrying O_2, it also reduces the dissociation of oxyhemoglobin. When air containing about 1 l of CO has been breathed by an average man, he is in danger of collapse.[37] Symptoms of poisoning preceding unconsciousness include headache, nausea, lassitude and mental impairment; the latter may persist even after initial recovery. Based on the usual work week (8 hr/day, 5 days/wk), 100 ppm has been set as the maximum allowable concentration of CO in the atmosphere.[38] Traffic officers exposed daily to about 70 ppm of CO in the Holland Tunnel showed no abnormalities attributable to this gas over a 13 yr period of intermittent exposure.[39] No harmful effects were found in dogs, rats and rabbits exposed continuously for 3 mo to 50 ppm of CO.[40] The concentration proposed by the U. S. Navy for continuous, prolonged exposure of personnel in nuclear-powered submarines is 25 to 30 ppm.[29]

Ozone is present in the atmosphere at an altitude of about 60,000 ft, and its use as the oxidizer in liquid-fueled rockets makes it possible that it could contaminate the air breathed by personnel engaged in space flight operations. Its odor varies from a sweet scent in low concentrations to an acrid, pungent scent at high concentrations. Between 4 and 5 ppm breathed for 1 hr produced signs of decreased pulmonary function in exposed men. A concentration of about 25 ppm was found to be the LD 50 (median lethal dose necessary to kill 50 per cent of exposed animals) for guinea pigs. Ozone poisoning produces pulmonary edema and hyperemia, eventually resulting in death from asphyxiation.[41] Concentrated liquid ozone is extremely reactive, and will explode upon contact with even minute amounts of many organic substances.

Air Ions

Atoms, molecules and particles in the air can become charged by either loss or gain of electrons, and when so charged, are called air ions. High-energy particles like alpha and beta rays from radio-active sources, cosmic rays, ultraviolet rays, coronal discharges, charge separation brought about by rapid relative movements of surfaces, and thermionic emission are the principal methods of producing air ions, both naturally and artificially. The efficiency of producing air ions by these methods varies; thus a corona discharge may produce particles, each of which has, on the average, about forty-five charges, while alpha rays may produce singly charged particles. Only about one molecule in 10^{16} is ordinarily ionized or charged, and these charged molecules frequently clump together forming groups. The sizes of the charged particles vary from a fraction of a micron in diameter to many microns, and it is the larger particles which have many hundreds of charges per particle. The dust, smoke and salt which ordinarily may be suspended in air act as condensation nuclei for rain formation, and are also very effective deionizers of the atmosphere.

Unipolar, small air ions have been shown to be biologically active under certain conditions. Molecules and perhaps atoms of O_2 in the air have an affinity for electrons, and thus form negative ions. Only fluorine and chlorine molecules seem to have the same capacity for forming negative ions as do the O_2 molecules. Positive ions are formed primarily by CO_2 molecules. Ion mobility studies indicate that small ions in the air are not single molecules, but probably are combined with molecules of water. These studies also show that positive ions have lower mobilities than do the negative ions, presumably because of the additional water molecules attached to the former. Ion counters measure the ion current flow produced when ionized air flows at a metered rate between electrodes. Some modern counters employing micromicroammeters are said to have an accuracy of 20 ions/cc of air, and currents as small as 10^{-17} amp can be measured by commercially available instruments.

TABLE 5

SMALL BIOLOGICAL EFFECTS OF AIR IONS

	Negative Ions	Positive Ions
Animal Subjects		
Blood pH	Marked increase	Small decrease
Growth:		
Embryonic cells	Enhanced	Depressed
Tissue cells	Enhanced	Depressed
Newborn litters	Enhanced	None
Bacteria	Inhibited	Inhibited
Tracheal ciliary activity	Increased	Depressed
Vasomotor activity	Dilation	Constriction
Human subjects		
Performance	Improved	Decreased
Work capacity	Increased	
Disposition	Cheerful	Depressed
Reaction time	Decreased	Decreased
Equilibrium	Improved	
Vitamin metabolism	Enhanced	
Pain	Relieved	
Allergic disorders	Relieved	
Burn recovery & healing	Enhanced	

In general, experimental results seem to indicate that negative air ions have a beneficial biological effect. Table 5 shows some of the more detailed effects attributed to the presence of air ions. Of the effects shown, those obtained with healthy human subjects are probably the most questionable. Much of the difficulty associated with air ionization experiments concerns the techniques used to produce effective ion concentrations. It is known, for example, that ion density decreases very rapidly with distance from the source, with time, and with atmospheric contaminants, such as dust. Because of the poor distribution of small air ions, which are those having the greatest biological effect, it has been difficult in many cases to estimate the concentration of ions actually inhaled. Attempts to produce high levels of air ion density have demonstrated that levels above 5000–10,000 ions/cc are very difficult to achieve in practice, except in small localized air streams.[42] Yet some believe that millions of ions/cc are required before consistent biological effects can be expected.

Within a sealed compartment in space, it is likely that cosmic ray bombardment of the walls of the capsule could produce high concentrations of air ions. If the internal environment were rich in O_2, the likelihood of an increase in negatively charged ions would be considerable.

PRESSURE

One of the major distinctions between conditions on the surface of the earth and those in space is the presence of an almost constant pressure of 14.7 psi here on earth and the complete absence of atmospheric pressure in space. The biological effectiveness of the gases necessary for life depend to a large extent on their partial pressure, and this, of course, is directly dependent upon the total pressure. Certain relationships between gas pressures and respiration have already been pointed out. The following discussion will therefore be primarily concerned with the mechanical effects upon the living body produced by various pressure levels and by changes in pressure.

In general, the body can tolerate pressure without structural failure as long as the pressure is uniformly applied. If steps are taken to assure that pressures applied to the body result in no imbalance of forces, no tissue deformation can result and consequently the integrity of the body is maintained. On the other hand, if pressure differences occur so that the magnitude and direction of forces applied to the tissues are not opposed by forces of equal magnitude and opposite direction, displacement of the tissues occurs. Within limits, a certain amount of tissue displacement can occur without permanent damage, although pain and reversible changes may be produced which limit an individual's performance. If these limits are exceeded, the relative displacements between adjacent parts can produce severe injuries and death.

From Boyle's Law, it is known that when the temperature remains constant, the pressure and volume of a gas are inversely related. At 18,000 ft, therefore, where the barometric pressure is one-half that at sea level, a given quantity of gas at a fixed temperature would be expected to occupy twice its sea level volume. In the case of gases contained in spaces within the living body, a correction must be introduced for the partial pressure of water vapor at body temperature, which maintains a constant value of 47 mm Hg at all altitudes. The correction mentioned is made by subtracting 47 mm Hg from the total pressures producing the gas volume change. Therefore, a saturated gas at body temperature, when exposed to a barometric pressure of $1/2$ atm, occupies 7 per cent more volume than would an equivalent dry gas. At an altitude of 39,000 ft, the saturated gas at body temperature occupies about 40 per cent more volume than does an equivalent dry gas.

The significance of the expansion of gases contained within the body relates to imbalances of pressures which can cause tissue deformation. Cavities in the body which are usually partly or wholly air-filled include the chest, middle ear, paranasal sinuses, stomach and intestines. Tooth cavities which are incompletely filled represent a non-physiologic type of cavity but one that is extremely common. All of these cavities are usually opened to the ambient atmosphere, although the openings in certain cases are relatively long and tortuous, or are protected by coverings which retract only under certain conditions. An imbalance of forces is set up when the pressure within a cavity differs from the ambient pressure around it. If the ambient pressure is reduced, such as occurs upon ascent to altitude, and the opening of one of the body cavities is blocked, a pressure differential is produced across the cavity walls. The block does not have to be accompanied by an actual change in the configuration of the opening, but can represent an inability of gas to move into or out of the cavity with sufficient rapidity to maintain pressure equilibrium. Such is the case with the thoracic cavity and the opening formed by the airways (trachea and associated structures) during explosive decompression. More will be said about this in what follows.

The gastrointestinal tract is filled with variable quantities of CO_2, O_2, N_2, H_2, CH_4 and H_2S in varying proportions arising from swallowed air and the processes of digestion, fermentation, decomposition and putrefaction. Gases not readily accessible to the openings formed by the mouth and the anus may become trapped in the transverse colon and small intestines during ascent to altitude, and expand as the ambient pressure decreases. Because the stomach and intestines are not closely surrounded by unyielding bony structures, they may undergo considerable deformation as the gas within them expands. No structural damage has been found, however, in the intestines of animals decompressed to 90,000 ft, nor in unprotected men taken to an altitude of 57,000 ft.[43] Incapacitating pain and shock, as well as interference with respiratory movements and impeded venous return through increased intrathoracic pressure, may result from unrelieved gastrointestinal gas expansion. An ascent rate to altitude of about 300 ft/min usually assures adequate opportunity for equalization of intra- and extra-gastrointestinal gas pressures, while an ascent rate of 2000 ft/min or faster apparently does not permit sufficiently rapid expulsion of expanding gastrointestinal gases to maintain pressure equilibrium. Proper eating habits and selection of foods which do not form gases tend to alleviate the occurrence and severity of the symptoms described.

The middle ear is a gas-containing cavity largely surrounded by bone, except for the tympanic membrane. The opening of this cavity is the Eustachian tube which connects the middle ear to the nasal pharynx. Equilibration between pressures in the middle ear and the ambient atmosphere are readily achieved in most individuals during ascent to altitude. Upon descent to lower altitudes, however, the flutter valve action of the Eustachian tube pharyngeal orifice resists the entrance of air into the middle ear cavity. Unless deliberate action, such as yawning or swallowing, is taken, a considerable pressure difference can be built up between the ambient atmosphere and the gases filling the middle ear. When the pressure difference reaches about 100 mm Hg, the walls of the Eustachian tube are so closely apposed that movements of the pharyngeal muscles can no longer force the tube to open. As the external pressure acting on the tympanic membrane becomes progressively greater, with respect to that in the middle ear cavity, the tympanic membrane moves inward toward the middle ear. Eventually, after the limits of deformation have been exceeded, the tympanic membrane ruptures and air enters the middle ear cavity to re-establish pressure equilibrium. The lower relative pressure in the middle ear produces pain when the pressure difference reaches 60–80 mm Hg. Rupture of the tympanic membrane is accompanied by very severe pain, hemmorrhage, vertigo, nausea and may be followed by collapse and shock.

The paranasal sinuses consist of air-filled, mucous membrane-lined cavities which communicate by narrow openings with the nasal passages. Blockage of these openings by swelling of the mucosa, commonly caused by inflammation or infection, creates a similar situation during change in altitude, as that described for the middle ear. Severe headache and pain result from pressure imbalances across the walls of these cavities. Cavities in the teeth or in the root canals resulting from disease processes may entrap gases which expand upon ascent to altitude. As in the other cases of pressure imbalance described, pain from the affected part may result.

Above an altitude of about 80,000 ft, it is no longer feasible to provide an internal atmosphere by compressing the ambient air, such as is presently the practice in pressurized aircraft cabins. The compressors required to compress air of such low density would be prohibitively large and weighty. If the ambient air at 100,000 ft were compressed to provide an atmosphere of a 10,000 ft altitude equivalent, the temperature of the compressed air would reach 550°C.[44] In addition, ozone in the air would be concentrated by compression and produce a toxic hazard. For these reasons, a hermitically sealed cabin designed to support life over prolonged periods must be relied upon for manned penetration and travel in space.

Masses of stone, iron or other material called meteoroids, traveling with speeds up to about 25 mi/sec, may collide with the hull of a space vehicle and either cause penetration or erosion. Danger from this source depends upon the size and speed of the meteoroid, the structure and strength of the vehicle hull and the duration of exposure. From present knowledge, it appears likely that a space vehicle exposed for long periods would be punctured by relatively small meteoroids. The amount of gases lost from the interior of the vehicle would then depend upon its volume, the size and number of orifices through which gases could escape, the pressure of the gases within and the rapidity with which leaks could be located and repaired. Decompressions have been arbitrarily classified as "rapid," if the pressure change occurs over a period lasting 1 sec or more, and "explosive," if the pressure change occurs in less than 1 sec. It has been estimated that a 500 cu ft volume would require about 1 min to decompress through a 1 sq in. orifice from a pressure equivalent to sea level to one equivalent to 25,000 ft.[43]

An unusual phenomenon occurring at very low ambient pressures is the "boiling" of body fluids. Boiling occurs when the total barometric pressure equals the vapor pressure of water. The vapor pressure of body fluids depends upon their temperature and upon the volatile and non-volatile solutes, and polymerized and colloidal suspensions they contain. In anoxia-resistant organisms, such as frogs, insects, worms and protozoa, exposure to an altitude of 79,000 ft (where the barometric pressure equals the vapor pressure of water at room temperature) was found to cause tissue water evaporation without active formation of bubbles. At even higher altitudes, the continuous stream of water vapor removed from the surface of the animals' bodies resulted in death from dehydration and freezing.[45] In warm-blooded animals, boiling of body fluids begins at altitudes ranging from about 63,000 ft to about 67,000 ft, and occurs most actively over the moist surfaces of the gastrointestinal tract, in the eye, thorax and cardiovascular system. Vigorous vaporization begins in the venae cavae (where pressure is ordinarily only a few mm Hg above atmospheric pressure), extends through the venous vessels to the tissues and then continues up the arterial side of the circulatory system to the left heart. Acute right heart failure, mental disorientation and ocular disruption will precede death resulting from circulatory or respiratory failure.[46]

When the effects of explosive decompression upon the body structures are considered, the lungs are the primary organs of interest. Not only are they gas-filled, but the bulk of their mass consists of an extensive network of alveolar-capillary membranes which are extremely thin and delicate. Sudden expansion of the gases contained in the lungs, resulting from an explosive decompression, could produce injurious or fatal intrapulmonic pressures, if the resistance of the airways were too great, or if the airways were obstructed, such as by inadvertent closure of the glottis.

Two factors have been related to the injury potential of explosive decompression, the decompression coefficient and the pressure ratio.[47] The decompression coefficient is the ratio of the area in sq m of the opening through which the gases flow during decompression to the volume in cu m of the space being decompressed. The pressure ratio is the ratio of the initial pressure (before decompression) to the final pressure (after decompression). Two successive decompression coefficients were measured for the respiratory tract: about $1/40$, due to the tracheal orifice, and $1/80$, due to the glottal orifice. In order to assure that no pressure excesses occur within the lungs during an explosive decompression, the maximum decompression coefficient of the cabin must remain below that of the glottal coefficient. A value of $1/200$ has been proposed as an adequate design criterion for pressurized cabin spaces containing men. For pressure ratios of 4 or below, a decompression ratio of $1/50$ causes only a temporary intrapulmonic pressure increase which is well tolerated. Experimental results have indicated that a decompression coefficient of $1/100$ is the maximum producing no change in the lungs, while pressure ratios of 2.3 and lower cause no lesions, no matter what the decompression coefficient may be.[47]

During explosive decompression, the lung initially acts like a container of fixed volume. Consequently, there is an abrupt pressure increase which can be measured in the pulmonary artery, cerebrospinal fluid, extra-pleural space, vena cava, jugular vein and carotid artery. The increase in cerebrospinal fluid pressure may give rise to the blown-up feeling reported by decompressed subjects. Pulmonary, cardiac, intracranial and retro-tympanic hemorrhagic lesions found in explosively decompressed animals may be produced by the collapse of venous capillaries due to the severe and rapid oscillations of venous pressure transmitted from the thoracic vessels.[47]

Intrapulmonic pressures of the order of 30 to 60 mm Hg were found to be sufficient to rupture mammalian lungs which had been removed from the body, while lungs *in situ*, and thus supported by the thoracic and abdominal walls, tolerated pressures from 50 to 100 mm Hg before rupturing.[48] The increased amounts of air and blood in the lungs during inspiration and the first third of expiration contribute to the frequent incidence of pulmonary hemorrhage after decompression, as compared to the relative infrequency of pulmonary hemorrhage after decompres sion during other phases of the respiratory cycle.[49] Since the hilus of the lung has no pleural covering, air which has escaped from ruptured alveoli can easily pass beneath the visceral pleura to the hilus, and thence into surrounding areas. It may infiltrate the anterior mediastinum and interfere with the coronary circulation; it may invade the subcutaneous tissues of the neck, face and axilla, or travel retroperitoneally and pass into the thighs. Should the air from ruptured alveoli enter the pulmonary veins, it would pass into the heart, emulsify the blood with air bubbles and travel as aeroemboli throughout the general circulation. Lodging of these emboli in the cerebral vessels could produce a wide variety of neurological symptoms.

From the viewpoint of the physiological hazards involved, decompression to an altitude of 72,000 ft is equivalent to decompression to the vacuum of space. Animal experiments have shown that one of the major dangers from decompression to 72,000 ft is the fulminating anoxia which ensues. In fact, because of the low barometric pressure, the direction of O_2 diffusion through the pulmonary membranes is reversed, and O_2 is removed from the blood and passes into the alveoli. After explosive decompression to 72,000 ft, dogs were found to have pulmonary lesions including atelectasis, hemorrhage and emphysema, as well as widespread hemorrhages in other organs. The atelectasis was considered to have resulted initially from vapothorax. Its persistence after return to ground level was ascribed to occlusion of small respiratory passages by hemorrhages, thereby preventing reinflation of the collapsed lung areas.[50]

SUMMARY

The integrity of man's physiological state during all phases of space flight depends directly upon the adequacy of the gaseous environment with which he is surrounded. The physiological effects of excesses and deficiencies in the environmental constituents of oxygen, carbon dioxide, nitrogen, toxic substances and air ions have been discussed. The effects of total pressure levels and changes in pressure have been related to structural and functional changes in body organs and systems. Consideration of these factors is important in determining the gaseous environment of man in space.

REFERENCES

1. RAHN, H.:   The gas stores of the body with particular reference to carbon dioxide.   In *Studies in Pulmonary Physiology*, Wright Air Development Div., Tech. Report 60-1, April, 1960.
2. FOWLER, W. S. and J. H. COMROE, Jr.:   Lung function studies.   I. The rate of increase of arterial oxygen saturation during the inhalation of 100 per cent oxygen.   *J. Clin. Invest.*, 27:327, 1948.
3. GESELL, R.:   On the clinical regulation of respiration.   I.   The regulation of respiration with special reference to the metabolism of the respiratory center and the coordination of the dual function of hemoglobin.   *Am. J. Physiol.*, 66:5, 1923.
4. SCHMIDT, C. F.:   Part II.   The respiration, in *Medical Physiology*.   St. Louis, C. V. Mosby Co., 1956.
5. HAGEN, H., W. HIRSCHBERGER, and W. SCHLOZ: Electron microscopic changes in brain tissue of syrian hamsters following acute hypoxia.   *Aerospace Med.*, 31:379, 1960.
6. THOMPSON, A. B.:   *Physiological and psychological considerations for manned space flight*.   Dallas, Tex., Chance Vought Aircraft Inc. Report No. E9R-12349, June 1, 1959.
7. DRIPPS, R. D., and J. H. COMROE, Jr.:   The effect of the inhalation of high and low oxygen concentrations on respiration, pulse rate, ballistocardiogram, and arterial oxygen saturation (oximeter) of normal individuals.   *Am. J. Physiol.*, 149:277, 1947.
8. VAN LIERE, E. J.:   *Anoxia, Its Effect on the Body*.   Chicago, University of Chicago Press, 1942.
9. HOUSTON, C. S., and R. L. RILEY: Respiratory and circulatory changes during acclimitization to high altitude.   *Am. J. Physiol.*, 149:565, 1947.

10. Otis, A. B., H. Rahn, M. A. Epstein, and W. O. Fenn: Performance as related to composition of alveolar air. *Am. J. Physiol., 146*:207, 1946.
11. Swann, H. G.: The principles of resuscitation. *Anesthesiology, 14*:126, 1953.
12. Henderson, Y., and H. W. Haggard: The maximum power and its fuel. *Am. J. Physiol., 72*:264, 1925.
13. Hallwachs, O.: Sauerstoffverbrauch und Temperaturverhalten des unnarkotisierten Hundes bei Lufttemperaturen von −10°C bis + 35°C. *Pflügers Arch. f.d. ges. Physiol., 271*:748, 1960.
14. Froese, G.: Effect of breathing O_2 at one atmosphere on O_2 consumption of rats. *J. Appl. Physiol., 15*:53, 1960.
15. Astrand, I., P. O. Astrand, E. H. Christensen, and R. Hedman: Intermittent muscular work. *Acta Physiol. Scand., 48*:448, 1960.
16. Christensen, E. H., R. Hedman, and I. Holmdahl: The influence of rest pauses on mechanical efficiency. *Acta Physiol. Scand., 48*:443, 1960.
17. Campbell, J. A.: Oxygen-want and its alleviation. *Lancet, 1*:914, 1938.
18. Hock, R. J.: The potential application of hibernation to space travel. *Aerospace Med., 31*:485, 1960.
19. Balke, B., and J. Gordon Wells: Ceiling altitude tolerance following physical training and acclimitization. *J. Av. Med., 29*:40, 1958.
20. Clark, R. T., H. G. Clamann, B. Balke, P. C. Tang, J. D. Fulton, A. Graybiel, and J. Vogel: Basic research problems in space medicine: a review. *Aerospace Med., 31*:553, 1960.
21. Comroe, J. H., Jr., and R. D. Dripps: *The Physiological Basis for Oxygen Therapy.* Springfield, Thomas, 1950.
22. Becker-Freysang, H., and H. G. Clamann: Zur Frage der sauerstoffvergiftung. *Klin. Wchnschr., 18*:1382, 1939.
23. Comroe, J. H., Jr., R. D. Dripps, P. R. Dumke, and M. Deming: Oxygen toxicity. *J.A.M.A., 128*:710, 1945
24. Ohlsson, W. T. L.: A study on oxygen toxicity at atmospheric pressure. *Acta Med. Scand., 128*: Suppl. 190, 1947.
25. Michel, E. L., R. W. Langevin, and C. F. Gell: Effect of continuous human exposure to oxygen tension of 418 mm Hg for 168 hrs. *Aerospace Med., 31*:138, 1960.
26. Rahn, H. C., R. C. Stroud, S. M. Tenney, and J. C. Mithoefer: Adaption to high altitude: respiratory response to CO_2 and O_2. *J. Appl. Physiol., 6*:158, 1953.
27. Bartlett, R. G., and N. E. Phillips: *Problems of Nitrogen-free and Carbon Dioxide-rich Extraterrestrial Atmospheres.* Pensacola, Fla.: U. S. Naval Sch. of Av. Med., Res. Proj. MR005.12-3100, Subtask 4, Report No. 3, July 7, 1960.

28. STEIN, S. N., H. E. LEE, J. H. ANNEGERS, S. A. KAPLAN, and D. G. McQUARRIE: *The Effects of Prolonged Inhalation of Hypernormal Amounts of Carbon Dioxide. 1. Physiological Effects of 3 Per Cent CO_2 for 93 Days Upon Monkeys.* Bethesda, Md.: Naval Medical Research Institute. Res. Report. NM 24 01 00.01.01, August 31, 1959.

28a. LAMBERTSEN, C. J.: *A Philosophy of Extremes for the Gaseous Environment of Manned, Closed Ecological Systems.* Proc. Manned Space Station Symposium. New York, Institute of Aeronautical Sciences, 1960.

29. SCHAEFER, K. E.: A concept of triple tolerance limits based on chronic carbon dioxide toxicity studies. *Aerospace Med., 32:*197, 1961.

30. SCHMIDT, C. F.: *The Cerebral Circulation in Health and Disease.* Springfield, Thomas, 1950.

31. HALDANE, J. S., and J. G. PRIESTLEY: *Respiration.* New York, Oxford University Press, 1935.

32. BEHNKE, A. R.: Decompression sickness following exposures to high pressures. In *Decompression Sickness,* ed. by J. F. Fulton. Philadelphia, W. B. Saunders Co., 1951.

33. HALL, A. L., and R. J. MARTIN: Prolonged exposure in the Navy full pressure suit at "space equivalent" altitudes. *Aerospace Med., 31:* 116, 1960.

34. SCHAEFER, K.: Selecting a space cabin atmosphere. *Astronautics, 4:*28, 1959.

35. COOK, S. F., and H. A. LEON: *Physiological Effects of Inert Gases.* Holloman Air Force Base, New Mexico, USAF Aeromedical Field Laboratory. Report AFMDC 59-26, June, 1959.

36. KELLER, D. M.: Cabin atmospheres: their physical and chemical control. In *Review of Lectures in Aerospace Med.,* Brooks Air Force Base, Tex., School of Aviation Medicine, USAF Aerospace Medical Center (ATC), 1960.

37. PETERS, J. P., and D. D. VAN SLYKE: *Quantitative Clinical Chemistry.* Baltimore, Williams and Wilkins Co., 1931.

38. *American Standard Allowable Concentration of Carbon Monoxide.* New York, American Standards Association, January, 1951.

39. SIEVERS, R. F., T. I. EDWARDS, A. L. MURRAY, and H. H. SCHRENK: Effect of exposure to known concentrations of carbon monoxide: a study of traffic officers stationed at the Holland Tunnel for thirteen years. *J.A.M.A., 118:*585, 1942.

40. MUSSELMAN, N. P., W. A. GROFF, P. P. YEVICH, F. T. WILINSKI, M. H. WEEKS, and F. W. OBERST: Continuous exposure of laboratory animals to low concentration of carbon monoxide. *Aerospace Med., 30:*524, 1959.

41. KING, M. E.: Toxicity of ozone. *Frontier, 23*:10, 1961.
42. KRANZ, P., and T. A. RICH: *The Physics of Small Air-borne Ions.* Philadelphia, Pa., Franklin Institute. First International Conference on Ionization of the Air. Oct. 16–17, 1961.
43. KONECCI, E. B.: *Decompression events in bio-satellites.* New York, American Rocket Society ARS No. 638–58, June, 1958.
44. BURGESS, E.: *Satellites and Spaceflight.* New York, The Macmillan Co., 1957.
45. BEISCHER, D. E., and S. BORN: The "boiling" phenomenon of living tissues at low atmospheric pressure. *J. Av. Med., 28*:154, 1957.
46. WARD, J. E.: The true nature of the boiling of body fluid in space. *J. Av. Med., 27*:429, 1956.
47. VIOLETTE, F.: Les effets physiologiques des décompressions explosives et leur mécanisme. *La Méd. Aéronautique, 9*:223, 1954.
48. HENRY, J. P.: *A Determination of the Mechanical Limits to Safe Pressurization of the Mammalian Lung.* Washington, Committee on Aviation Medicine, NRC, OSRD. Report No. 463, May 30, 1945.
49. BERG, W. E., J. P. BAUMBERGER, F. CRESCITELLI, S. RAPAPORT, and P. O. GREELEY: *Explosive Decompression: Lung Damage Correlated with Respiratory Cycle.* Washington, Committee on Aviation Medicine, NRC, OSRD. Report No. 173, August 16, 1943.
50. HITCHCOCK, F. A.: Physiological and pathological effects of explosive decompression. *J. Av. Med., 25*:578, 1954.

4

FOOD REQUIREMENTS IN SPACE

John R. Brobeck, M.D., Ph.D.

MAN'S NUTRITIONAL NEEDS

In something less than one hundred years the science of nutrition has reached a notable landmark, namely, that when foods are available in a reasonable variety, what a man should eat can be stated specifically. How much protein is required to maintain the metabolic machinery of an adult; how much extra protein is needed for growth; what are adequate amounts and sources of energy; how much of each mineral "trace" element is necessary; which molecular patterns must be provided as "essential" amino or fatty acids, or as vitamins—all of these questions have been answered for men, women and children, and for most laboratory and domestic animals. Having reached this goal, nutrition now enters a new stage in its development as a science, at a time when the challenge of providing food for men on space missions will stimulate further progress. From this effort may come a more thorough understanding of the physiology of food intake.

Where previous research was concerned with food requirements in a biochemical sense, the newer approach recognizes that a need cannot be met unless the proper food is eaten. If the older question was, "What *should* a man eat?," the newer one is, "What *will* a man eat?" or "What will he *want* to eat?" Now the selection of foods, choices or preferences are of interest; acceptability is important; feeding behavior is relevant; the phenomenon of "regulation of food intake" requires an explanation. Perhaps the difference between the old and new can be illustrated by reviewing one of the classic paradoxes of nutrition, as follows: In a growing animal where the protein requirement is known to be, for example, 16 per cent of the diet, if the protein concentration in the food is reduced to 12 per cent, the animal grows more slowly. Why does it not respond to this dietary change by increasing total food intake by one-third? If it did so, it would once again have an optimal intake of protein, and could grow at the previous rate. Instead, it eats less—not more—than previously. (Our own data on this phenomenon suggest that with only a moderate reduction in dietary protein concentration, a slight increase in food intake can occur. These particular animals may weigh the same as controls, but only because they convert the extra energy into fat in place of the protein which they cannot synthesize. But with a further decrease in dietary protein level, food intake as well as weight gain begins to fall.) The paradox is stated in the question, "Why do the animals not gain the necessary protein by eating more food?" This question is often asked in a manner implying that the animals are stupid, or that they are stubborn. No doubt at times this idea has entered the mind of everyone (including parents) in charge of feeding babies, children, patients in a hospital, college students, soldiers or laboratory or farm animals. The truth of the matter is that for purely physiological reasons the body is sometimes unable to eat food that seems perfectly adequate by the standards of classical nutrition. The physiological and psychological mechanisms that evoke this behavior are the subjects of the newer research. Why does an animal eat now, drink then? Why is this food acceptable, that refused? What limits the intake on this diet? Instead of asking what food an astronaut will need on the one hundred and third day of his voyage, we must know also what menu he will wish to select and what he will be able to eat.

The following discussion is organized as a review of the importance of three subjects, viz., (i) biochemical nutritional needs, (ii) feeding behavior and (iii) influence of food intake upon behavior. For each of these three an attempt is made to decide whether data to answer critical questions are already at hand, or whether they must be discovered through research before a space mission is undertaken. In certain instances where the data are not known and cannot be obtained in the time available, the flights will have to be planned in a manner which does not depend upon them. In general, for shorter flights where food can be taken along we know most of what we need to know about feeding; the questions remaining are of a practical nature, how to do it. For intermediate flights one can plan experiments to make the discoveries necessary to make the missions successful. But for extended flights we know very little, indeed. Stated in another fashion: As to man's biochemical need for food the theoretical foundation is all but complete, although a few practical questions remain to be answered. With reference to food acceptability and related phenomena, almost nothing is known theoretically, but it may be possible to minimize this ignorance by utilizing a few common sense principles. Regarding the impact of food upon behavior, neither theoretical nor practical research has been undertaken, and one can only trust that no major mistakes will be made.

FOOD REQUIREMENTS

Tables published by the Food and Nutrition Board give amounts of dietary constituents recommended for males and females, infants, children or adults, and for conditions such as pregnancy or lactation, or for heavy physical work. These requirements are not expected to be altered during space flight, except for the minor influence of the zero gravitational condition (Lawton, 1961). Exactly how much a lack of gravity may alter a man's daily energy requirement is not known. This ignorance, however, is of little importance for three reasons. First, shorter flights always precede longer ones, and provide data for more precise planning when this is necessary. Second, energy balance does not need to be very exact from day to day or even from week to week. A man who exchanges 2800 kcal/day has stored in his body, theoretically, 145,000 kcal of energy. Much of this cannot be used and remains in the bodily substance even after death from prolonged starvation. But a surprisingly large part of the reserve can be used, and serves as a "cushion" between irregularities of intake and energy output. It will compensate for the inability to predict exactly how much energy an astronaut will spend in doing his job under zero G. Third, food is relatively light in weight. A daily exchange of 3000 kcal requires only 750 g of dehydrated protein or carbohydrate, or about 330 g of pure fat. Lawton recommends one pound (450 g) of concentrated food per day, of a diet containing 32 per cent fat and 16 per cent pro- tein (1960). With proper selection of type of protein and pro- vision of vitamins and minerals, such a diet could be prescribed for indefinite use so far as biochemical requirements are con- cerned. (Whether a man can and will eat it indefinitely is another question.) On a space mission lasting ten days, an over- supply of dry food of 25 per cent will add only 2.5 lb to the load, while an undersupply of the same percentage will result in only an insignificant loss of body fat on the part of the astronaut.

Interestingly enough, most of the individual components of the diet do not need to be balanced up exactly on shorter flights, either Deficiencies are slow to develop in a man initially well nourished. One can say that for flights of possibly a week in duration, the com- position of the diet is of little nutritional significance. So far as possible it should be similar to his preflight menus. If it provides energy, if the subject eats it willingly, and if it satisfies hunger and appetite without any resulting discomfort such as nausea or ab- dominal discomfort, it will do. The period mentioned, 1 wk, can- not be precisely timed, of course, since nutritional inadequacies appear gradually. I confess that I do not know how soon the earli- est sign of deficiency will appear if thiamine, for example, is abruptly taken out of the diet of a well nourished adult male. An estimate of 1 wk is used because in animal experiments, and during fasting or starvation of men, 1 wk seems to be a period where ir- regularities in a biochemical sense are of little import. Because it is so easy, however, to make a balanced diet, there is no reason to plan for anything less, and a diet serving well for short missions will doubtless have a place in longer ones. At the moment, the main hazards seem to be those of packaging and preservation, rather than of nutrition (see Lawton, 1960).

Food-water Relations: Water is lost from the body via vaporization from moist surfaces of lungs, respiratory passages and skin; in formation of urine and feces; and in sweat. These losses are made up by ingestion of water in food and beverages, and by water of oxidation of foodstuffs. The amount of water needed per day can be estimated rather exactly. Two interesting features of water turnover have been pointed out. Clamann notes that because the body uses the water of food for other physiological processes, there is no saving of weight in short flights when food is dehydrated; the water has to be taken along in any case (1959). If water is recycled, however, then dehydrated food becomes advantageous, since the same water can be used over and over in reconstitution of food. The second feature is that if water is only recovered physically or chemically, it will accumulate. Thus, in an aircraft with 100 per cent recovery of water lost from the body in sweat, vapor, urine and feces, and this recovered water available for eating and drinking, the conversion of oxygen and the hydrogen of food into water by metabolic processes will continually increase the water supply. This will not occur when complete regeneration is accomplished, with photosynthesis or some other process as a converter of water and carbon dioxide back into foodstuffs. The "molecular bookkeeping" needed to monitor these conversions has been reviewed in one of the classic papers of this field, the 1958 paper of Clark.

If one compares a fasting man with one having food available, other interrelations of food and water become evident. Food intake increases water intake for three types of reaction, as follows:

1. Digestion and absorption of food;

2. Renal excretion of extra electrolyte, and of extra urea and other nitrogenous compounds derived from the food in excess of fasting turnover;

3. Dissipation of heat of metabolism of food, the so-called S.D.A. or "specific dynamic effect" (Kleiber, 1961).

Of these three, the last can be minimized or abolished by techniques including the adjustment of clothing and of air temperature so as to prevent sweating after eating; if the environment is already a bit cool, the S.D.A. will not appreciably enhance the cutaneous water loss. The second, excretion of osmotic load, can also be minimized; from studies already published one can predict just how much protein and electrolyte should be present in the diet to give the most efficient possible turnover of these materials. The amount of protein yielding maximal efficiency will be less than the customary intake in our culture. Finally, there is some reason to believe that the amount of water utilized for digestion may be likewise subject to modification. Definite interactions of feeding and drinking have been described (Adolph, 1947; Adolph, *et al.*, 1954). It is conceivable that by controlling size of meals and frequency of feeding, a schedule can be discovered which will permit optimal food intake with minimal water consumption. Nevertheless, in short flights any attempt to do this will be of little value. Ten pounds of dry food for a ten-day flight will require 50 lb of water for reconstitution to usual food consistency. This amount of water will serve nicely for purposes of water balance, and it will provide more than 1 ml of water for each kilocalorie of food, a ratio not unusual in more ordinary living conditions. Any serious attempt to decrease this 50 lb of water by a few per cent seems unwarranted.

Worf has emphasized, however, the urgent need for efficient water use in longer flights, those of more than 4 wk (1960). A flight of thirty days will take 30 lb of food and 150 lb of water—a weight equal to or exceeding that of the astronaut. Here the recovery of water and recycling of respiratory gases begins to become more practicable than exclusive use of stores. In logical sequence one may expect to see the planning of flights so as to achieve: (i) shorter flights like those of Project Mercury where food is not needed but where food as well as water can be taken from storage; (ii) longer flights of several days where storage is more than adequate; (iii) flights of a few weeks or a month with ample storage but with testing of equipment for recovery or recycling; and, finally, (iv) flights with recycling and with food and water reserves for only supplementation or emergency use. Worf's graph shows that missions of 12 wk are unwise until complete and dependable regeneration is possible.

Yet even for flights of this latter duration or longer, there is little risk that a space mission will fail because of any failure to understand the food requirements of the metabolic processes of the body.

ACCEPTABILITY OF FOOD

Shorter Flights: A different matter entirely is the question of how long an astronaut will eat the food supplied. Experience in World War II with combat and emergency rations revealed the distinction between food made available and food eaten. One has only to mention the phrase, "K rations" to evoke memories of unacceptable food. Dehydrated foods were especially troublesome, as were original and even unique mixtures and combinations. No soldier had ever eaten what he found when he opened his first combat packet. Why did these difficulties arise at that particular time? Probably, for reasons both of transport and food processing. In place of the rather immediate "feed back" situation of a conventional mess hall, where at the next meal a cook can alter the menu in response to complaints or compliments, a highly efficient system of food supply was in operation in a fashion which took months or even years to change. Usually a cook depends upon natural foods, available locally; in a given area at a certain season of the year, items of food are not diverse. Cooks serve what they can get, and their customers are used to eating what is served. During the war all of this was affected by the artificial manipulations of transport and processing of food. Another complication was perhaps caused by nutrition experts who are likely to think in terms of laboratory diets. No one had inquired whether laboratory animals really liked these diets, or whether they preferred something else, or whether they would feel like killing the cook if the same old mixture was served once more. Consequently, when food packets were made similar to these experimental diets, it is not surprising that under many conditions soldiers either would not or could not eat them.

These problems together with the rise of experimental psychology, have now led to research on food acceptability. Preferences of laboratory, domestic and farm animals have been studied, the roles of taste and odor are under investigation, and studies of consumer, preferences are sponsored by food merchants. A general conclusion of this research is that men prefer foods they are used to, possibly even foods to which they were accustomed as children. This suggests the principle, therefore, that diets for space missions should be similar to civilian diets. It will be unfortunate if the bungling of the war is repeated by "experts" who believe that they can easily concoct synthetic foods or mixtures of foods, and that men with motivation strong enough to qualify them as astronauts will docilely eat whatever they are given. Both of these propositions may be true. Yet there are better ways of meeting the situation.

For missions up to 4 wk, where food will be taken from stores, the "T-V dinner" supplied by American supermarkets seems to be the diet of choice. It is similar to what is served by airlines to passengers in flight. Precooked, it is stored frozen, then thawed and heated before it is served. Usually it includes a meat, vegetable and a serving of potatoes, and may include appetizer, salad, roll or bread and dessert. Preparing, packaging, storing and serving of these foods are well understood. A provision of four packages each of six different T-V dinners, plus miscellaneous standard foods for breakfast, lunches and snacks, is probably better than any kind of artificial diet blended scientifically. Some of the items will need special packaging so that they can be served without the aid of gravity, but the processes of eating, per se, do not need gravity once the food reaches the mouth. This can be demonstrated by the ease with which one can eat either prone or supine, with head down or head up. Liquids must be served in squeeze bottles. Foods usually brought to the mouth with a spoon—such as cereals, vegetables in small pieces and salads—are excluded. But if the food can be carried by a fork, or manually, it can be managed without gravity.* Crumbs are said to be troublesome when they are suspended in space within the cabin. No doubt they can be disposed of by the technique used in many labora-

---

* Worf (1960) seems to have overestimated these difficulties, possibly misled by data of Ward, *et al.* (1959), whose observations were complicated by unavoidable changes in force of gravity during each experiment.

tories for recovering spilled mercury—a vacuum cleaner. In addition to his plastic mittens (Finkelstein, 1960), and whatever other aids the astronaut is given for cleaning up after a meal, he should have a small, hand type vacuum cleaner or a vacuum hose with which he can tidy up the cabin and his uniform when he has finished eating.

If the first recommendation is to select foods to which the crew is accustomed, the second is to select men who are in the habit of eating what can be provided. Regional differences accounted for many of the complaints about food in the army twenty years ago. Perhaps they are less important now because rapid transit of food, high mobility of population and general prosperity tend to even out local peculiarities of diet. One can imagine a situation, however, where it becomes convenient to expect an astronaut to eat a fortified milk shake for lunch each day for twenty days, after a breakfast of cereal and fruit, and followed by a T-V style dinner. It should be relatively easy to locate among our younger generation a rather large number of young men whose usual diet is not far removed from this. Feeding them in space for a few weeks should be a straightforward task.

Longer Flights: For physiology as for engineering, the real problems of space missions begin when food regeneration is needed (Clark, 1958). Worf places this point at 12 wk. No doubt the first flight intended to require recycling will be preceded by intensive experimentation on the ground, as well as by testing of equipment in flights where other food can be made available from stores. In general, food regeneration will be attempted through photosynthesis in simple organisms such as algae (Clark, *et al.*, 1960; Bates, 1961). They yield organic material with plentiful carbohydrate, which can be high in protein or in fat (Lawton, 1960), and which needs to be supplemented with methionine. The products of such cultures have been used as dietary supplements, although not with complete success (Powell, Nevels and McDowell, 1961). To my knowledge, the use of algae or any other simple plant or animal as the only source of food for men has not been achieved.

Research in this field, however, should be encouraged. If it is true, as noted earlier, that the biochemical, nutritional requirements of man are well understood, then one can predict from the chemical analysis of a given organism the extent to which it can serve as a complete diet. Evidence already at hand shows that with efficient means of culture, with perfection of techniques for separating the several constituents of the organism, and with development of processing so as to create acceptable foods, this whole endeavor can be a successful one. Without being specific, I will attempt to outline the objectives of this undertaking. If the material is to serve as a longterm substitute for more usual foods, it is obvious that it cannot be served as algae; it will have to be converted into other forms. I propose that it should be converted into the equivalent of T-V dinners, milkshakes, cereal, bread, etc. Instead of asking the question, "How can algae be made into a substance that a man can eat for an extended time?" one should ask, "How can algae be made into beefsteak?" If this latter question is not taken seriously, the experience of the war twenty years ago will be repeated—a food substance nutritionally adequate will be provided, but the men will not eat it. The diet of "enriched sugar water thickened with shredded paper towel" described by Clark is something less than ideal (1958).

To develop methods for processing algae into other foods appears at first to be an impossible task. Fortunately, three types of industrial success support the conclusion that this, too, can be achieved. First, the use of previously inedible oils in manufacture of shortening and margarine shows how the fats can be upgraded. Second, the creation of the new, so-called "formula" diets, either for weight reduction, for infant feeding, or for replacement of conventional meals, points the way to enhancing the acceptability of otherwise inacceptable foods. Third, the invention of synthetic fibers for use in fabrics (nylon, rayon, etc.) implies that synthetic foods can be manufactured from protein sources now regarded as inedible. Patents have already been granted for this purpose. One is for the manufacture of meat-like fibers from solutions of protein (Giddey, 1960a). The other is intended "to provide an improved protein composition for use as foodstuffs for animals or human beings, for example, as synthetic meat or meat-like food." The resulting product can be flavored or colored, can be cut into pieces like meat, and can be modified so as to achieve a "chewiness" appropriate for the "synthetic meat (Giddey, 1960b). In order to take advantage of these discoveries or others related to them, the space vehicle should have not only the facilities for growing the photosynthetic organism, but also for recovering the harvest, purifying it, separating its constituents, and from them synthesizing the materials to be used in the diet. Clamann estimates that the apparatus will weigh one ton per man to be fed (1959). Energy from the sun, or from thermonuclear reactions, will not be lacking. What is needed is a great research effort designed to reveal how materials now unused as food, particularly, protein, can be transformed into the finest type and most desirable form of high protein foods.

A principle advantage of this type of research is that it will benefit, in addition to space travelers, millions of other persons now in need of food here on the earth. The use of physical or chemical energy to create preferred foods out of organisms low down in the cycle of food production, or out of protein now wasted, with the resulting by-passing of intermediate stages in the natural chain of synthesis from plants to man, will make better food available more economically everywhere. It will provide desirable foods where they simply do not exist. This is an exciting goal, and one which promises to benefit much of the world's population.

IMPACT OF FOOD UPON BEHAVIOR

How feeding modifies behavior is a subject almost untouched in the scientific literature, and yet familiar to a degree to all of us. If the question is phrased, "Is the behavior of a starving animal different from that of the same animal well fed?" or "Does a baby behave differently before and after nursing?" or even "Does the office staff act differently after lunch?" the answer can only be, "Of course." I am reminded of an experience of some years ago when a book on the influence of hormones on behavior—a fine account of laboratory research—nowhere mentioned what every farmer knows about the differences in behavior between a cow, steer or bull, or a mare, gelding and stallion. So it is with food and behavior. The interaction is obvious; but not in the scientific literature.

Perhaps the most striking effect of feeding upon behavior is the sedative action of food. This is apparent in the slumber of a fed infant, in the sleepiness which follows lunch, and in the attention usually given to after dinner speakers. Food has been called the oldest tranquillizer—it is the first one given to every individual and so is oldest in terms of personal experience, and it was used by the human race before alcohol, narcotics, or other sedative agents were discovered. It is not only old, its use is universal by animals of all types, although its sedative action is more obvious in some than in others. Many psychiatrists believe that patients can become addicted to its tranquillizing action just as others become addicted to alcohol or other drugs. When a patient has this type of addiction, obesity follows. Unlike the sedative drugs which are eventually destroyed or otherwise eliminated from the body, the extra food accumulates in the form of fat as an evidence of the addiction.

A second important point is that food sometimes cannot be used as a tranquillizer because the gastro-intestinal tract will not accept or retain it. Sedative drugs given by injection do not present this complication although any medication given by mouth may do so. The subject is of some importance in feeding of men in space, in that one can predict that food will have a sedative action, but one cannot plan to use food for this purpose as a means of relieving anxiety or tension under all circumstances. The uneasy stomach of athletes before or during contests is a familiar illustration of this point. In a track meet, food is not recommended to reduce the tension of a high jumper just before his event. If he does eat or has eaten recently, he will more than likely empty his stomach by vomiting before his turn to jump. Similar experiences were common for men entering combat during the war, and they led to a fair amount of research as to what soldiers should be fed just before they fight. My opinion is that they should not be fed;

there is no harm in fasting for a few days, and if a man is not hungry under these conditions he will easily live off the reserves he has already accumulated within his body. (Whether a hypoglycemia will ensue during this fasting has been questioned, and methods for preventing it by providing "snacks" of food have been recommended. But if the snacks are not desired by the men, even they are unnecessary. The preferable means of avoiding the hypoglycemia is to make sure that the diet fed for some weeks previously is reasonably high in fat, since fasting hypoglycemia is a sequel to the eating of a high-carbohydrate diet, Roberts, *et al.*, 1944). The explanation for the inability of the digestive tract to retain food under these conditions is not certain; perhaps it follows a breakdown in the usual patterns of visceral activity. Normally, with the onset of feeding there begin secretion and motility of the stomach and intestine and its glands, which, together, ensure the digestion of the food. During fright or anxiety, the motility and secretion are prevented. There is failure of activation of the parasympathetic nervous system, and inhibition of motility and secretion via the sympathetic nerves. Yet in spite of this visceral paralysis, the voluntary muscles of mouth, jaw and upper pharynx can be "commanded" to cooperate in eating. So the usual synergism of voluntary and of automatic activities is disrupted. If the automatic stasis is severe enough, it will carry the day and the food will be ejected by vomiting. A less drastic autonomic quiescence will simply allow the food to remain in the stomach undigested. In either event, the response of the digestive tract seems to illustrate what Cannon called, "the wisdom of the body," and indicates clearly that one cannot administer food as a sedative or tranquillizer when the body is not prepared to receive it. In flights of the shorter durations, therefore, men do not need to be encouraged to eat unless they feel like it; and if they are persuaded to eat against their wishes one should not be surprised if nausea and vomiting follow.

Thirdly, food is widely used in psychology and in animal training for its value as a reward. Whether for pressing a bar in a Skinner box, or for mastering some circus stunt, food is the pay received by the animal. The converse of the situation, however, is equally or even more fascinating. Most animals will not work "spontaneously" unless they are in a fasting state, and when food is used as a reward, it must be used sparingly lest the animal pass over into satiation and so fail to perform as desired. The number of experiments where fasting has been used, knowingly or unknowingly, as a technique for inducing "motivation" is beyond counting. In human cultures, the phenomenon of food reward is less obvious (for example in a home), but it may become dominant (for example, in a prison camp). This possibility should not be overlooked in planning of space missions. Perhaps an astronaut who is not asked nor expected to eat during the count-down nor in the tenseness of establishing a flight path or checking the operation of the ship, will later on accept a snack and a tube of coffee as a minor reward for finishing his "chores."

Finally, one must consider the opposite of the sedative effect of food, namely, the stimulant effects of fasting. Laboratory animals and also animals living naturally are more active when they are fasted, or fed limited amounts of food. Stevenson found that exposure to cold intensifies this hyperactivity of fasting (1955). It is interesting to discover that Sherrington observed something like this when he was studying spinal reflexes (1900, p. 845). He found that if the animal was well nourished and recently fed, the reflexes he wished to analyze could be obtained only with some difficulty. The animal of choice was one previously well nourished, "hungry and expecting food." What is true of the spinal cord seems to be true of the whole animal, and of man. Physical work is accomplished more easily before, rather than after, a large meal (Young, 1959; Young, *et al.*, 1959). Another phenomenon seems to complicate the situation, however. Most men who do heavy work say that they are unable to work effectively unless they have had, for example, a good breakfast. This is something of a puzzle, in that work is done more easily during fasting, but working men prefer to be well fed. Perhaps the onset of hyperglycemia in the middle of the morning plays a part in the desire for an ample breakfast; or perhaps the discomfort of the hunger contractions simply distracts the man from his job. Even modern man is not far removed from a fear that he will starve to death. Whatever the explanation, these observations together suggest the following conclusions:

i. Irritability and possibly activity can be decreased by feeding;

ii. Overfeeding is to be avoided;

iii. Appetite is an adequate guide in short-term exposures (up to a few days);

iv. When appetite fails and food is not desired during an interval of longer than a few days, the situation justifies a thorough study from both a psychological and a physiological point of view. In other words, the food (and water) intake must be considered as critical factors in assuring both the "habitability" of any space craft (Celentano and Adams, 1961) and the performance of its crew (Lawton, 1960).

TECHNICAL INFORMATION ABOUT FEEDING MEN IN SPACE

Information more specific and more complete than what is given in this review is gradually becoming available in the form of official publications of the government, and other scientific reports. One of the more imaginative and yet also practical essays is by Hursh (1960), in which he estimated the cost of a round trip to the moon for one man as $815,000 for the man's fare and $350,000 for his oxygen and food. A good discussion of the use of algae is also given. Two other reviews which are invaluable were published anonymously in Nutrition Reviews, both in the year 1960. To about this same period belong Clamann's survey of the metabolic problems of space flight (1959), and Lawton's thorough and systematic appraisal of metabolic and nutritional requirements of food reserves for space travelers (1960). All phases of the problem are considered, with quantitative data where they are available and pertinent.

More general and consequently less informative accounts are found in the 1959 Staff Report of the Select Committee on Astronautics and Space Exploration of the U. S. House of Representatives (Feldman and Sheldon, 1959). According to my notes, this document is made up mainly of "engineering, physics, astronomy and philosophy." The chapter by Sells and Berry on requirements for space travel is a briefer introduction to much of the same material (1961). As to techniques and machines for supporting life off the earth, Feldman and Sheldon (1959a) describe methods of food preservation, while Clark, *et al.*, (1960) and Clamann (1961) give useful introductions to the maintenance of closed systems, including photosynthetic reclamation of oxygen, water and food. Lastly, the recent paper by Whisenhunt (1961) summarizes recent thinking about life support systems in a highly informative manner. All of these others, of course, are to be interpreted with the insight provided by the astronauts of Project Mercury. An account of John Glenn's flight is available as a report of the National Aeronautics and Space Administration describing the results of the first U. S. manned orbital flight of February 20, 1962.

REFERENCES

ADOLPH, E. F.: Urges to eat and drink in rats. *Am. J. Physiol., 151*:110–125, 1947.

ADOLPH, E. F., JUNE P. BARKER, and PATRICIA A. HOY: Multiple factors in thirst. *Am. J. Physiol., 178*:538–562, 1954.

ANONYMOUS: Nutrition for man in space. *Nutrition Rev., 18*:100–101, 1960.

ANONYMOUS: Nutrition of man in space. *Nutrition Rev., 18*:325–328, 1960.

BATES, J. H.: Recent aspects in the development of a closed ecologic system. *Aerospace Med., 32*:12–24, 1961.

CELENTANO, J. T., and B. B. ADAMS: Habitability and maintenance of human performance in long-duration space missions. *Advances in Astronautical Sci., 7*:349–361, 1961.

CLAMANN, H. G.: Some metabolic problems of space flight. *Fed. Proc., 18*:1249–1255, 1959.

CLAMANN, H. G.: The engineered environment of the space vehicle. In *Human Factors in Jet and Space Travel*, ed. by S. B. Sells and C. A. Berry, Ronald Press Co., New York, 1961, pp. 330–344.

CLARK, C. C.: A closed food cycle atomic conservation for space flight. *J. Aviat. Med., 29*:535–539, 1958.

CLARK, R. T., H. G. CLAMANN, B. BALKE, P. C. TANG, J. D. FULTON, A. GRAYBIEL, and J. VOGEL: Basic research problems in space medicine: a review. *Aerospace Med., 31*:553–577, 1960.

FELDMAN, G. J., and C. S. SHELDON, II: *Space Handbook: Astronautics and its Applications.* Staff report of the Select Committee on Astronautics and Space Exploration, 1959a, House Document No. 86, U. S. Government Printing Office, Washington.

FELDMAN, G. J., and C. S. SHELDON, II: *The Next Ten Years in Space, 1959–1969.* Staff report of the Select Committee on Astronautics and Space Exploration, 1959b, House Document No. 115, U. S. Government Printing Office, Washington.

FINKELSTEIN, BEATRICE: Nutrition research for the space traveler. *J. Am. Diet. Assoc., 36*:313–317, 1960.

GIDDEY, C.: *Artificial fibres.* U. S. Pat. 2,947,644, 1960a, U. S. Patent Office.

GIDDEY, C.: *Protein compositions and process of producing the same.* U. S. Patent 2,952,542, 1960b, U. S. Patent Office.

HURSH, L. M.: Nutrition in space. *Mil. Med., 125*:567–569, 1960.

KLEIBER, M.: *The Fire of Life.* John Wiley & Sons, Inc., New York, 1961, xxii + 454 pp.

LAWTON, R. W.: *Food reserves on space trips: A review of metabolic and nutritional requirements.* Technical Information Series R60SD400, 1960, General Electric Co., Missile and Space Vehicle Dept., Life Support Systems, Philadelphia.

LAWTON, R. W.: *Physiological considerations relevant to the problem of prolonged weightlessness: A review.* Technical Information Series 61SD202, 1961, General Electric Co., Missile and Space Vehicle Dept., Biosciences and Human Factors, Philadelphia.

NATIONAL AERONAUTICS AND SPACE ADMINISTRATION: *Results of the First United States Manned Orbital Space Flight, February 20, 1962.* U. S. Government Printing Office, O-634401, 1962.

POWELL, R. C., ELIZABETH M. NEVELS, and M. E. McDOWELL: Algae feeding in humans. *J. Nutrition, 75*:7–12, 1961.

ROBERTS, S., L. T. SAMUELS, and R. M. REINECKE: Previous diet and the apparent utilization of fat in the absence of the liver. *Am. J. Physiol., 140*:639–644, 1944.

SELLS, S. B., and C. A. BERRY: Human requirements for space travel. In *Human Factors in Jet and Space Travel,* ed. by S. B. Sells and C. A. Berry, Ronald Press Co., New York, 1961, pp. 166–186.

SHERRINGTON, C. S.: The spinal cord. In *Textbook of Physiology* by E. A. Schafer, Vol. 2, Young J. Pentland, Edinburgh, 1900, pp. 781–883.

STEVENSON, J. A. F.: Diet and survival. In *Cold Injury, Third Conference.* Josiah Macy, Jr., Foundation, New York, 1955, pp. 165–188.

WARD, J. E., W. R. HAWKINS, and H. D. STALLINGS: Physiological response to subgravity. I. Mechanic of nourishment and deglutition of solids and liquids. *J. Aviat. Med., 30*:151–154, 1959.

WHISENHUNT, G. B., Jr. A life support system for a near earth or circumlunar space vehicle. *Advances in Astronautical Sci.*, 7:325–348, 1961.

WORF, D. L. Advanced biomedical programs. In *Space Research in the Life Sciences. An inventory of related programs, resources, and facilities.* Report on the Committee on Aeronautical and Space Sciences, 1960, U. S. Government Printing Office, Washington, pp. 15–24.

YOUNG, D. R. Effect of food deprivation on treadmill running in dogs. *J. Appl. Physiol.*, 14:1018–1022, 1959.

YOUNG, D. R., A. IACOVINO, P. ERVE, R. MOSHER, and H. SPECTOR: Effect of time after feeding and carbohydrate or water supplement on work in dogs. *J. Appl. Physiol.*, 14:1013–1017, 1959.

5

ACCELERATION

James D. Hardy, Ph.D.

INTRODUCTION

It has been only within recent years that the problems associated with in-flight acceleration have become important to humans. In an early reference to this subject, Henry Head, in writing on *The Sense of Stability and Balance in the Air*,[1] reported that a British aviator in making tight turns observed "the sky appeared to go gray; a mist gradually arose like going under an anesthetic" . . . . and the pilot fainted. When he regained consciousness (about 20 sec later) he was flying over a village about a mile distant from his maneuver area. The pilot reported the general sensation as "not unpleasant." The report describes very well the phenomena of "gray-out," "black-out," and unconsciousness which today are well known conditions associated with the accelerations of certain aerial maneuvers. As the problems of acceleration and high speed are in so many respects inseparable, the growth of interest in acceleration problems parallels the changes in man's speed capabilities. In 1903, when Orville and Wilbur Wright made their first powered airplane flights, the flying speed was about 30 mph, and in 1961, when the Russian "Cosmonaut Gagarin made the first human Earth-orbiting flight, the average speed was near 18,000 mph. Thus, in his continuing search for increased speed of transport, man has achieved a 600-fold improvement in less than 60 yrs and now can travel at a speed of more than six times that of a bullet as it leaves the muzzle of a rifle! Thus, one of the major problem areas of aero-space medicine covers the effects of acceleration. As noted by Stewart in 1958,[2] "Speed, originally seen as a useless 'craze,' is now seen as the key to man's liberation from his gravitational cage. The pattern of the future has been outlined in unmistakable terms by Esmault-Peltrie, in 1907, by Goddard in 1919, and by Oberth in 1923 . . . . It has all arisen out of aviation and, although it will be no longer aviation in the exact sense, it will still owe its existence to aviation and to those inventors, pioneers and designers who made aviation the fastest developing form of human endeavor yet known."

APPLIED AND INERTIAL FORCES

When a steady force is applied to the surface of a body at rest, it first compresses the structure and, if the force be large enough to overcome friction, the body will move. Also, if the body is in motion, an applied force will change the motion either by slowing down, speeding up, or perhaps by changing direction. The change in velocity divided by the time of action of the force is called acceleration. That is,

$$a = \frac{v - v_0}{t} \qquad (1)$$

in which

a = the acceleration
v = the velocity after time, t
v_0 = the initial velocity

The magnitude of the acceleration is in direct proportion to the magnitude of the force and is in the direction of the force. Although rapid changes in velocity are the dynamic manifestation of the forces, it is really the force as applied to the man which is of importance to the aerospace medical problem. The force can be defined in terms of the acceleration as

$$F = ma \qquad (2)$$

in which m is the mass accelerated. If applied forces were all that the physiologist had to concern himself about it is probable that aerospace medicine would not have to do with acceleration at all but would talk about forces. However, there are inertial forces which are of major importance, particularly in cardiovascular and respiratory functions, and the simplest way of dealing with these mysterious forces is by measuring the acceleration. The exact origin of the inertial forces is not clear to the physicist even today, although there is a tendency to think of these forces as being the result of the gravitational attraction of all the matter in the universe acting on the various Earth-bound masses.[3] Newton identified gravitational force with mechanical forces and indicated that gravitational and other forces could be added, multiplied and otherwise treated in the same way. Mach (of mach number fame), has suggested the principle that inertia is not so much a "property of matter" as of gravitational attraction of the distant stars, nebulae, etc., which make up the universe. Thus, if a man were far out in space where the gravitational attractions of the sun and planets were small, he would because of inertial forces have to use force (perhaps fire his rocket motors) to change his velocity either in direction or magnitude. From Mach's principle it is clear that no place in space is free of gravitational forces and thus inertial forces will remain problems for aerospace medicine. An important characteristic of gravitational force is that there is no known shielding for it as there is for electric and magnetic forces. The gravitational field penetrates all solids and liquids so that every atom and molecule is affected and so far as is known this force extends to the outermost boundaries of our expanding universe. We can imagine ourselves surrounded by a shell of matter extending practically to infinity with a mean density of 1 hydrogen atom for each 10 liters of space and that it is the gravitational attraction of this great mass which gives rise to inertial forces.

Gravitational force is familiar to us mainly through the Earth's attraction for the movable objects on its surface. However, the old saying, "Everything that goes up must come down," is now no longer true! An example may serve to illustrate the action of these two forces, inertial and gravitational. In the "boost" phase of a rocket flight, the astronaut facing towards the nose of the rocket will have a contact force applied to his back due to the rocket thrust which is transmitted through the astronaut's seat. (Figure 1). At the same time, the man's heart and other organs

will be displaced from their normal position towards his back (in
the opposite direction to the thrust) due to the inertial forces and
gravitational forces.   All of the forces are important to the man
since the first compresses his peripheral tissues and the latter cause

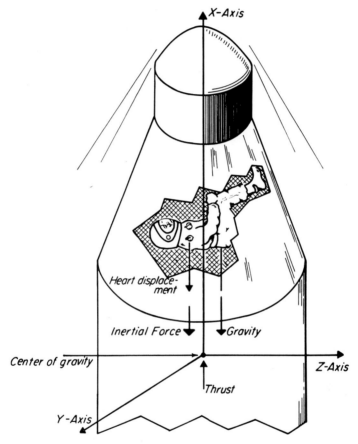

Fig. 1.   Relation of inertial, gravitational and thrust forces to
astronaut during rocket boost phase.

distortions and strains in the visceral organs.   Since the problems
of man arise mainly from these tissue distortions, it is necessary to
specify the forces as to direction, and magnitude, and for the contact forces, the point of application.

WHAT IS G?

Any physical body which is being accelerated can be regarded as under the action of an unbalanced force. Such forces are looked upon as a means of getting up speed by overcoming the "inertia" of the body. As noted above (eq. 2), this force can be related by Newton's second law to acceleration. However, force is required not only to accelerate a body but also merely to keep it at a constant speed when traveling through any medium (air or water, for example) other than a perfect vacuum. Such a force is overcoming the resistance of the medium and is generating frictional heat. Also, forces distort a semi-rigid system such as the human body and thus can be considered as overcoming the *elastic* reactance of the body. These forces are usually proportional to the amount of displacement they produce so long as the elastic limits of the tissues are not exceeded. Thus, force may be concerned in three distinctly separate functions in its action on man: (1) distortion of tissue, (2) overcoming of frictional forces and (3) production of velocity change. We can write the force equation as follows:

Total force = displacement force + frictional force + acceleration force

or

$$F \quad = \quad \alpha x \quad + \quad \beta \frac{dx}{dt} \quad + \quad \frac{\gamma d^2 x}{dt^2} \quad (3)$$

in which

α, β and γ = factors representing the compliance, and the viscoelastic and inertial properties of the body, respectively

x = the displacement

$\dfrac{dx}{dt}$ = the velocity

$\dfrac{d^2 x}{dt^2}$ = the acceleration

F = the total force

From a physiological point of view the importance of the displacement force and frictional force is evident but the acceleration force is less clear in its effects. To explore this further, let us assume that an astronaut in a capsule is being boosted in space in a vertical direction from the Earth's surface with a thrust, T. The thrust is the force applied and as shown in equation 3, it will displace the structures of the rocket, overcome the air friction and also overcome the inertial and gravitational forces as shown in Figure 1. For convenience, the thrust is spoken of in terms of pounds of force and the acceleration in terms of multiples of the gravitational acceleration at the Earth's surface (g_0) instead of feet per second "Squared".[4] Neglecting the air friction and displacement forces, we can write equation 3 for the rocket boost as

$$\text{Thrust} = F = \text{Weight} + \text{acceleration force}$$
$$= Mg + M \cdot \text{upward acceleration}$$

In this equation, M is the mass of the system, and g is the gravitational acceleration at any height above the earth's surface. Then we can write, since Weight $= Mg_0$

$$\frac{F}{Mg_0} = \frac{Ma}{Mg_0} = \frac{M(g + \text{upward acceleration})}{Mg_0} = \frac{a}{g_0} \qquad (4)$$

Since a/g_0 is the acceleration in terms of g_0, this can be taken to be the definition of acceleration in g units.

Force has both *magnitude* and *direction* and so also does acceleration and this requires a consideration of, what is the direction? Usually, we refer directions to the earth's surface as the horizontal plane and the direction of the gravitational force as the vertical. However, in space, one does not have these references and thus it is necessary to set up new "directions" for reference. This was a problem in aircraft flight and the reference axes shown as System 1 in Figure 2 are those used by the National Aeronautics and Space Administration. This system is designed for aircraft and space vehicles,[5] to describe all the combinations of applied linear and angular forces acting on the aircraft to *move* the vehicle; however, as the airplane sitting quietly on the ground is not moving, the gravitational force on the aircraft is omitted in many aerodynamic calculations. It is seen from Figures 1 and 2 that the space craft or aircraft can be accelerated along or around any of the three axes, and complex forces can be resolved along these axes at each instant of flight and their accelerations estimated. These linear and angular accelerations can then be applied to a test seat on a human centrifuge, spinning device, vibration device or other simulator to observe the effects on the man. Thus, it is always necessary to have a good measure of the forces applied to the man's seat because these are measures of the physical simuli which evoke the physiological responses. If man were a rigid body instead of a viscoelastic mass built about a semi-rigid skeleton with air spaces included, the applied forces would be a sufficient description, but

BODY ACCELERATION – COMPARATIVE TABLE OF EQUIVALENTS

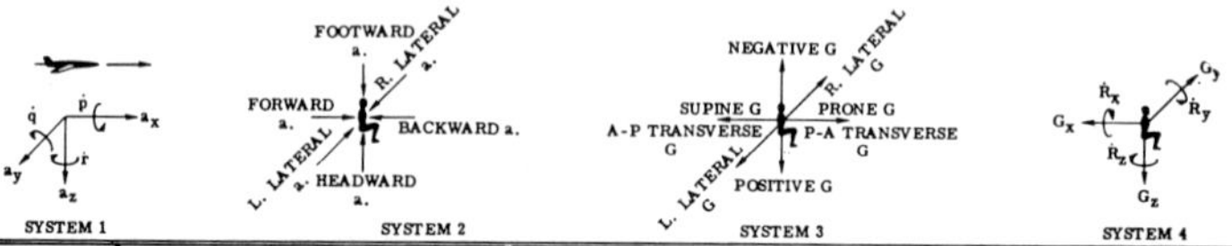

LINEAR MOTION	TABLE A — Direction of Acceleration		TABLE B — Inertial Resultant of Body Acceleration		
	Aircraft Computer Standard (Sys. 1)	Acceleration Descriptive (Sys. 2)	Physiological Descriptive (Sys. 3)	Physiological Computer Standard (Sys. 4)	Vernacular Descriptive
Forward	+a_x	Forward accel.	(1,2) Transverse A-P G / Supine G / Chest to Back G	+G_x	Eye Balls In
Backward	-a_x	Backward accel.	Transverse P-A G / Prone G / Back to Chest G	-G_x	Eye Balls Out
Upward	-a_z	Headward accel.	Positive G	+G_z	Eye Balls Down
Downward	+a_z	Footward accel.	Negative G	-G_z	Eye Balls Up
To Right	+a_y	R. Lateral accel.	Left Lateral G	+G_y	Eye Balls Left
To Left	-a_y	L. Lateral accel.	Right Lateral G	-G_y	Eye Balls Right
ANGULAR MOTION					
Roll Right	+$\dot{p}$		Roll	-$\dot{R}_x$	
Roll Left	-$\dot{p}$			+$\dot{R}_x$	
Pitch Up	+$\dot{q}$		Pitch	-$\dot{R}_y$	
Pitch Down	-$\dot{q}$			+$\dot{R}_y$	
Yaw Right	+$\dot{r}$		Yaw	+$\dot{R}_z$	
Yaw Left	-$\dot{r}$			-$\dot{R}_z$	

FOOTNOTES:
1. Large letter, G, used as unit to express inertial resultant to whole body acceleration in multiples of the magnitude of the acceleration of gravity. Acceleration of gravity, g_0, = 980.665 cm/sec^2 or 32.1739 ft/sec^2.
2. A-P, P-A refers to Anterior-Posterior, Posterior-Anterior.

Fig. 2. Airplane and human axis systems for describing accelerations due to applied and inertial forces. (With permission of Dr. C. F. Gell.)

as the blood and other body tissues move with respect to the skeletal framework, and these movements cause profound physiological effects, it is desirable to consider the skeleton as the basis for describing "physiological" accelerations.

Consider a man seated in his automobile. His heart under the gravitational force is pulled down slightly in his thorax as is his diaphragm, lungs, etc. If he starts his car forward he is pushed back against his seat and his heart and other organs are displaced towards his spine; thus, the movement of the heart and viscera is in the *opposite* direction from the applied force and is *in* the direction of the inertial force. For this reason it is customary to define the physiological acceleration G in terms of the inertial forces or, from equation 4,

$$G = -\frac{a}{g_0} \qquad (5)$$

As shown in Figure 2, the axes of reference for the man (Systems 3 and 4) are parallel to the aircraft and space craft axes in Systems 1 and 2, if the man is seated in the usual position in these vehicles. The axes are referred, however, to the center of gravity of the man rather than that of the vehicle and the directions are opposite except for the z axis. For example, during a space vehicle boost, the applied force may produce an $+a_x$ acceleration of $+5$ g units and the astronaut experiences $+5$ G_x physiological acceleration. At burnout of the rocket engine, the applied force disappears, i.e., the thrust is zero and the upward acceleration is zero; from equation 5 one sees that now the astronaut is under "zero G."

A summary of the various terms which have been used to de-scribe the in-flight accelerations by engineers and physiologists is shown under the various systems in Figure 2. The use of the standard aircraft or space craft system of coordinates is, of course, essential for a description of the "applied" or "driving" force, and the use of the inertial or coordinate system 4 is desirable for describing many of the physiological effects. Transformation of the origin of the physiological coordinate system from the center of gravity of the body to some other location can be made for special situations such as for studies of the head, with its sensitive acceleration detectors, the otolith organs and semi-circular canals. The angular accelerations have to do with changes in angular velocity about the pitch, roll and yaw axes and are included in the acceleration descriptions. These accelerations are considered positive when the circular motion is in a direction that is indicated by the fingers of the closed right hand when the thumb of hand is pointed along the positive direction of the axis involved (the "right-hand" rule).

From the point of view of aerospace physiology, two problem areas are of major importance, namely, tolerance to acceleration and ability to perform in acceleration environments.   These two areas will be discussed in order.

HUMAN TOLERANCE TO ACCELERATIONS

Accelerations may be classified for convenience because of their different effects on man as follows:

a) Vibration and oscillation—continued periodic forces of various magnitudes, directions and frequencies.

b) Impact—suddenly applied linear forces and torques of relatively large magnitude ($G > 30$) acting for times shorter than 1.0 sec are usually involved in impact.

c) Sustained linear and angular accelerations—forces acting for times longer than 1 sec are usually considered in this category.

d) Weightlessness and subgravity—these terms are applied to acceleration environments of magnitudes less than 1 G.

VIBRATION AND OSCILLATION

Although vibration is a common enough experience, few individuals during their lifetime experience the pain and general unpleasantness of the effects of vibration near the tolerance limits. These high levels of vibration can occur in high speed aircraft in low level flight and in spacecraft when the rocket is attaining supersonic speed, and when the capsule is re-entering the Earth's atmosphere.   The driving forces for vibration can vary in frequency amplitude and the total time during which the man is exposed.   The forces may be in simple harmonic motion or, as is more common, may vary irregularly so that many harmonic components are included in the force pattern.   For sinusoidal motion we can represent the relationship of frequency and amplitude to G as

$$G = n^2x \tag{6}$$

in which n is the frequency and x the amplitude of the driving force.   Thus, for any frequency the G is proportional to the amplitude and to the square of the frequency.   All frequencies are not equally damaging, as shown in Figure 3, for mice being vibrated along their X and Z axes. In this experiment the acceleration was constant and the time to death measured at various frequencies between 5 and 50 cps. A frequency of 12 cps killed the animals more than six times as rapidly as the same acceleration at 5 or 50 cps. The reason for this is that the mouse absorbs more energy and "resonates" at 12–17 cps as a result of the elastic

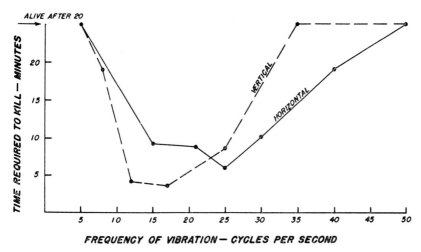

Fig. 3.   Average duration of vibration at constant acceleration required to kill test animal as a function of frequency of vibration. Vertical = vibration along Z axis; Horizontal = vibration along X axis. (Roman, *et al.*: *J. Av. Med.*, 30:118, 1959.)

properties of its tissues and the conformation of its thoracic and abdominal organs and attachments. A similar finding appears in the tolerance of man to vibration at different frequencies. Figure 4 shows the voluntary tolerance limits for 15 young men who were exposed to a sinusoidal acceleration at various frequencies between 1 and 20 cps. The exposures were limited by the severity of the pain and general discomfort in the chest, abdomen, pelvis and head. The tolerance limits shown in Figure 4 were thus generally below the limits which are indicated by obvious damage. However, in some experiments, bloody stools indicated that the limits shown were very near to the damage threshold. Of importance in Figure 4 is the fact that the seated man appears

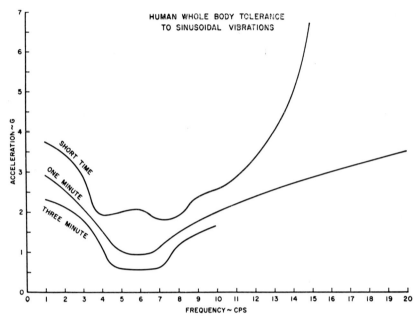

Fig. 4.   Voluntary tolerance of seated human subjects exposed to vibration along the Z axis.   (Magid, *et al.: J. Av. Med., 31*:915, 1960.)

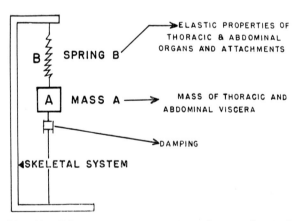

Fig. 5.   Schematic representation of a mechanical simulation of the human thorax-abdomen system for low frequency vibration.   (Roman, *et al.—Ibid.*)

to have a resonance in the 4–8 cps range which is associated with the movement of the abdominal and pelvic viscera with respect to the more rigid bony and muscular structures. Thus, the body can be considered as a vibrating system with properties of mass, elasticity and damping as postulated in equation 3. Such a system, shown in Figure 5, can be denoted as a spring, a mass, and a dashpot (damping) suspended in a more or less rigid frame. The approximate values of the over all damping, elasticity and moving mass can be determined from visual observations and x-ray studies and can be substituted in the equations of motion of the system (eq. 3). The results can be compared to the subjective tolerance curves as shown in Figure 6. While none of the calculated curves fit the tolerance curve exactly, there is general agreement especially for the absorbed energy curve. At 13 cps the absorbed

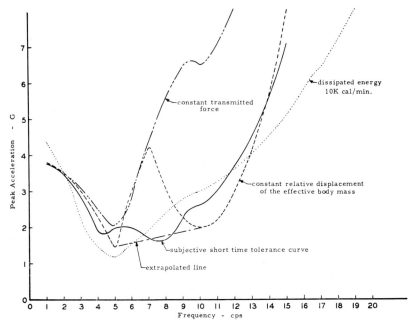

Fig. 6. Human tolerance curve for vibration along Z axis (solid line) compared to calculated curves for constant transmitted force, constant relative displacement of the effective body mass, and constant dissipated energy. Low tolerance for humans at 6–8 cps may be due to contributions from heat superimposed on the thorax-abdomen system. (Roman *et al.–Ibid.*)

energy is 600 kcal/hr or about ten times the basal heat production and thus will cause a marked hyperthermia after a few minutes. Such a hyperthermia has been observed in experimental animals during periods of vibration on a shake table. The relative mass displacement curve agrees with the tolerance curve only in the 1–5 cps and 10–15 cps ranges and there is a marked peak at 7 cps which is not seen in the human tolerance curve. Statements of the subjects indicate that chest pain is marked in this region and thus a second system is effective here. Apparently an organ or organs (i.e., the heart and lungs) have resonances in this range and the bouncing up and down may cause stretching of the large arteries, veins and connective structures, thus giving rise to intense pain.

The symptoms of the human subject exposed to a sinusoidal vibration at different frequencies along the Z axis are shown in Figure 7 and are believed related to specific distortions of pain sensitive tissues as follows:

Head pain may be partly due to displacement of facial skin and subcutaneous tissues about their bony attachments. Vision is blurred although the resonance for the optic globe within its bony socket is probably in the 50–100 cps range. The movement of the brain and cerebral spinal fluid is probably important but has not been evaluated. The jaw resonates at 6–8 cps making speech impossible. The sensations in the throat are described as a "tug" or painful lump due, possibly, to movement of the trachea and the main stem bronchi.

Chest pain at 5–9 cps may be associated with movement of the diaphragm (which may also cause the marked dyspnea experienced by the subjects), but is more likely due to the displacements; of the heart and lungs. Pain from the chest was one of the most common causes of discomfort to the subjects.

Abdominal pain occurring at 4–10 cps may have been due to stretching of the terminal ileum, cecum, hepatic flexure, transverse colon, and their supporting structures. In animals killed by vibration, tearing of these tissues and massive abdominal hemorrhage were common findings.

Pelvic pain was common and associated with severe urge to defecate and micturate. These symptoms disappeared immediately after exposure. One series of experiments was followed by bloody stools indicating the severity of the mechanical distortion of the pelvic tissues.

At the end of an experimental series, the subjects experienced facial flush, disphoresed and were euphoric. Two to four hours later most subjects experienced marked weariness and were somewhat depressed. These symptoms suggest alterations in metabolic and hormonal balance during and following exposure to vibratory accelerations at the tolerance limits.

For the higher frequency ranges the body does not move as a whole and the vibratory energy is propagated in the tissues as waves which are much affected by bony interfaces where the

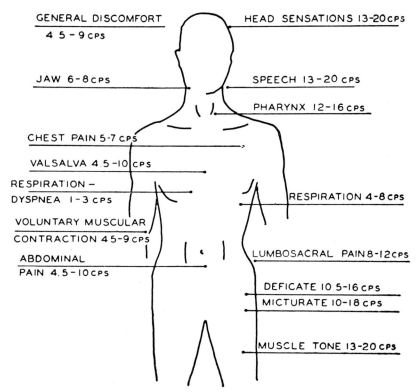

Fig. 7. Symptoms and sites of reference of various sensations evoked by vibration at frequencies between 1 and 20 cps at tolerance limits. (Magid, et al.—Ibid.)

energy is absorbed as heat.   Above 100 kilocycles/sec, compression waves predominate and are propagated in the tissues as beams of energy which are converted to heat.

IMPACT

High magnitude forces which are encountered when a rapidly moving object strikes a barrier is often termed "impact." Such forces are met with in a large variety of situations, such as automobile collisions, aircraft accidents, and other uncontrolled situations in which there is a large velocity change in a very short time. There are also controlled impacts such as that which the pilot of a jet aircraft experiences when he fires his ejection seat. From the point of view of the space traveller, due to the very high speeds, impacts of considerable magnitude can be anticipated in some phase of deceleration of the space craft or himself in coming to rest on the Earth, Moon or any other object. As impacts are associated with bruises, broken bones and ruptured organs, a study of this type of acceleration is of paramount importance.

If the duration of an acceleration is less than the natural frequency of man, the acceleration pulse will be over before the body as a whole begins to move at all. As was observed in the last section, man has a resonant frequency beween 5 and 10 cps and thus impacts are often considered as accelerations lasting less than 0.1 sec. In such a short time there is tissue displacement without the "hydraulic" or inertial displacements of blood and visceral masses. To appreciate the dynamic aspects of impact forces it is again desirable to consider the man as a mass, spring and viscous system, just as was done for the vibratory accelerations. Structurally, the body consists of the hard bony skeleton, the pieces of which are held together by tough, fibrous ligaments. The muscles and connective tissues overlay this framework and give it added cohesiveness and strength. The rib cage contains a considerable air space together with soft visceral organs and blood vessels. The abdomen can for most purposes be considered as a solid mass, equivalent in many of its properties to water, supported by the pelvis.

Mechanical Properties of Human Tissue (Goldman and von Gierke)[6]

	Soft Tissue	Bone
Density (g/cm³)	1–1.2	1.93–1.98
Youngs modulus (dyne/cm²)	7.5×10^4	2.26×10^{11}
Volume compressibility (dyne/cm²)	2.6×10^{10}	
Tensile strength (dyne/cm²)		9.75×10^8
Shearing strength (dyne/cm²)		4.9×10^8

A comparison of the mechanical properties of the soft body tissues and bone show the incompressibility but low resistance to distortion of soft tissue and the remarkable tensile strength (about the same as cast iron) and relatively high rigidity of bone. These differences in mechanical properties and the distribution of bone and soft tissue in the body determine the response to impact, because in the final analysis it is the distortion and relative displacement of tissues that is the cause of the damage to the body from mechanical forces.

We can conveniently divide our considerations of impact accelerations according to length of time the force is applied. For short period impact, the application of the force is brief, i.e., less than 0.1 sec, and for long period impacts the force application is less than 1 sec. The reason for making such a distinction is that for short period impact the body behaves as a solid viscous mass, whereas in the longer duration impacts the spring-like characteristics of the body cause considerable *overshoot* of the acceleration of parts of the body. The body is thus much more "tolerant" of the short period impact forces than of the longer period forces. This dynamic overshoot is also affected by the suddenness with which the force is applied or the rise-time of the acceleration. This "jolt" factor can be visualized from a consideration of Figure 8. In the figure, the rise-time is denoted at t_R and the duration as Δt. For values of duration of the applied force much less than the natural body frequency, body overshoot will be minimized. However, if the rise time is short, in relation to the natural period of the body, a maximum of 100 per cent overshoot may occur if the duration is fairly long as compared to the natural body resonances (i.e., 0.5 sec). The importance of overshoot is emphasized particularly at the limits of tolerance, because if a man can tolerate a certain maximum acceleration when rise time is long, he can

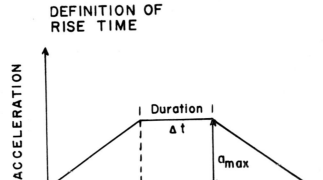

DEFINITION OF RISE TIME

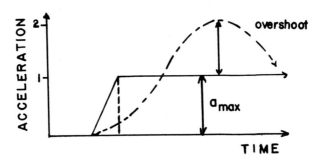

SHORT RISE TIME

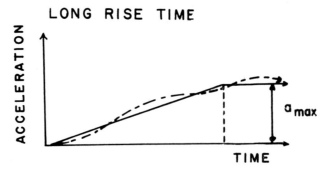

LONG RISE TIME

Fig. 8. Effect of force rise-time upon the acceleration of the mass in a single mass-spring system with damping. (Redrawn from P. R. Payne: Dynamics of Human Restraint Systems, Nat. Acad. Sci. Symposium on "Impact," November, 1961.)

tolerate only half this amount if the rise time is short. The effects of putting a cushion under the man can also be seen affecting overshoot. If a force of 0.01–0.1 sec duration is applied upward on the seat of a man without a cushion the overshoot may be as much as 20 per cent. However, with a cushion which slows the force and thus increases its duration, the overshoot may be as much as 100 per cent and thus increase the danger of damage to the man. The overshoot problem, in studies of impact, makes it necessary to mount accelerometers on the subject as well as on the mechanical device which applies the force to the man.

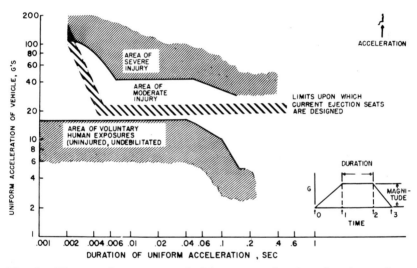

Fig. 9. Human tolerance to applied impact accelerations $(-a_z)$ as a function of magnitude and logarithm of duration. (From Eiband, M.: NASA Memo 5-10-59E.)

As the tissue displacements are in the same direction as the applied force and as inertial effects do not become important in impact, it is usual to use the applied accelerations a rather than the inertial accelerations G to describe the situation. We shall now describe the effects of impact along various body axes.

Impact on the Seat ($-a_z$): The study of the effects of high forces applied to the bottom of the seat is closely associated with the development of upward ejection seats for escape from high speed aircraft. The "jolt" or dynamic overshoot in the ejection seat situation is minimized by using rise times of 0.1 sec and dura tions of 0.2 sec at 20 g. Figure 9 shows the tolerance of human subjects to impact on the seat for the seated human subject well aligned in his seat so as to control the flexion of the spine and neck. Since the vertebrae between the eighth thoracic and fifth lumbar segments are fractured at about the same static load (i.e., 25 g), the tolerance limit of 20 g is generally assumed to allow for the possibility of some minimal overshooting.

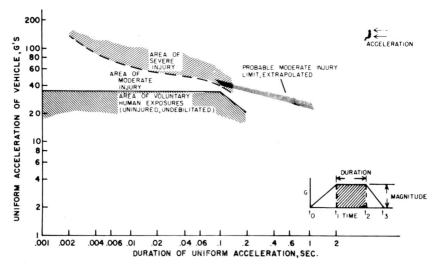

Fig. 10. Human tolerance to applied impact accelerations $(+a_x)$ as a function of magnitude and logarithm of duration. (From Eiband, *Ibid.*)

Accelerations along the X axis $(\pm a_x)$ are the most frequently encountered in surface transport crashes. Human tolerance to these forces has been studied extensively on high speed tracks, drop towers, experimental automobile crashes, and by analysis of various accidents including non-fatal falls. With force durations of about 0.1 sec no overshoot is observed in the head or chest, but with durations of 0.3 sec overshoot of chest accelerations of 30 per cent results. However, such results depend to a great extent on the type of body restraint which is used in the test. The data for human tolerance to $\pm a_x$ accelerations is shown in Figures 10 and 11.

Head Responses: The elastic shell of the skull is filled with tissues of low compressibility and other properties similar to water. The reaction of the head to a blow is a function of the velocity, duration and area of impact and the transfer of momentum. Near the point of application of the blow, there will be an indentation of the skull which will cause shear strains in the brain substance in a region close to the indentation. Compression waves

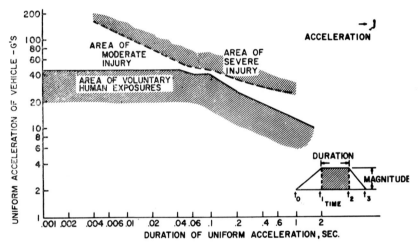

Fig. 11. Human tolerance to impact accelerations $(-a_x)$ as a function of magnitude and logarithm of duration. (From Eiband, *Ibid.*)

emanate from this area which normally have small amplitudes since the brain is highly incompressible. The distribution of the shear strains has been studied using high speed photography on models made of plastic and containing special solutions to show the strain patterns. The maximum strains are concentrated at regions where the skull has a good "grip" on the brain owing to inward projecting ridges, especially at the wing of the sphenoid bone of the skull. Shear strains must also be present throughout the brain and in the brain stem. If the blow is sufficiently great the skull response will exceed the elastic deformation limit and

fracture occurs. High velocity impacts result in localized circumscribed fracture and skull indentation whereas low velocity blows
insufficient to cause a permanent depression (occurring frequently
in falls) cause inward bending of the skull at the contact area and
at a considerable distance an outbending of the skull of the "con-
trecoup" type which may cause fracture. The total energy required to fracture the skull is estimated between 400–900 in-lb
and this is equivalent to having the head hit a hard flat surface
after a free fall of about 5 ft. Dry skull preparations require only
about 25 in.-lb for fracture, mainly because of the lack of the
protection afforded by the attenuating properties of the scalp.

Neck Response: The limitations for forward and lateral bending of the neck are, for most purposes, the anterior chest wall and
the shoulders, respectively. Since the head is almost entirely held
by the neck muscles, the absence of their supporting action gives
any blow to the head or neck a relatively long distance through
which to act with the result that fractures and dislocations are
likely. Dislocations involving the first and second vertebral joints
are usually less severe if the odontoid process is fractured (i.e.,
less damage to the spinal cord). If this is not the case, the spinal
cord may be severed or crushed.

The study of automobile and aircraft crashes and experiments
with dummies and living subjects show that complete body support and restraint of extremities which minimized tissue distortions and displacements provide maximum protection against the
effects of impact and give the best chance for survival. If the subject is restrained to his seat he makes full use of the moderating
action of the collapsing of the vehicle structure and is in a position
to distribute the impact load over as large body area as possible,
thus avoiding local force concentrations. A rigid envelope around
the body would protect it to the maximum extent, at least theoretically, by preventing tissue deformation.

SUSTAINED ACCELERATIONS

Applied forces which are maintained for periods longer than 1
to 2 sec produce, in addition to movement of the body, marked

displacements of the internal body fluids and organs with respect to the skeletal framework; these "hydraulic" shifts in blood and organ positions are the factors which set the physiological limits of tolerance for the sustained accelerations. Sustained accelerations are those which are often termed "in flight" accelerations due to maneuver loadings and thrust. They have been an important factor in aviation medicine since the advent of high speed flight and because of the extremely high velocities involved in space travel these accelerations are of great importance in aerospace

HUMAN TOLERANCE TO ACCELERATION

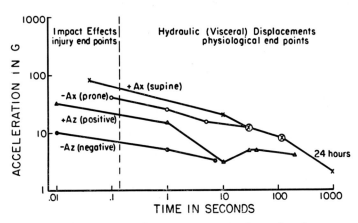

Fig. 12. Human tolerance to sustained accelerations.

medicine. The accelerations which can be expected during the catapulting of a manned vehicle from Earth into orbit will depend upon the type of propulsion rocket used and at present these accelerations are within tolerance limits. Figure 12 depicts the relationship between the magnitude of acceleration and the time of exposure for impact and sustained accelerations along the Z and X body axes. These data have been obtained from many laboratories using impact devices and human centrifuges. In Figure 13 is shown the interior of the large human centrifuge laboratory at the U. S. Naval Air Development Center. The Centrifuge is an instrument which can be used to apply desired levels of acceleration on the subject for indefinite periods but has the disadvantages of producing rotations which disorient the individual. The very long arm of this centrifuge (50 ft) tends to minimize the gradients of acceleration across the subject's body but this artifact still persists in all centrifuges and more especially in those for which the arm length is short in comparison with the dimensions of the man. These conditions must be considered as artifacts because they are not characteristics of in-flight accelerations.

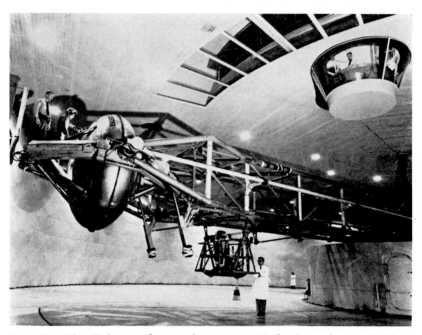

Fig. 13.   The 50-ft centrifuge at the Aviation Medical Acceleration Laboratory, Johnsville, Pa.

Using the symbol w to represent the angular velocity of the centrifuge arm and L as the length of the arm, the forces applied to a man seated in the gondola at the end of the arm can be calculated if his orientation relative to the direction of rotation is known. Suppose the pilot is intially sitting vertically facing the direction of motion of the arm. As the centrifuge starts, the applied forces result in the "applied" accelerations as follows:

$$+a_x = \frac{L\dot\Omega}{g_0} \qquad (7)$$

in which $\dot\Omega$ is the starting angular acceleration and a_x is the starting linear acceleration of the pilot's seat;

$$+a_y = \frac{L\Omega^2}{g_0} \qquad (8)$$

Ω = instant angular velocity and the pilot is sitting so that his right side is furthest from the center of rotation;

$$-a_z = 1 \qquad (9)$$

that is the earth's gravitational attraction.

If the man remains fixed in his orientation, the resultant acceleration is the vector sum of the above components, or

$$a^2 = a_x^2 + a_y^2 + a_z^2 \qquad (10)$$

and

$$a = \frac{L}{g_0}\sqrt{\frac{g_0^2}{L} + \Omega^4 + \dot\Omega^2} \qquad (11)$$

For a constant angular velocity ($\dot\Omega = 0$) and neglecting the gravitational acceleration of 1 g_0, equation 11 becomes

$$a = a_y = \frac{L\Omega^2}{g_0} \qquad (12)$$

Equation 12 indicates that for high levels of G it is desirable to have a rapidly rotating centrifuge with a short arm because the acceleration depends on the square of the angular velocity and only on the first power of the length of centrifuge arm. However, the pilot's disorienting effects increase in proportion to the angular velocity and the acceleration gradients within the man's body increase as the length of the arm is decreased. From many physio - logical points of view it is desirable to reproduce the conditions of aero-space accelerations on the centrifuge and thus in many modern human centrifuges an arm length of not less than 50 ft is used.

In Figure 14 is shown a schematized acceleration pattern which might be expected from a three-stage liquid fuel rocket capable of achieving orbital speeds. The accelerations indicated for the boost phase are all within the tolerance limits for the astronaut is usually in the supine position ($\pm G_x$) in respect to the thrust vector. If rockets with solid propellants should be used, much higher accelerations would be expected, reaching perhaps 20–30 G_x for the boost, and a man in a capsule propelled by such a rocket would require special measures for his protection. At the burnout of the last stage of the three-stage rocket shown in Figure 14, the

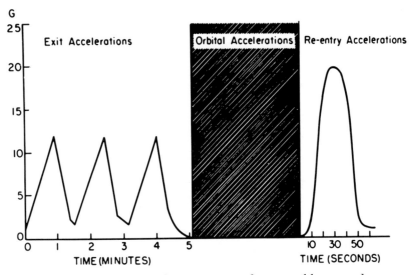

Fig. 14.   Schematized acceleration pattern for a possible manned space capsule.

astronaut will be in a state of zero gravity or weightlessness except for the rotational effects which may have been induced by the rocket engine or by the occupant. The return from orbit would require the firing of retro-rockets to slow the vehicle and thus permit the Earth's gravity field to pull the capsule into the upper atmosphere. As the vehicle comes in contact with the very low density gas at extreme altitudes, more or less slowing will be encountered due to the drag of the atmosphere on the vehicle. It is, of course, necessary to use the atmosphere to absorb all of the kinetic energy which has been stored in the capsule by the booster rocket. Should the astronaut choose to bring the capsule in very rapidly, a really high acceleration will be experienced, as shown in Figure 14. This maneuver has the advantage of pinpointing the landing area more exactly. On the other hand, there is the choice of circling the earth while being gradually slowed by the upper atmosphere and finally landing with a much decreased kinetic energy and acceleration. In the limiting case of a capsule

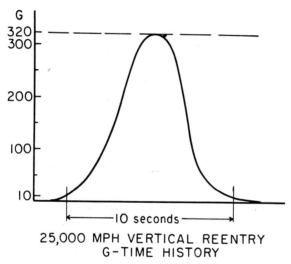

25,000 MPH VERTICAL REENTRY
G-TIME HISTORY

Fig. 15.   Acceleration pattern for an object entering the Earth's atmosphere with maximum drag.

entering the Earth's atmosphere and heading directly toward the Earth with a cosmic speed of 25,000 miles an hour, an acceleration as high as 300–400 G could be developed as indicated in Figure 15. Although this acceleration would be associated only with an emergency type of maneuver, it represents a possible in-flight acceleration for an astronaut. At the present time, methods for protecting man against the effects of such high forces have not been studied.

Accepting the fact that large accelerations must be expected during both the boost phase and re-entry phase of a space flight, and that unusually high accelerations (as measured by aviation standards) may face the space traveler wherever he goes in space, it is worthwhile to review some of the effects of gravitational forces. In Figure 16 are shown four effects of high gravitational fields which are physiologically important and may have effects which are as yet unknown, particularly in long exposures of man. They are:

(1) Change in total weight since Weight = mass × acceleration

(2) Change in internal pressure gradients

(3) The tendency of suspended solids of different densities to separate with a velocity which is proportional to the acceleration

(4) The distortion of elastic tissues of the body with time.

These effects may be so profound physiologically as to make life impossible for prolonged periods as, for example, the exploration of the surface of Jupiter with a gravitational field of 2.6 *g*.

Each of the above effects become important physiologically when the acceleration is sustained sufficiently long or is of high

EFFECTS OF GRAVITATIONAL FIELD

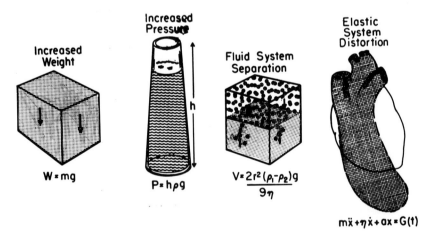

Fig. 16.   Important effects of acceleration.

magnitude. Increased weight of the chest wall and the forcing of the abdominal viscera against the diaphragm will embarass breathing and at about $+10\ G_x$ the vital capacity is reduced to about 500 cc; at acceleration levels near $+20\ G_x$ respiration is impossible. In Figure 17 is shown the changes in respiratory capability in 15 healthy young airmen when exposed to increasing acceleration loads up to $+5\ G_x$. The marked decrease in total vital

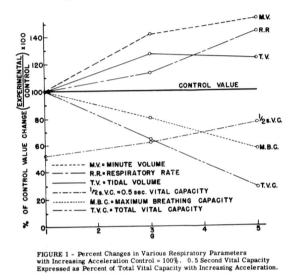

FIGURE 1 - Percent Changes in Various Respiratory Parameters with Increasing Acceleration Control = 100%. 0.5 Second Vital Capacity Expressed as Percent of Total Vital Capacity with Increasing Acceleration.

Fig. 17. Average changes in various respiratory parameters with increasing $+G_x$ accelerations in fifteen subjects. 0.5 sec vital capacity expressed as percent of total vital capacity. (After Cherniac, *et al.*: WADC Tech. Rpt. 59–347.)

capacity together with the increasing 0.5 sec timed vital capacity indicates according to Cherniac a "restrictive" type of defect in pulmonary function analogous to that observed in patients with paralysis of respiratory muscles (i.e., poliomyelitis). This condition can be alleviated to some extent by increasing the pressure within the chest during the G_x loading. This positive "pressure breathing" with pure oxygen has been found to increase comfort, visual acuity and total performance of subjects, particularly at loads of $+10\ G_x$ and higher.

In the supine or prone position, i.e., the $\pm G_x$ directions, man can accept relatively large acceleration loads due to the minimizing of the intravascular pressure differences which cause serious effects in the erect or G_z direction. Thus, in the $+G_x$ direction difficulty of breathing and chest pain due to deformations of the pericardium and large vessels set the tolerance limits. As shown in Figure 12, although man's tolerance to $\pm G_x$ accelerations is great enough to sustain any of the boost or re-entry accelerations shown in figure 14 for a space vehicle, the safety factor is small and unless protective measures are taken some damage to body tissue can be anticipated at levels of acceleration greater than 10 G_x. Carefully molded couches designed to fit exactly the body contours have been developed which afford much protection against external tissue displacements under $+G_x$ loads. In spite of this there will be internal displacements; for example, a tendency for blood and extra vascular fluid to pool in the posterior thorax under $+G_x$ accelerations. A result of this pooling is the distention of the large veins in the thorax and the associated reflex action which causes decreased release of the anti-diuretic hormone and a temporary increase in urine flow. Also, with pure oxygen breathing at one atmosphere there results an adelectasis which can be detected by x-ray examination and by rales, shortness of breath, and coughing of the subject. This effect is not so quickly developed when air is breathed or under positive pressure breathing of oxygen, indicating that the nitrogen in the air and increased pressure of oxygen tend to keep alveoli open whereas the oxygen alone under low pressure, being rapidly absorbed, allows collapse of the alveoli under high acceleration loading.

One of the principal differences in the body response to $+G_x$ (supine) and $-G_x$ (prone) accelerations is the movement of the large mass of the abdominal viscera. Under $-G_x$ loadings the clothing and other external supports such as belting may serve to prevent large tissue displacements and thus to give protection. However, straps and other supports which go around the abdomen and fasten to seats or other fixed structures may, because of the throwing forward of the body, compress the abdominal viscera up against the diaphragm and may cause excessively high venous pressure. This pressure may rupture small and large veins locally or in remote body areas such as the nose or conjunctiva. These conditions were described in human subjects after exposure to $-G_x$ accelerations on high-speed sleds. With $+G_x$ accelerations, the viscera are compressed against the posterior peritoneum and the diaphragm and the possible effects of increased venous pres-

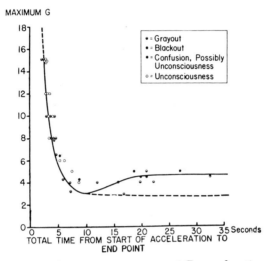

Fig. 18. Human responses to $+G_z$ acceleration. (After Stoll: U. S. Naval Air Dev. Center Report No. MA-5508-1955.)

sure have been reported from sled tests. These include a mild or marked bradycardia possibly due to a vagal reflex initiated by receptors in the large vessels of the thorax. In one preliminary study, atropine was observed to abolish the mild bradycardia observed at $-15 G_x$.

The $\pm G_z$ accelerations are characterized by large shifts in blood volume with respect to the heart and the consequent changes in rate of perfusion of blood through vital tissues such as the brain.[7] The long fluid columns and the elastic vessels which contain them respond under $+G_z$ with the tendency to drain the arterial system and the pooling of the blood in the venous side of the vascular tree below the heart level. The first symptoms of increased $+G_z$

on the seated man is increased proprioception and a dimming of peripheral vision. This endpoint of loss of peripheral vision is used in many laboratories as an endpoint for G_z acceleration tests. Following "gray out" there is a complete loss of vision, or "black out," although the subject may be conscious and can report his

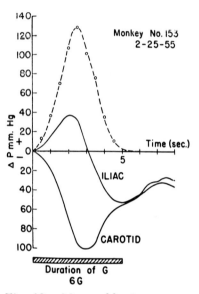

Fig. 19. Mean blood pressure changes as a function of time in the iliac and carotid arteries of the seated monkey under +6 G_z. The dotted line represents the change in hydrostatic pressure between the arteries; the open circles = the instantaneous acceleration values. (After Lawton, *et al.*: U. S. Naval Air Dev. Center Report No. MA-5611, 1956.)

sensory deficits. Following closely on black out is unconsciousness which in about 20 per cent of subjects is followed by a prolonged recovery period (up to 40 sec) of vigorous muscular paroxysms, or fit, which is similar to that seen in subjects recovering from brief exposures to the hypoxia associated with high altitude. How quickly these events follow each other depends to a great extent upon how rapidly is the onset of the acceleration. In Figure 18 is shown the time tolerance curve for the seated subject under $+G_z$ acceleration. It is seen that for short exposures to high G_z grayout and unconsciousness merge so rapidly that a blackout phase is not always observed. With exposures to lower G_z levels the effects are more easily distinguished and the pilot at 3–4 G_z can observe the grayout going into blackout and then returning to grayout and even to full vision as the exposure is continued for 10–20 sec. The best evidence at present is that

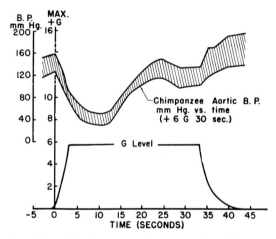

Fig. 20.   Blood pressure changes in the chimpanzee exposed to $+6\ G_z$.   (After Stoll, *Ibid.*)

the failure of visual function (before other sensory modalities such as hearing) is due to the fall of arterial blood pressure below the level of the intra-ocular pressure. However, as the consensual light reflex can still be elicited in the visually blacked out subject, some retinal function is still active even though the subject can not see. The fall in blood pressure is due to the increased hydrostatic pressure of the blood in the column between the heart and the eye. As shown in Figure 16, the differential pressures in a liquid column are a function of the strength of the gravitational field, g. In Figure 19 is shown the changes in mean blood

pressure in a seated monkey under +6 G_z measured at the levels
of the carotid sinus and the iliac artery, a distance of about 22 cm.
The pressure differential, i.e., the dashed curve, is seen to follow
the level of instantaneous G_z (open circles) very closely. The
changes in pressure in this experiment are for the most part the
result of the passive changes in the vascular system as the reflex
actions in response to increased G_z are not developed in 5 sec.
The carotid sinus and other reflex effects which act to restore
the arterial blood pressure can be visualized from Figure 20 which
shows an experiment on a chimpanzee exposed to +6 G_z for 30
sec. The initial fall in aortic blood pressure is followed after
about 10 sec with a recovery and a return to the pre-run blood pressure level in about 25 sec even under continued loading. The
weight of the blood at 7 g is about that of molten iron and thus,
the ability of the vascular system to perform its function under
such conditions irrespective of the orientation of the body is note-
worthy.

These dislocations in the cardiovascular system affect many
elements of the circulatory system and these have been studied
by Wood and his associates at the Mayo Foundation.[8] As shown
in Figure 21a, the cardiac index decreases as the level of +G_z
in the sitting subject is increased so that at +4 G_z the cardiac
index is about 80 per cent of the control value. A decrease of
venous return to the right heart due to increased weight of blood
may partially account for this. An increase in heart rate (Figure
21b) and in aortic blood pressure (Figure 21c) were associated
with a marked fall in stroke volume (Figure 21d) as the acceleration load was increased. The increase in "peripheral resistance"
(Figure 21e) may result from compensatory reflexes assisting
maintenance of blood pressure. The effect of inflating a "g suit"
(Figure 21f) in increasing peripheral resistance may explain in
part the usefulness of this equipment in providing aviators with
a "protection" of 1–2 g.

For the few seconds required for boost and re-entry, the possible use of water submersion has been explored as a protective
device which offers uniform and complete support for the body
exterior. Experiments on animals have been conducted by many

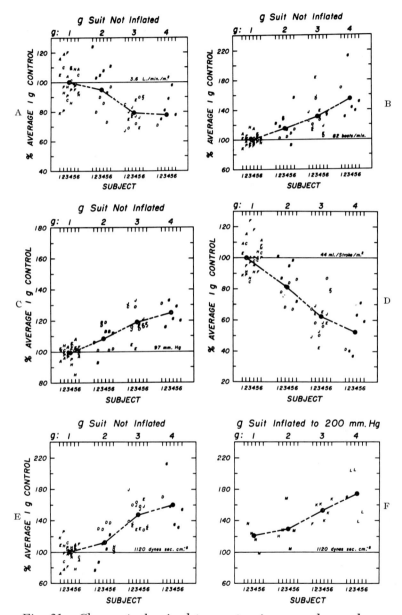

Fig. 21.   Changes in the circulatory system in man under accelerations of +1 G$_z$, +2 G$_z$, +3 G$_z$, and +4 G$_z$.   Measurements shown were made about 30 sec after reaching a steady acceleration level. (After Wood, *et al.*: Ref. 8)

investigators and it has been shown that if an animal be surrounded by water extremely high acceleration loads can be tolerated. For example, rats can tolerate for several seconds loads as high as 1000 *g* providing the animal be surrounded with a fluid medium of approximately the same density as the tissue of

SUBJECT SUBMERGED IN MAYO TANK
FOR POSITIVE G STUDY

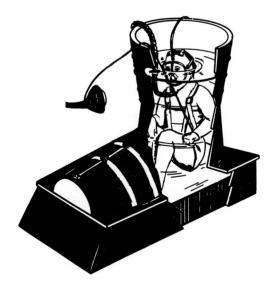

Fig. 22.   Experimental tank for $+G_z$ acceleration tests with partial water immersion.

the animal. The limiting factor in this instance is the air-filled space of the thorax which permits distortions of the heart, lungs and major vessels, as shown to the far right in Figure 16. If experiments are done on pregnant rats about to deliver, it is found that the fetus will survive without damage accelerations as great as 10,000 *g*, although the mother will die. Increasing the pressure in the thorax provides considerable protection for the animal although this will not prevent distortion of the heart and large vessels of the thorax. For example, mice placed in plastic bags

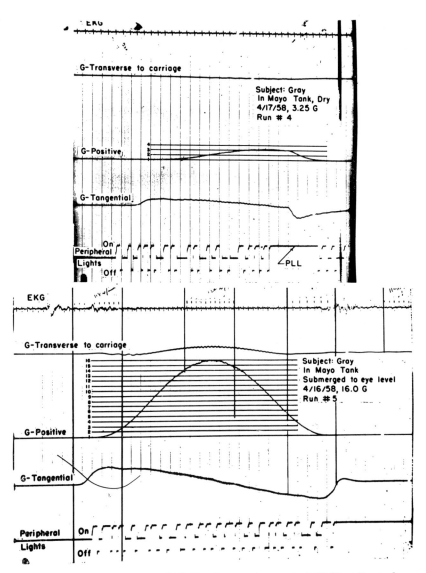

Fig. 23. Experimental record of Gray's experiment at $+16\ G_z$. Control run with tank empty at top; peripheral lights lost (PLL) at $+3.25\ G_z$. Bottom record showing G_y, G_z, and G_x records with subject submerged. Note no loss of peripheral lights.

with a supply of oxygen and the whole submerged in water have been observed to survive 1300 g for 60 sec.

The use of water to protect man against the effects of sustained acceleration by balancing the fluid columns inside and outside the body was demonstrated during World War II. It was found that immersion of the body up to the level of the third rib would provide an increased acceleration tolerance of approximately $+1.5$ to $+2$ G_z, about that offered by the pneumatic g suits. Immersions to higher levels caused considerable chest pain and discomfort due to squeezing of the thorax by external hydrostatic pressure under 4–6 G loads.

In 1958, tests were made using complete submersion to above the eye level with the subject holding his breath during the test. The experimental tank is shown in Figure 22 with a provision for making the usual tests for grayout or blackout. Elastic cords were arranged as a safety measure so that the subject had to forcibly hold himself submerged, and should he become unconscious he would be automatically raised above the surface of the water. The protocol of an experiment with this tank is shown in Figure 23. The control experiment is shown at the top of the figure with the acceleration pattern for positive G shown along the middle line. At the bottom of the protocol is the record of responses to the peripheral lights and the loss of this response when the acceleration had reached 3.2 G_z. At this time the centrifuge was stopped, thereby inducing the tangential acceleration and the immediate fall in positive G. The acceleration pattern followed a haversine function of time requiring 12.5 sec to reach maximum G and the same length of time to come to rest. In the lower part of the figure is shown the exposure to $+16$ G_z and during the run there were small changes in G_x and G_y. Peripheral vision was not lost although there were changes in heart rate and some of the air was forced from the chest due to the high external hydrostatic pressure. An occasional abdominal pain was reported during this run with variable location and the possibility of gas compression seemed a likely explanation. No chest pain, coughing or other indication of thoracic cavity involvement was observed.

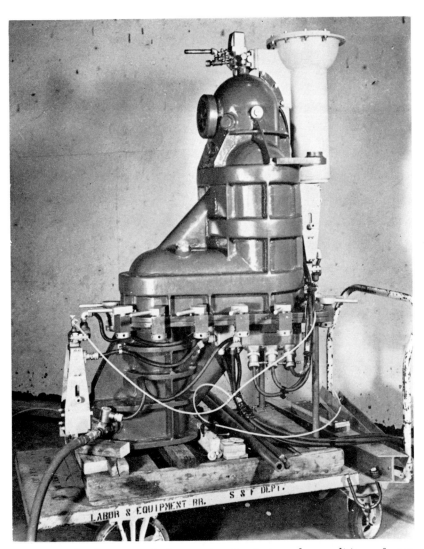

Fig. 24. The Gray capsule for acceleration tests under conditions of complete water submersion.

A series of experiments was carried out in a completely closed system exposing the subject to $-G_x$ acceleration. The shell of the experimental capsule shown in Figure 24 was of reinforced cast aluminum tested to ensure small expansion under several atmospheres of internal pressure. The subject was placed in a seated position and the upper shell lowered into place and mounted on the centrifuge. The top and bottom of the capsule were forced together by a series of pressure locks forming a tight

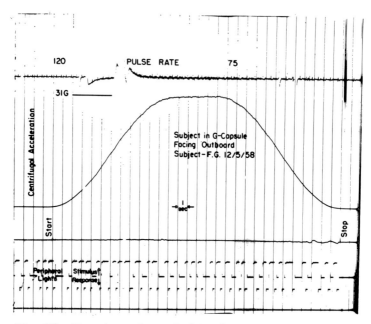

Fig. 25.   Experimental record of Gray's run at -31.5 G_x for five sec.   No loss of visual function was observed during run.

seal. Pressure seals were provided for electrical connections so that the subject's reaction to the usual visual stimuli could be followed. At the beginning of an experiment the chamber was completely closed and the subject held his breath during the 20–30 sec of acceleration.

The record of one experiment in this capsule is shown in Figure 25. In this experiment the subject had no loss of visual field and his motor function was not impaired. Chest pain, which is a limiting factor in exposure to acceleration of $-G_x$, was absent although the subject reported some abdominal pain, possibly from intestinal gases. There were no untoward effects on the subject from exposure to acceleration which might otherwise have been lethal.

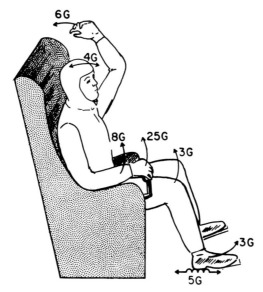

MOVEMENT OF THE BODY, AS INDICATED
BY THE ARROWS, IS JUST POSSIBLE AT
THE VEHICLE ACCELERATIONS LISTED

Fig. 26. Some human performance limitation under acceleration.

The experiments just described have indicated that with proper support, human tolerance to sustained acceleration can be considerably expanded. The limiting factor is likely to be the distortion of the heart and large vessels within the thorax. A possible solution which has been suggested for this difficulty is providing a method for quickly filling and emptying the lungs with fluid so as to allow the human to react in a fashion which is similar to that of a fish. A practical method of accomplishing this maneuver in man has not as yet been devised. It is, however, encouraging that most of the sustained accelerations which are anticipated in *normal* space flight operations at this time can be tolerated by the human with supports and restraints which are now available.

As sustained accelerations may last for several minutes, a factor of major importance is the ability of the astronaut to perform useful functions under these high loads. In Figure 26 is shown movements of the body which are just possible at various ac-celerations. For example, it is not possible for a man to maintain control of his head at accelerations higher than $+4\ G_x$ and he can just barely raise his arm under an acceleration of $+6\ G_z$.

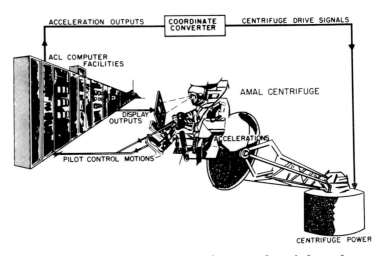

Fig. 27.   The human centrifuge with powered gimbals used as a 3 degree of freedom flight simulator.

Movements of the wrist and fingers are possible at accelerations as high as $-25\ G_x$ and fairly skilled control movements can be performed even at this loading. The variations in loading are, of course, important in determining the ability of the astronaut to control his vehicle because account must be taken of the possi-bility of the involuntary inputs by the man into his control sys-tem caused by combinations of vibration, oscillation and sus-tained acceleration. The general situation is so complicated that it is not possible to define the performance of a man under every conceivable acceleration loading, and thus resort must be had to simulation. Simulation can be accomplished on centrifuges providing the angular accelerations which are required by the centrifuge operation to produce the high linear loads in space flight are not unacceptable. A simulator which has been found valuable in the testing and training of astronauts is shown in Figure 27. This simulator consists of the Johnsville centrifuge controlled by

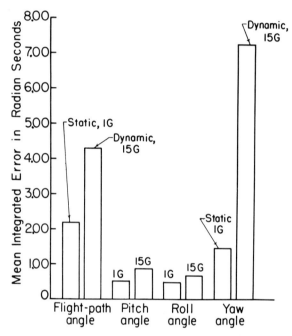

Fig. 28. Analysis of pilot performance under static conditions and under a load of +15 G_x.

the large analog computer at the U. S. Naval Air Development Center. In this simulator the astronaut, together with his complete spacecraft instrument and control system, is mounted in the gondola of the centrifuge and the control motions are fed directly to the analog computer. On this computer are programmed the dynamic characteristics of the aircraft or spacecraft and its control system. The computer makes an instant-by-instant calcula-

tion of the accelerations as well as the appropriate readings of
the indicating instruments on the astronaut's panel. The acceleration outputs from the computer are fed into a coordinate converter so that the centrifuge controls are driven to furnish as close
an approximation of the in-flight accelerations as is possible. This
system permits the introduction of mechanical and electrical
failures into the system and the testing of pilot reaction to such
emergencies. The effects of high acceleration loadings on pilot
performance can be seen in Figure 28 in which the control situation with no load is designated as static, or 1g, and the dynamic
loading as 15 g. The mean integrated error during the flight was
determined for the pilot's ability to maintain flight path, pitch
angle, roll angle and yaw angle. The greatest error was observed
for the maintenance of yaw angle and the least error for the maintenance of roll angle. Simulation procedures have great advantages in answering specific questions about a particular system but they suffer from the lack of general applicability of the
results. In testing and training astronauts for various space programs it was possible to say with reasonable confidence whether
or not the astronaut could control his vehicle under a variety of
emergencies. It is thus likely that a wide variety of simulators
will be required for setting up as nearly as possible space conditions on the Earth and testing and abilities of the man and his
machine in the space environment.

REFERENCES

1. HEAD, HENRY: *The Sense of Stability and Balance in the Air.* Med. Res.
Council Report, Special Series No. 28, London, 1919.
2. STEWART, O.: *First Flights.* Pitman Publ. Corp., New York, 1958.
3. HESSE, MARY B.: *Forces and Fields.* Philosophical Library, New York,
1962.
4. DIXON, F., and J. L. PATTERSON: *Determination of Accelerative Forces
Acting on Man in Flight and on the Centrifuge.* U. S. Naval School
of Aviation Medicine, Report No. NM 001-059. 04.01, July, 1953.
5. CLARK, C. C., J. D. HARDY, and R. CROSBIE: *A Proposed Physiological
Acceleration Terminology with an Historical Review.* Publ. 913, National Academy of Sciences and National Research Council, Washington, 1961.

6. Goldman, D. F., and H. von Gierke: *The Effects of Shock and Vibration on Man.* Naval Med. Research Inst., Report No. 60-3, Bethesda, Md., 1960.

7. Gauer, O. H., and G. D. Zuidema: *Gravitational Stress in Aerospace Medicine*, Little, Brown Co., Boston, 1961.

8. Wood, E. H., W. F. Sutterer, H. W. Marshall, E. F. Lindberg, and R. N. Headley: *WADD Tech. Report No. 60-634*, 1961.

6

WEIGHTLESSNESS* AND SUB-GRAVITY PROBLEMS

James D. Hardy, Ph.D.

INTRODUCTION

With the advent of the unpowered flight above the atmosphere, producing weightlessness throughout a non-rotating space vehicle or along the axis of rotation of a rotating vehicle, man can explore the relative merits and problems of living weightless. Freed from the series of parallel levels to which on Earth he is bound by gravitation, and also freed from the massive construction required to support static loads on the Earth's surface, he can experience living with zero G or with an artificial gravity produced by rotation or other means. Conclusions based on these comparisons as to the mode of life to select in a space station must await further human experience in space. Present data cannot provide the assurance that important factors, particularly among long duration effects, have not been neglected. For systems as complex as man, predictions of performance by extrapolations from the limited experience of a few hours or days may be hazardous. Four points may be emphasized: (a) Restraint systems both for man and for movable objects will have to be developed for use at zero G. (b) In a rotating space station, velocities of linear or angular motions of the head may have to be kept of low magnitude by using restraints and possibly eye prism devices, mirror walls, etc., to reduce the need for head motions, to avoid

---

* Gerathewohl[1] has suggested that, for the sake of clarity, the term "weightless" be reserved for the physiological responses and psychological experience of the man under conditions of zero G.

196

disorienting illusions and nausea. (c) Normal growth of the embryo and the young and normal repair of adult tissues, such as bone and muscle, which are affected in cellular patterns by force distributions, may require artificial gravity. (d) it may be necessary to develop exercises and other procedures to use prior to changes of acceleration level to restore or develop tolerance to the new gravity level in spite of acclimatization to the old level.

GENERAL PROBLEMS OF WEIGHTLESSNESS

These problems may be analyzed according to Lawton[2] in terms of physical consequences of weightlessness: a) Static effect: Loss of structural distortions due to weight. A corollary of this is that there will be the loss of pressure gradients due to depth. Another corollary is that there will be a loss of frictional contact forces due to gravitation b) Dynamic effect: Loss of gravitational acceleration effects on displacements. A corollary is the loss of convection or stratification of separate bodies due to density differences. Another corollary is that gases, liquids and solids will tend to randomize their positions in the presence of other distorting forces, or intermix, so that homogeneous volumes will tend to diminish. Another corollary is that there will be a loss of flight path direction deviations due to gravitation. Objects once in motion with no further forces acting will move in straight lines with regard to the vehicle coordinate system at zero G. These consequences of the loss of gravitational forces on living systems have been surmised and partially examined by experiment.

Even with the absence of gravitational forces, other forces remain, such as inertia, mechanical or molecular structure, magnetic fields, electrical fields, etc. The effect of weightlessness on a biological system may be significantly related to the relative importance of gravitational forces to other forces acting on the system. As an example, although the circulatory system is affected by increased gravitation by the altering weight of the blood and other tissues, for accelerations less than one G in magnitude the force of the heart's contraction may be of equal or greater significance than the force, or weight, due to the sub-gravity. Hence,

in the Russian experiments, Laika's heart rate became normal a
few minutes after the animal was in orbit, although it took three
times as long to return to normal in orbit as it took following cen-
trifugation.

At zero G the control of skeletal muscles in the absence of
weight is rapidly learned, for an arm pointing task, for body maneuvers while free-floating in the cabin of a large aircraft, for
walking with magnetic shoes on a steel-plate surface, and for
certain other body functions. The concern that muscle tone, due
to its dependence on the vestibular apparatus, might be modified
at zero G has not yet been substantiated in any of the human space
flights. This is an area for further exploration possibly by studies
in an orbiting laboratory over periods of weeks or months. An
implication is that the absence of external proprioceptive stimulation does not result in the complete absence of internal stimulation
of neural pathways. As discussed in a later chapter, the muscular support of the skeleton may be represented by a system of
springs obeying Hooke's law, with voluntary action or changes
of muscle tone represented by variations of the spring constants
and changes in length. Thus, for such a spring system (within its
elastic limits) the deformation produced by a given load and the
frequency of oscillation are more or less independent of the level
of subgravity. In this framework, it can be predicted that external loads applied to the body will have similar effects at zero G
and at 1 G and that muscular action to control these loads will be
quite similar. However, the action of a mass as a load is quite
different in the two cases. At 1 G both inertial (dynamic effect)
and weight (static effect) forces operate. At zero G inertial
effects alone operate; when the mass is no longer accelerated, the
load disappears. Very large masses may be displaced, although
care must be used in providing deceleration for the masses.
Because of the greater ease in effecting body displacements at
zero G, the Astronaut may find it desirable on trips of more than
several days duration to maintain his strength by programmed
exercises. Vigorous rhythmic tensing of the muscles for several
minutes each day may provide sufficient exercise for maintenance
of physiological function.

METABOLIC EFFECTS

Lawton[2] has called attention to the lowering of the metabolic rate which may be expected in weightlessness, and the importance of the gravitational field of the Earth in man's energy balance. In Table I are shown data demonstrating the elevation of metabolic rate for men under conditions of variable rest under 1 G. As the musculature assumes more of the gravitational load from

TABLE I

Condition	Energy Output, kcal/hr	%
Lying down	68.4	100
Sitting	71.4	104
Standing at ease	75.0	109
Standing passively		118
Space cabin activity (30 days)	57–60 estimated	82

the lying to the standing position the metabolism rises with increase in muscle tone. The conditions of space cabin activity (simulated altitude 18,000 ft, 40 per cent oxygen and 60 per cent nitrogen), as indicated by the rate of energy exchange, suggest that space flight may be characterized by an inactivity and a lack of exercise comparable with the immobilization produced by body plaster casts. If to this be added the effects of lack of gravity forces the metabolic rate may decline even further so that it is worth considering the effects of recumbency and bed rest confinement as somewhat analogous to space flight. Bed rest has been studied under a wide variety of conditions including the voluntary restriction of normal individuals for periods up to seven weeks in body plaster casts from the umbilicus down. Under these conditions the basal metabolic rate declined 7 per cent, the subjects went into negative nitrogen balance, and there was a partial wasting of the lower extremities. There was an associated loss of muscle strength and loss of ability to stand up. Complete recovery of function occurred slowly, requiring as much as 6 weeks in some subjects. No such effects have been observed in the human space flights up to a few days. However, for prolonged flights of weeks or months duration, especially designed daily exercises may be required to preserve body function so that re-entry accelerations and life of 1 G will be tolerable to the astronaut.

CARDIOVASCULAR EFFECTS

Space flights up to date have not indicated severe or troublesome effects of weightlessness upon the cardiovascular system in man or animals. It is thus necessary to use data from simulated conditions of weightlessness such as prolonged bed rest or water submersion for an evaluation of the *possible* effects of prolonged weightlessness. It is widely believed that the postural hypotension which develops during prolonged inactivity reflects a loss to some degree of vascular reflexes. However, other effects, such as decreased circulating blood volume, alteration of the blood electrolytes and possible changes in the elastic and mechanical properties of the blood vessels, may be even more important factors in the loss of vascular responses in the production of hypotension.

Thus, the conditioning of the astronaut to accept gravitational loads of 1G or more after being exposed for hours or days to subgravity or zero G conditions presents difficulties of as yet unknown proportions. Until recently it has been generally thought that suitable "protection" would be provided by maintaining muscular strength through exercise routines such as manipulation of spring and tension devices and muscle tensing, etc. Undoubtedly, such exercises will be of benefit in maintaining muscular strength but, as Graveline[3] and others have pointed out, this activity may not ensure against vascular collapse, due to the differential hydrostatic pressures in the long venous channels, when the returning astronaut attempts to stand or walk under 1 G conditions. In order to study these effects separately, Graveline carried out the following experiments.

Five subjects were evaluated before and after a 2-wk period of bed rest by means of the tilt-table test (sensitive test of cardiovascular antigravity reflexes) and muscle strength tests. Three of the subjects exercised daily in bed by doing strenuous exercises of the "set-up" and "push-up" variety; the two other subjects rested quietly in bed. At the end of the period both groups showed the same degree of cardiovascular reflex impairment when placed on the tilt-table or walking on a treadmill, although the tests indicated that there was no impairment of the muscular strength in the subjects who exercised in bed daily.

In another test done under water—a situation simulating the condition of weightlessness—subjects exposed for 6 hr showed definite impairment of the antigravity cardiovascular reflexes by the tilt-table test even though there was no impairment of muscle strength. These data point to the hydrostatic pressure gradients normally existing in the body under 1 G as being an essential component of the cardiovascular reflexes which counteract the tendency to pool blood in the lower extremities when a man stands erect under the Earth's gravitational field. Thus, the subgravity conditions of orbital flight may possibly impair these important reflexes in spite of programmed muscular exercise, especially if the flights are of long duration.

Whedon and his associates[4] have shown that a patient on an oscillating bed will not suffer the marked impairment of vascular reflexes that is observed in other patients on bed rest. The intermittent tilting of the feet several inches lower than the heart provides sufficient gradients of hydrostatic pressure to stimulate the vascular reflexes and thus the patient retains considerable ability to prevent blood pooling when he attempts to stand or walk. Extending this idea, Graveline has proposed that intermittent occlusion of venous return from the arms and legs by means of pressure cuffs inflated to 60 mm Hg might also prevent the loss of vascular reflexes. Tests were carried out on subjects while completely submerged in water, by inflating pressure cuffs on a cycle of 1 min pressure and 2 min deflation, for a period of 6 hr. Following immersion, orthostatic tolerance was estimated by tilt-table testing, using a 90° tilt for 10 min. The results of tests on one subject are shown in Figure 1; this subject fainted and was removed from the tilt-table 5 min after beginning the test following submersion for 6 hr. However, the same submersion with cyclical occlusion of venous return from legs and arms did not produce the loss of vascular reflexes. All subjects tested showed marked improvement of these reflexes following submersion with the use of the cyclic venous occlusion.

It is possible that a combination of exercises which include both skeletal and smooth musculatures may provide the necessary conditioning for the astronaut on his return from the weightless

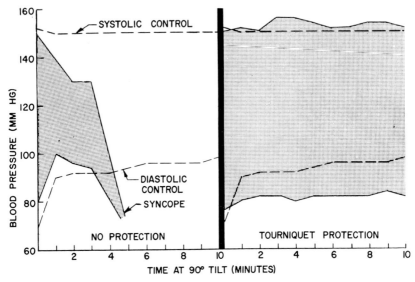

Fig. 1. Blood pressure responses to tilt-table testing in one subject following 6 hr total submersion in two experiments. Experiment at left—unrestricted activity; experiment at right—unrestricted activity with 1 min on—2 min off pressure cycling in tourniquets.

state to the Earth. However, for short periods of weightlessness (up to 6 hr for Glenn and even several days for others) such measures will probably not be required.

MUSCULAR AND BONE EFFECTS

The possibility of skeletal muscular weakness and even atrophy occurring during very long periods of weightlessness has been recognized. However, disuse atrophy occurs very slowly when compared to the atrophy which follows motor nerve section. In experimental studies a gradual decline in electromyographic response to stimulation of splinted limbs is seen during 101 days of immobilization; on the other hand, following motor nerve section a loss of as much as 86 per cent of total muscle weight may occur in a similar time. Graybiel[5] from his studies of prolonged submersion, found that muscle strength and endurance were maintained, possibly by the muscular activity involved in getting in and out of the water, moving in bed, etc. If activity exceeds one third of the maximum muscular effort muscular strength will be maintained and thus, for short space missions, planned exercises by the astronaut may be expected to maintain his muscle strength. However, under zero G, certain antigravity muscles might not be called into play by space cabin duties and very long periods of exposure may possibly present problems of muscle weakness.

Bone is a tissue in dynamic equilibrium in which the activity of mineral deposition (osteoblastic) is in balance with the activity of mineral absorption (osteoclastic), and thus a change in either activities will affect the bone structures of the body. Diminution in bony mass may result from either increased bone resorption (characteristic of hyperparathyroidism) or decreased bone formation. Mechanical stress on the bony members is required for normal osteoblastic activity and thus the effects of prolonged weightlessness in reducing these stresses may be important. Deitrick[4], in his study on normal men in body casts and on a constant diet, showed calcium losses from 9 to 24 gm during the 6 to 7 wk test. This loss may have resulted from the under-activity of the osteoblasts in laying down bone matrix or the failure to deposit bone calcium at the resorption rate.

Studies of calcium metabolism indicate that the great body store of calcium is in the bones and that of the total blood calcium, 10 mg/100 ml of blood, about 3 mg/100 ml is under the control of the parathyroid. These glands regulate the blood calcium level under ordinary circumstances mobilizing calcium as required from the bones. The interplay between the bones and the blood is very active indeed, at least in the young, since radioactive studies indicate that a 100 per cent turnover can take place in as short a time as 1 min. Mechanical stresses such as weight-bearing stimulate bone growth and repair, and relief from these stresses

promotes bone rarefaction in experimental animals. Thus, prolonged weightlessness may cause some changes in the bones and
may retard repair of fractures. However, studies of paraplegics
have indicated that muscular contraction itself is a potent stimulus
to osteoblastic activity so that the space crewman with a good
exercise regimen will probably be able to maintain satisfactory
bone metabolism and avoid any appreciable bone demineraliza-
tion.

OTOLITH AND SEMICIRCULAR CANAL EFFECTS

Because of the importance of gravity in producing sensations
which affect our orientation it has been thought that weightlessness would result in varying degrees of disorientation. Humans
are easily disoriented with respect to the direction in which they
are facing following rotation about their vertical axis. Such disorientation, is attributed to the effects of angular acceleration in
stimulating the semi-circular canals. On the other hand, rotating
a man about an horizontal axis does not result in the loss of the
sense of "up" and "down." Even without visual cues, the stimulation of the kinesthetic sensations by shifts in pressures against the
body and within the body and the stimulation of the utricles of the
vestibular apparatus provide a keen awareness of the sense of the
vertical. In the weightless state restraints of various sorts will
provide kinesthetic sensations. Experiments, involving attempts
to walk during weightlessness on a steel plate while wearing mag-
nets on the shoe soles, have shown that the subject has an immediate sensation of "down" towards the plate regardless of the orientation of the surfaces. Using visual and kinesthetic sensations
together it appears that the astronaut will be able to orient him·
self without difficulty with respect to his spacecraft. In the absence of vision, sensations of touch and pressure provided by
restraints should prove sufficient. There remains, however, the
lack of stimulation of the utricles and its effects over long periods
of time.

Linear accelerations stimulate the utricles. In 1942, Adrian[6]
demonstrated a prolonged discharge in the afferent nerve fibers to

the utricles in animals following changes in linear acceleration. The utricles seem to signal changes in the orientation and magnitude of linear accelerations. Thus, during weightlessness there should be little or no simulation of this sense with change in the astronaut's position in the spacecraft. However, the threshold for utricular simulation is small, 0.00344 g for sitting human subjects, and thus turning on the atomic engines of a spacecraft could be expected to give some sensations of linear acceleration. Usually with weak stimuli the awareness of stimulus change is keener and thus it is possible that the astronaut will be more sensitive to changes in linear accelerations near zero g than he is at 1 g. Also, although there seems to be little doubt of the existence of an utricular sensation, its normal function is in conjunction with sensations arising in the semicircular canals rather than an independent sensation.

During weightlessness there should be no impairment of the stimulation of the semicircular canals upon rotation of the head. These sensations are not specifically dependent upon the Earth's gravity and thus the position of the head relative to the body will be accurately reflected at zero G. However, it is likely that during prolonged space flights some form of artificial gravity will have to be provided at least from time to time. Dust, liquids, water vapor and all loose objects large and small will tend to move about the space cabin and mix in confusion unless there is some small force which will tend to settle everything in one direction. The turning on of space propulsion machinery if power be available could provide a linear acceleration and rotation of the space cabin about some center can produce a radial acceleration. Since rotation can be continued for long periods without use of power this method of producing artificial gravity has been widely considered. In a rotating space station the stimulation of the vestibular apparatus may induce unusual and undersirable effects. When a subject is passively rotated about one axis and turns his head about another he feels as if he were being rotated about a third axis which is roughly at right angles to the first two. The total sensation is complex and usually unpleasant giving rise to visual illusions, nausea and disorientation. The visual effects, termed oculogyrol illusions, will be discussed in detail in Chapter 7. They seem to have their origin in the stimulation of the semi-circular canals by the Coriolis acceleration which is the vector product of the linear velocity of the head and the angular velocity of the rotating space station. To minimize these effects the speed of rotation of the space station can be kept minimal or the angular accelerations, (i.e., movements) of the head can be limited. The magnitude of the Coriolis force per unit mass can be expressed in g units as

$$F = \frac{2\omega \times V}{g_0}$$

F = the Coriolis force per unit mass
ω = the angular velocity of the space station in radians per second
$\times$ = represents the vector product
V = the linear velocity of the head with respect to center of rotation
   of the space station
g_0 = 32 ft/sec²

Thus, in the rotating space station the Coriolis forces on the vestibular apparatus will be small if head is moved very slowly or not at all. Also, by rotating the space station very slowly the effects can be reduced. The forces per unit mass that can be attained within the space station in g units can be expressed in a similar manner to the centrifuge radial acceleration (p. 158).

$$F = \frac{\omega^2 R}{g_0}$$

in which ω is the angular velocity of the space station in radians per second, and R is the radius of rotation of the station.

It has been estimated that a space station with an angular velocity of not greater than 0.01 radian/sec would permit normal head movements without disconcerting illusions due to Coriolis accelerations. For a radial force in the space station of one hundredth that on the Earth's surface the radius of rotation of the station as calculated from equation 2 would have to be about 0.6 miles. Such a situation might be provided by the rotation of the space cabin and the final boster engine tied together and rotating about a common center of gravity. However, the complexity of such a system and its inconvenience might be balanced against the ability of the astronaut to accommodate after prolonged exposure to the rotation about a much shorter radius. Graybiel[7] has shown that a marked degree of adaptation is possible for some individuals.

SUMMARY

There appears to be few instances in which physiologic function is truly gravity-dependent. The stresses of gravity contribute to backache, flat feet, varicose veins and bed sores. Also, the vascular system of the body is sufficiently marginal in some of its functions so that prolonged sitting may result in swollen feet and rigid standing may cause fainting. With proper exercise routines there seems to be little reason to feel that the astronaut will be in danger from weightlessness per se. The physiological systems likely to be affected by weightlessness include the musculo-skeletal and cardiovascular systems and the equilibrium senses. Inactivity on the part of the astronaut must be avoided and space for exercising within the space craft must be provided. From time to time during a prolonged space flight some form of artificial gravity will have to be provided to keep the spacecraft orderly. It is useful in this connection to consider a possible lunar mission. Following the launch accelerations, the crew must pass into weightlessness. Although there has been indication that this transition may be associated with nausea in some individuals, the U. S. astronauts have not reported any significant effects of this kind. Some time later, the spacecraft may be set into rotation. During this early phase of the mission to the moon, critical guidance corrections must be made or a decision made to abort the mission. The rotation will thus have to be stopped and a period of several hours of weightlessness experienced while the course corrections are made. The cabin can then be rotated again if desired but course corrections may call for as many as five or more periods of no rotation. Rotation must be stopped also in order to insert the craft into lunar orbit, and visual observation and study of the lunar surface may require a non-rotating platform. The return journey will similarly require periods of non-rotation for course corrections and thus the astronaut may prefer to make much of the journey without resort to rotation. There is some evidence that the changes from acceleration to weightlessness may be more disturbing than continued weightlessness. However, much additional information is needed concerning weightlessness, and data on metabolic, biochemical and sensory changes brought about in man by very long periods of weightlessness will be sought in the coming years as the length of space journeys increases from periods of a few hours or days to several weeks.

REFERENCES

1. RITTER, O. L., and S. J. GERATHEWOHL: *The concept of Weight and Stress in Human Flight.* Report No. 58-154, USAF School of Aviation Medicine, 1959.
2. LAWTON, R. L.: *Physiological Considerations Relevant to the Problem of Prolonged Weightlessness—A Review.* Report No. 61SD202, General Electric Co., Philadelphia, 1961.
3. GRAVELINE, D. E.: *Maintenance of Cardiovascular Adaptability during Prolonged Weightlessness.* ASD Tech. Report No. 61-707, Aero-Space Med. Lab., Dayton, Ohio, 1961.
4. DEITRICK, J. E., WHEDON, G. D., and SHORR, E.: Effects of Immobilization upon various metabolic and physiological Functions of Normal Men. *Am. J. Med., 4*:3, 1948.
5. GRAYBIEL, A., and B. CLARK: Symptoms Resulting from Prolonged Immersion in Water: The Problem of Zero G Asthenia. *J. Aero-Space Med., 32*:181, 1961.
6. ADRIAN, E. D.: Discharges from Vestibular Receptors in the Cat. *J. Physiol., 101*:389, 1942.
7. GRAYBIEL, A., B. CLARK, and J. J. ZARRIELLO. Observations on Human Subjects Living in a Slow Rotation Room for Periods of Two Days: Canal Sickness. *AMA Archiv. of Neurology, 3*:55, 1960.

7

SENSORY AND PERCEPTUAL PROBLEMS IN SPACE FLIGHT*

JOHN LOTT BROWN, PH.D.

INTRODUCTION

At this stage in our space program it seems evident that the men who man our space vehicles should play an active role in the performance of their missions. Man has a variety of valuable capabilities and it would be wasteful of valuable space and fuel to send him on any mission if his capabilities were not somehow utilized. When some of the functions which must be performed in space and the completely automatic equipment required to perform them are considered objectively, it is clear that man can play an important role. Estimates of the over-all reliability of space systems, with and without the inclusion of a man as an essential element, suggest substantially higher reliability when man is included. The first American orbital flight made by John Glenn provided a dramatic example of the way a human pilot can take over control and successfully complete a mission when automatic equipment functions improperly.

If man is to play more than a passive role in space, it is necessary to provide him with considerably more than the essential physiological requirements. His sensory and motor capabilities and the demands which may be imposed on them must also be evaluated. Man must be provided with the equipment required to match his

* The preparation of this chapter was supported by U. S. Public Health Service Award No. GM-K3-15277-C2.

capabilities to the characteristics of other elements of the system.[4] He must be provided with information via his senses. This he will evaluate in relation to other current information and his knowledge of the mission. Then, when necessary, he will act upon that information via his motor response capabilities.

It is the purpose of this chapter to consider the sensory and perceptual capabilities of man in relation to the possible tasks which he may be called upon to perform during space flight.[7] Some of the hazards to sensory processes which may be encountered are also discussed.

VISION

Vision will be the principal available distance receptor in space in the absence of a sound transmitting atmosphere. Its importance in this capacity will therefore be greater than ever. It will be of equal importance for the receipt of information from displays within the space vehicle, however. Its various applications can best be reviewed by considering them in relation to the various stages of space missions.

Launch

During initial stages of the launching of a space flight mission, man may be called upon for the performance of several tasks. He will undoubtedly be required to monitor the progress of the launch with respect to changing velocity, altitude and flight-path angle during successive stages of rocket firing. He may also be called upon to monitor and possibly control vehicle attitude in roll and yaw and to make corrections in pitch in order to achieve the desired flight path angle at burnout.[5] He could conceivably be called upon to time initiation and termination of firing of a given rocket stage. Such activities, if required, will probably be accomplished by reference to panel indicators within the space vehicle. External references such as horizon will be of limited value by reason of the high order of precision which will be required. For example, in order to come within 6000 miles of the planet Mars, a rocket launched from the earth may require a velocity at rocket burnout which is accurate to within 1 fps and a flight path angle which is accurate to within 0.001°.[37] The exact requirement will depend upon the precise relation of the two planets at the time of launch. Even under optimum conditions, precision requirements will be so high at this stage, however, that man will probably perform only a "back-up" function in case of emergency. The nature of space flight for some time to come will be such that all stages of flight will be carefully pre-planned.[1, 37] The crew of space vehicles will not exercise discretion as to the course to be followed. There will only be one correct course for a given destination, and once the launch has been initiated the crew will be committed either to follow this course or to "abort" the mission.

Visual problems which arise during launch will relate to the selection of appropriate methods of displaying information so that it can be interpreted rapidly and accurately. Information will include vehicle speed, altitude, attitude and flight-path angle, in addition to engineering information on the status of various components in sub-systems of the vehicle. The crew of a rocket may also be required to look for external indications of proper vehicle function during launch such as steam clouds which will indicate proper function of reaction control nozzles. Deleterious effects of acceleration on vision may represent a hazard during this stage of flight. Such effects must also be considered during recovery and landing. They are discussed further in a subsequent section.

Orbit

On orbital missions, once the launch has been completed, the space vehicle will be rotating about the earth at a speed such that centrifugal force developed will balance the gravitational attraction of the earth. The altitude of an orbital flight will probably fall within 100 and 500 miles. The minimum is determined by the retarding effect of the earth's atmosphere which will be encountered at lower altitudes. The maximum altitude is imposed by the dangerous amounts of radiation exposure (Van Allen Belt) which may be encountered at altitudes above 500 miles.

Reconnaissance: During orbital flight man may be called upon to make observations of the surface of the earth. It must not be supposed that he will be able to observe human activities, however. The resolution capacity of the eye is such that a minimum angular separation of between 1 and 10 min of arc can be discriminated for a wide range of illuminations. Thus, for an object to be identified, the dimensions of its distinguishing characteristics must be sufficiently great that they will subtend a visual angle of between 1 and 10 min of arc at the eye of an observer in orbit. The required length in feet to meet the criterion of 10 min of arc is equal to fifteen times the distance of the observer in miles. Thus, at an altitude of 100 miles, the distinguishing elements of clearly recognizable objects must have dimensions of 1500 ft. Many manmade objects, including fairly large buildings, will be too small to be detected. After his recent orbital flight, Glenn remarked that an object such as a bridge could not be picked out with any certainty. A river can be seen from an altitude of 100 miles, however, and when a spot is seen on the river there is a tendency to assume there is a bridge.

With the aid of a telescope, objects can be magnified but there will be a concomitant reduction in the size of the over-all field of view and a substantial reduction in the time during which any particular object remains in the field of view. It has been found experimentally that the probability of detecting an object in a stationary pattern increases appreciably with duration of viewing for up to 12-sec.[3] If relatively small objects (20 to 30 ft in length) are magnified sufficiently to be identified, the time for which they are visible may be reduced to 1 sec or less. Identification will be rendered even more difficult by reason of the fact that objects will be part of a moving, constantly changing pattern. It may be concluded that a man with unaided vision will not be capable of performing any important reconnaissance function from an orbital altitude of 100 miles or greater.[43] He will be able to discriminate such things as lakes and rivers, coastlines and islands which may enable him to localize his position, however. These observations will provide a method of noting the time at which various check points are reached.

Attitude Control: During orbit it will be possible for a man to control the attitude of his craft by external visual reference. In the

Mercury capsule, the normal attitude is such that there is a direct view of the horizon. This provides a reference for control of roll. A wide-angle periscope provides a view of the ground below out to the horizon in all directions. At an altitude of 100 miles the horizon is at a distance of approximately 900 miles. Thus, the visible surface of the earth represents a circular area with a diameter of 165° of visual angle subtended at the vehicle. In the Mercury cap- sule the periscope field is so positioned that vehicle attitude in pitch and roll are correct when the earth's visible surface is centered in the field. At 18,000 mph, at an altitude of 100 miles, the vehicle will be traversing 5 miles on the earth's surface every second. If any pattern is discriminable on the earth's surface as seen in the periscope field, orientation of the vehicle in yaw may be observed in terms of the relative motion of the pattern. If no surface pattern is discriminable, control of yaw may be accomplished by reference to star patterns. Outside observation will be complicated during orbit by a daylight and darkness cycle of approximately 90 min. The horizon may be visible continuously, either as a band of light or as a discontinuity between star patterns and the blackness of the earth, but in general the earth's surface will only be visible during the daylight half of the cycle. Light from population centers may be seen, and occasionally in the case of a city located on the shore of a lake or ocean the light pattern may have a distinctive contour.

During the dark part of the cycle the observation of stars will be of increased importance as a basis for controlling vehicle attitude. Continuing reference to instruments within the vehicle will also be required, however. Thus, a system of illumination which permits instrument visibility but at the same time does not reduce sensitivity of the eye excessively is essential. This has been provided in the Mercury capsule.[30] When red instrument illumination is employed, it is possible to observe stars of the fifth magnitude without difficulty. Some precautions must be taken during the daylight portion of orbital flight to prevent excessive light adaptation. In the Mercury vehicle this is accomplished with the aid of a red filter and an opaque screen which can readily be positioned over the window.

Detection: The possibility of detecting other space vehicles or objects in space during an orbital flight may be considered remote, except where contact has been specifically planned. The relative velocity between two objects will be considerable unless they are in similar orbits. Relative velocity will increase with increased deviation of orbits and the time during which an object the size of a space vehicle would be visible will decrease commensurately. Some of the problems associated with the detection of objects moving in space both transverse to the line of sight[38] and in depth[2] have been studied experimentally. Vehicles will not be placed in orbit to search for other vehicles that are not already known to be in a specific orbit.

Detection of objects in space will not necessarily be limited by their size in relation to the resolution capacity of the eye. An object will be visible as a point source of reflected light against a dark background. The distance over which it may be detected will therefore depend solely on the total amount of luminous energy which is reflected or emitted. There is no minimum resolvable visual angle for a point source of light against a dark background. Detectibility of point sources of light will be improved by the fact that the outside atmospheric luminance of the sky background will be only 10 per cent of the luminance of the sky on a moonless night.[41] Results of a recent experiment suggest that detection of a light spot against a dark sky within a pattern of stars will not be a simple matter unless it is markedly brighter than the surrounding stars.[26]

At least one of the visibility problems which confront the pilot of a high altitude aircraft should not exist for the occupant of a space vehicle. That is the problem of space myopia.[12, 50] During daylight at altitudes between 40,000 and 60,000 ft there may be nothing visible outside an aircraft other than the homogeneous sky illumination. Under these circumstances, with no external cue for distance accommodation, the eye tends to accommodate for near objects. It is thus effectively myopic in relation to the problem of detecting objects in space. As altitude is increased, however, and the atmosphere becomes thinner, the ambient sky illumination is reduced. At an orbital altitude of 100 miles, sky illumination will be sufficiently reduced that stars will be visible and these will provide adequate cues for distance accommodation.

Astronomical Observations: Observations of stars from an orbital vehicle may be of importance for the purpose of fixing position and controlling vehicle attitude.   An orbital vehicle which is above the earth's atmosphere will receive approximately 30 per cent more visible light from the stars than the amount which reaches the earth's surface, and observations will not be subject to atmospheric shimmer.[41]   There are other factors which will minimize the importance of astronomical observations for scientific purposes, however.   It will not be possible to include telescopes which begin to approach the size of large terrestrial telescopes in orbiting vehicles.   The degree of stabilization required for precise astronomical observation will also be difficult to achieve in a manned orbital vehicle of moderate size.

Direct observations of stars through a window will be limited by the transmittance of the materials from which the window is constructed.   These will be dictated to some extent by the structural integrity requirements of the vehicle.   It will also be desirable to attenuate ultra violet light and direct sunlight for the protection of the man.   Following his orbital flight, Glenn reported that he was able to see fewer stars than he had expected.   He tentatively attributed this to the attenuation of light by the window of the Mercury capsule.   The transmittance of the window of this capsule is between 35 and 50 per cent in the visible spectrum for a normal viewing angle, but it is reduced to 15 or 25 per cent for a viewing angle of 60°.[30]

Rendezvous: One extremely challenging problem which will occur in future space flight missions will be that of rendezvousing with a vehicle which is already in orbit.   It will not only be necessary to achieve the same orbit, but the same point in that orbit. The accuracy required with respect to timing, control of trajectory and burnout velocity will be considerable.[20]   Corrections will undoubtedly be required even under optimum conditions.   Terminal rendezvous will require a system which can assess the error between the orbit of the rendezvousing vehicle and that of its target and compute the appropriate method of reducing the error to zero.

It is possible that a man, employing direct vision, might be able to play some role in the final stages of the problem. On the other hand, estimates of shape, size and the distance of objects are strongly dependent on familiarity of the object and its appearance in relation to other objects in the visual field.[28] In empty space, such estimates may be difficult to make with sufficient accuracy for control of precise maneuvers.

Lunar and Interplanetary Flight

Vision Outside the Vehicle: During earth-lunar and interplanetary flights, external visual observations of the stars and planets may be employed to determine position and course as a check on the stellar guidance system which probably will be used. Such observations will require training in the recognition of celestial patterns and the nature of changes in the relative positions of planets which will occur during a specific flight. The location of a space vehicle in its orbital path about the earth, the sun or some target planet can be determined by simultaneous or successive observations of two or more known bodies.[1, 31] Simultaneous, multiple observations will afford the highest precision. It will be necessary to develop special techniques and devices to aid him if man is to make such observations visually.

Orientation: For the major portion of lunar and interplanetary flights, there will be no available horizon or ground plane such as there is on orbital flights to provide a stable frame of reference. Occupants of a space vehicle will therefore be more dependent on points of reference within the vehicle. In the absence of any gravitational field, certain novel problems may arise. It has been suggested that the interior design of a vehicle to be used for a prolonged space mission should be conventional, i.e., with a floor, walls and ceiling, and with instruments and controls arrayed in much the same way that they would be for use in the presence of a field of gravity.[27] It is argued that a conventional environment will be easier to work in and more compatible because of the extensive training and experience which man has had in such an environment on the earth's surface. The use of magnetic shoes and adhesive materials could be employed to aid in the stabilization of the "up" and "down" character of the interior of such a vehicle. On the other hand, it will not be necessary for a vehicle which will be in a condition of zero gravity for extended periods to have any floors and ceilings as such. Occupants will be quite capable of moving in any direction within the vehicle, and not just with reference to a specific ground plane. Restrictions as to body positions which apply at the earth's surface will not apply. The most efficient design of work spaces and the integration of activities of several occupants of a compartment might lead to a design which is quite unique in relation to conventional terrestrial design. Stations of crew members may be oriented such that these individuals are at unique angles with respect to one another.

It is to be expected that man's training and experience in earthly surroundings will cause him some difficulty in such a novel environment. He is accustomed to a rectangular organization of the enclosures in which he lives on the surface of the earth and even minor deviations from such right-angle organization may result in considerable confusion. A good example is the disorientation experienced by most newcomers to the Pentagon. As the Ames demonstrations show very clearly[28] judgments of distance, size and shape of quite familiar objects may suffer remarkable distortion when they are observed in rooms which deviate from the usual rectangular design. These disorientations and distortions are greatest when the appearance of deviation from conventional design is least, however. The unconventionality of the most efficient interior design of a space vehicle may be sufficiently obvious that the interference effects of prior training and experience will be minimized. In any case, there is some evidence that man can compensate very rapidly for novel perceptual situations[32] even in the face of excessive prior training and experience which are not compatible.

Visual Display Problems: If a novel interior design is employed which does not provide a consistent "up," certain instrument display problems may arise as a result. The interpretation of conventional visual displays is frequently dependent to some extent on their orientation with respect to the environment, and particularly with respect to the observer. The possible location of observers in a variety of unique positions with respect to a visual display will require a display design such that its interpretation is not dependent on its position with respect to the background against which it appears or with respect to the observer. Individual elements within the display must have unique, recognizable characteristics which are independent of their position. Visual coding by color and shape will be of importance.

Landing

In many circumstances, landing will be initiated from a condition of orbital flight by firing a rocket which is oriented to reduce orbital velocity. Timing of the firing of a retro-rocket must be carefully controlled in order to land in a desired location. Such timing can best be controlled from ground stations where precise fixes of orbital vehicle position can be made. Ground support will not always be available, however. In its absence, rocket firing may be timed by an occupant of the vehicle in relation to the transit of some recognizable landmark on the surface below. With fairly simple sighting equipment, man should be able to accomplish this within an accuracy of 250 to 500 milliseconds.[51] For an earth orbit at an altitude of 100 miles, this corresponds to a variation in final landing point of 1.25 to 2.5 miles.

Landing from orbit upon a relatively unknown planet or moon will be somewhat more difficult than landing on earth. There won't be any recognizable landmarks. Several reconnaissance orbits may be necessary in order to obtain some basis for selecting a landing sight. Visual observation will be of only limited value in assessing the nature of the surface, however. Such observation may be aided by the use of low, off-set flares which will illuminate the surface in such a way that surface irregularities will cast long, discriminable shadows.

If there is a gaseous atmosphere and the landing vehicle is capable of maneuvering within it in the fashion of a conventional aircraft, then direct visual observation of the surface may be of considerable importance in the selection of a landing site and control of the vehicle during the final stages of the landing. On the other hand, if the landing is accomplished by deceleration of a "high-drag" vehicle such as the Mercury capsule, although some control of flight path will be possible by alterations of capsule attitude, there will be relatively little which an occupant can do to influence the landing. Parachute release will probably be automatic, but it may be timed on the basis of visual observations of the surface. This will be difficult over water and other areas with relatively homogeneous surfaces.

In the absence of a suitable combination of atmosphere, gravitational field, and vehicle design, landing will be accomplished with the aid of a deceleration rocket which will slow the vehicle as it approaches the surface. The vertical component of velocity must be reduced sufficiently at the moment of contact that there will be no damage to the vehicle or injury to vehicle occupants. It will be wasteful of energy to reduce it too rapidly. The satisfactory solution of this problem will require continuous information concerning altitude, velocity, and deceleration during descent. It seems unlikely that it can be solved by a man on the basis of direct visual observation of the surface, but given appropriate instrument information he may perform a significant role.

Hazards to Vision

High Illumination Level: Illumination of the sun, unattenuated by the earth's atmosphere, is approximately 12,000 to 14,000 ft candles in the region of the earth. [25, 29, 45] In the absence of any atmospheric dispersion the brightness of the sky is lower than that observed on the surface of the earth on a moonless night, however (on the order of 10^{-5} nit).[41] Therefore much greater contrast occurs between illuminated objects and their surroundings.[50] The range of luminances in the visual field may be expected to be greater and irritation from glare will be greater than that which occurs on the earth's surface.[36] High contrast effects need not necessarily be a problem within a space vehicle, however. They can be reduced by the use of painted surfaces of high reflectance which will scatter the light.

During observation outside a space vehicle there will be the possibility of injury to the eyes as a result of excessive exposure to sunlight.[6] Formation of an image of the sun on the retina by optical elements of the eye results in a concentration of visible and infra-red energy sufficient to cause a retinal burn after less than a minute's observation at the earth's surface.[16] Beyond the 30 per cent attenuation of the earth's atmosphere the required duration will be shorter, perhaps 15 sec, and the closer the sun is approached, the shorter will this time become. An exposure duration of seconds represents a fairly long time, however, and it should be possible to avert the eyes in ample time to prevent damage if they are suddenly exposed to the sun. Of course, the attenuation introduced by the window material of the space vehicle will provide a considerable margin of safety.

Eye injuries caused by exposure to excessive illumination may be of two kinds.[21] Thermal injuries may occur to any part of the eye with excessive exposure to visible and infra-red radiation. Non-thermal or abiotic effects may result from exposure to shorter wavelengths (365 mμ down to below 300 mμ). These effects include erythema with severe itching and burning sensations of the eyes which may last for several weeks. The retina is not affected because virtually all the energy of these shorter wavelengths is absorbed by cornea and lens. Effects of repeated exposures to short wavelength radiation may be cumulative over a 24 hr period. Fortunately, short wavelength radiation may be almost completely absorbed by the windows of a space vehicle.

Ionizing Radiation: It has long been known that excessive ionizing radiation can cause ocular damage.[17] Cataracts can readily be produced in normal eyes by irradiation with x-rays. The younger the organism, the greater is the susceptibility. Irradiation of the lens damages anterior epithelial cells, and if cells which are capable of division are damaged, i.e., those which lie in a ring about 1 mm in front of the lens equator, cataracts may result.[39] Cataract is actually formed when damaged cells, the fibers of which are opaque to light, are moved back toward the posterior pole of the lens and subsequent cell division occurs. The effects of irradiation may be cumulative for up to four months, which is the approximate time required for recovery from irradiation effects.

There will be a variety of possible sources of radiation hazard which may be encountered in space flight. These will include the Van Allen radiation belt, cosmic rays, auroral displays and possible solar sources[40] in addition to nuclear propulsion systems of the future.[33] Structural and chemical shielding should provide adequate protection of the crew of a rocket vehicle from radiation of its own power plant. In addition, it will be necessary to plan flights such that minimum amounts of time are spent in zones of high radiation.

Exotic Fuels: Some of the constituents of the chemical fuels which will be employed in rocket flight for some time to come may be extremely toxic when absorbed or inhaled. Specific effects on vision may occur if precautions are not taken to protect the occupant of the space vehicle from the fumes of such fuels.[42]

Acceleration: Man may be exposed to high levels of acceleration both during launch and landing of a space vehicle. When the acceleration includes a positive component, i.e., one which is oriented along the long axis of the body such that flow of blood to the head is impeded, impairment of visual function may frequently result. Definite subjective visual symptoms ranging from the apparent dimming of light up to complete loss of vision are noted in the range between 3.5 and 6.0 positive G. The level at which these effects occur is highly variable in different individuals and in a given individual from one time to another.[14] Reaction time to visual signals is prolonged by exposure to positive acceleration[9] in the same levels where subjective symptoms are observed. White and his colleagues have found increased errors in dial reading,[49] decreased visual acuity,[48] and an elevation of light detection threshold[46] with increases in positive acceleration. Visual acuity showed impairment with increased level of acceleration, independent of the orientation of the acceleration vector. Such impairment has been attributed to mechanical effects of acceleration on optical elements of the eye.[47] Increased errors in dial reading and elevations of visual threshold may reflect interference with retinal circulation.[18] To some extent, impairment of visual functions can be offset by an increase in the level of illumination provided for the performance of visual tasks.[47]   On space flight missions, visual impairment as a result of acceleration exposure should not be a serious problem.   Occupants of a space vehicle will be supported by special couches which will be oriented at right angles to the line of action of acceleration.   The positive acceleration component which gives rise to the most serious visual effects will therefore be kept sufficiently low that it should not cause difficulty.

HEARING

In space flight, hearing will depend almost entirely on artificial aids.   It will be a most important sensory modality, nonetheless, in that it will provide the most important link between man in space and the surface of the earth.   The maintenance of this link will be extremely important, not only for the exchange of information but also for the psychological support of the man.

Normal speech sounds may be altered in a variety of ways without becoming unintelligible, and it has been demonstrated that information capacity of speech is dependent on a relatively small proportion of the total band width occupied by normal speech.   Any method which can be employed to effect economies in the power requirements for communication in space will be of considerable importance.[7]   A careful evaluation of the effects of modification of speech sounds on intelligibility must accompany the introduction of any new methods, however.

In addition to its importance for communication, hearing may prove of considerable importance for purposes of recreation and relaxation.   For example, the ability to listen to music may assume an unimagined degree of importance for the occupant of a space vehicle on a protracted flight.

Hazards

Noise and vibration may constitute specific hazards for hearing within a space vehicle.   These effects can be expected to be prominent only during launch and recovery, and can be minimized during these phases of flight by appropriate engineering design.   The use of head-phones in sound-shielding mounts will afford additional protection. Acceleration apparently has no important specific effect on hearing and therefore does not constitute a specific hazard.[11]

VESTIBULAR SENSE

There has been much concern over the possible effects of exposure to zero gravity in space flight. One basis for such concern is the fact that the pattern of stimulation of the vestibular mechanism will be very different in the absence of the earth's gravitational field. The utricular system of the vestibular apparatus contains otoliths, calcareous "stones" which are of a greater density than surrounding tissue. Variations in the orientation of a gravitational field results in a variation of the way in which these otoliths are displaced with respect to the associated macula.[8] There is an accompanying variation in the pattern of discharge of the afferent neural connections of the utricles.[23] At zero gravity, changes in body position will no longer be associated with the same changes in the pattern of utricular discharge. In addition, the perceptual results of stimulation of the semi-circular canals may be altered in the absence of the terrestrial response patterns of the utricles. These effects will be manifested by their influence on visual perception and orientation. The stability of the visual world in spite of head and body movements is related to vestibular signals which effect a stabilization of visual perception.[44] Such stabilization is partly the result of compensatory eye movements but it also depends in part upon the integration of visual and vestibular inputs at some more central location. The evidence available at present indicates that although there may be individual differences, it probably will be possible for man to adapt to a zero gravity environment fairly quickly. When vision is not impaired good adjustment to complete destruction of the vestibular apparatus occurs rapidly.[35] Placing a man in a zero gravity environment represents a much less extreme situation.

The possibility of rotating a space vehicle in order to create an artificial "gravitational field" has been considered.[34] In addition to presumed physiological advantages, certain physical reasons are sometimes put forward in support of this kind of system. It has been said that liquids will be more readily manageable in a gravitational field, that convection currents which result in circulation of air will depend upon the presence of the gravitational field, and that the physics of the circulation of the blood require the action of a gravitational force during long term confinement. Man has difficulty tolerating rotational rates greater than 5 or 6 rpm. Although some adaptation occurs, nausea and disorientation are frequent results of exposure to a rotating environment.[13, 24] Illusory effects accompany any movement of the head. Unless the radius is substantial, only a relatively low acceleration component can be achieved by rotation at 5 or 6 rpm. Additional problems would arise in connection with external observations from a rotating vehicle.

The vestibular apparatus, by reason of differences in the density of its components, can be injured or destroyed by exposure to acceleration. In one experiment, subjects reported vertigo for up to 48 hr following exposure up to 15 transverse G for up to 5 sec. Edema of the vestibular apparatus was suggested as a tentative explanation.[19] In a later experiment[10] in which transverse accelerations of nearly 12 G were investigated, one of the subjects noted some disorientation following exposure which increased during the course of the experiment. Disorientation and vertigo persisted for some time after the completion of the experiment and disorientation was precipitated by sudden head movements for a period of several weeks. There is some evidence that disorientation following exposure to transverse acceleration of as high as 20 G may be reduced following repeated exposures.[15] The levels of acceleration required to cause irreversible damage are relatively high, and this should not pose a problem in space flight.[35]

OTHER SENSES

Kinesthetic Sense

The regulation of complex motor performance such as that which may be required by the occupants of space craft is dependent to a large extent on kinesthetic feedback from the muscle groups which are involved.[4] In a gravitational field the position of a limb, its orientation, and its component of motion in the direction of action of the gravitational field all influence patterns of tension on the musculature involved in a way which is dependent upon the strength and line of action of the gravitational force. It is difficult to predict the extent to which highly coordinated motions may depend on this kind of feedback. It is possible that certain types of motor performance may be extremely difficult when kinesthetic cues dependent upon gravity are absent. The problem may become particularly important in connection with the manipulation of objects and tools in the unusual ways which may be required for maintenance operations in space. Preliminary studies can be conducted on the surface of the earth in which changes in motor performance capabilities are observed when organisms trained at one level of acceleration are placed in an environment at a different level of acceleration. The important limitation of studies of this kind conducted on centrifuges lies in the fact that accelerations of less than 1 G cannot be achieved for any significant duration. "Weightlessness" can be achieved, within limitations, by immersion in water, however.[8] Although the weightlessness achieved in water immersion is radically different from that which will occur under zero gravity, water immersion may nevertheless be of considerable value for training purposes prior to actual space flight.

Tactual Sense

In recent years, tactual signal systems have received considerable attention. The efficiency of these systems has been demonstrated for the receipt of information at relatively high rates.[22a] Such systems may prove useful in space craft where large numbers of non-interfering information channels will be required. On long missions it may be desirable to make some provision for the presentation of tactual stimulation in the form of low amplitude vibrations. These could be applied as a form of massage to maintain peripheral circulation and muscle tone.

Olfactory Sense

Man is limited in the number of senses available to him but his integration as a component of a space vehicle system may require that his senses be employed in unique ways. Weight and space restrictions of a space vehicle are such that information flow to the man must be accomplished in the most efficient manner possible. This might require, for example, the use of olfactory cues for the presentation of discrete signals which may be widely spaced. Such signals might be employed to signify equipment component malfunction. Some equipment malfunctions may result in olfactory cues which do not occur by design. Olfactory signalling systems may be constructed of very small size with very low power requirements while at the same time they may encompass an appreciable number of discretely coded signals. Unpleasant odors derived from paint and other materials employed in the construction of a space vehicle, from equipment failure, or which are of the occupant's own production must be eliminated or controlled. Although there is usually fairly rapid and complete adaptation of the olfactory sense, the aversive effects of some odors may continue over a long period.

Gustatory Sense

The sense of taste may not play any direct role in man's performance in space flight but it will be of importance if he is to be kept well and happy on an extended mission. He must be provided with palatable food which is manageable in the zero G environment of outer space and which will not create unnecessary problems of waste disposal.

OTHER PROBLEMS

Time Perception

It has been speculated that in the absence of acceleration and the resulting lack of the requirement of continuous tension to maintain posture, the occupants of a space vehicle may require little or no sleep. This may grossly affect such things as the perception of the passage of time. The gross distortion of time perception may have severe effects, both practical and psychological, on an individual who has undergone extensive prior training at 1 G without time distortion. It may also render irrelevant work done at the surface of the earth in a 1 G environment on the subject of sleep-rest cycles.

Sensory Deprivation

Some concern has been expressed over the implications of studies of sensory deprivation for space flight. Although there has been considerable variability in the results of these experiments, some of them indicate that in the absence of the usual pattern of sensory inputs, man may suffer serious psychological and perceptual disruptions.[22] Although his environment will be severely limited within the confines of a space vehicle, man in space will not be deprived of sensory inputs in the same sense that subjects of sensory deprivation experiments have been deprived, however. It will be surprising if the restricted environment of the space vehicle and the limitations on the variety of sensory experience do not have profound psychological effects on the members of space missions. It seems highly improbable that these effects can be predicted from sensory deprivation studies, however.

REFERENCES

1. ADAMS, C. C.: .*Space Flight.* McGraw-Hill; New York, 1958.
2. BAKER, C. A.: *Man's Visual Capabilities in Space.* Proc. Seventh Annual East Coast Conference on Aeronautical and Navigational Electronics, October, 1960.
3. BOYNTON, R. M., ELSWORTH, C., and PALMER, R. M.: Laboratory studies pertaining to visual air reconnaissance. *WADC Tech. Rept. 53-304,* Part III. Wright-Patterson Air Force Base, Ohio, April, 1958.
4. BROWN, J. L.: The bio-dynamics of launch and re-entry. *Mil. Med., 124*:775–781, 1959.
5. BROWN, J. L.: Acceleration and motor performance. *Human Factors, 2*:175–185, 1960.
6. BROWN, J. L.: Flash blindness. *Tech. Rept. Missile and Space Vehicle Dept.* General Electric Co., September, 1961.
7. BROWN, J. L., editor: *Sensory and Perceptual Problems Related to Space Flight.* Washington, Nat. Acad. Sci.-Nat. Res. Council, Pub. No. 872, 1961.
8. BROWN, J. L.: Orientation to the vertical during water immersion. *Aerospace Med., 32*:209–217, 1961.

9. Brown, J. L., and Burke, R. E.:   The effect of positive acceleration on visual reaction time. *J. Aviat. Med.*, 29:48–58, 1958.
10. Brown, J. L., Ellis, W. H. B., Webb, M. G., and Gray, R. F.:   *The Effect of Simulated Catapult Launching on Pilot Performance.* Rept. NADC Ma 5719, U. S. Naval Air Dev. Cen., Johnsville, Pa., December, 1957.
11. Brown, J. L., and Lechner, M.:   Acceleration and human performance. *J. Aviat. Med.*, 27:32–49, 1956.
12. Brown, R. H.:   "Empty-field" myopia and visibility of distant objects at high altitudes. *Am. J. Psychol.*, 70:376–385, 1957.
13. Clark, B., and Graybiel, A.:   *Human Performance During Adaptation to Stress in the Pensacola Slow Rotation Room.* U. S. Naval School of Aviat. Med., Pensacola, Fla.   Proj. MR 005.13-6001, Subtask 1, Rept. No. 2, May, 1960.
14. Cochran, L. B., Gard, P. W., and Norsworthy, M. E.:   *Variations in Human G Tolerance to Positive Acceleration.* Rept. 001 059 02.10 U. S. Naval School of Aviat. Med., Pensacola, Fla.   August, 1954.
15. Collins, C. C., Crosbie, R. J., and Gray, R. F.:   *Pilot Performance and Tolerance Studies of Orbital Reentry Acceleration.* Letter Rept. TED ADC AE 1412.   U. S. Naval Air Dev. Cen., Johnsville, Pa., September, 1958.
16. Cordes, F. C.   Eclipse retinitis. *Am. J. Ophthal.*, 31:101, 1948.
17. Culver, J. F., and Newton, N. L.:   *Early Ocular Effects of High-energy Proton and Alpha Radiation.*   USAF Sch. Aviat. Med., Brooks AFB, Texas, 1961.
18. Duane, T. D.:   Observations of the fundus oculi during blackout. *Arch. Ophthal.*, 51:343–355, 1954.
19. Duane, T. D., Beckman, E. L., Ziegler, J. E., and Hunter, H. N.:   *Some Observations on Human Tolerance to Exposures of 15 Transverse G.* Rept. NADC Ma 5305.   U. S. Naval Air Dev. Cen., Johnsville, Pa., July, 1953.
20. DuBridge, L. A.:   *Introduction to Space.*   New York, Columbia Univ. Press, 1960.
21. Duke-Elder, W. S.:   *Textbook of Ophthalmology*, Vol. I.   C. V. Mosby Co., 1942.   pg. 815 ff.
22. Freedman, S. J.:   Perceptual changes in sensory deprivation: Suggestions for a conative theory. *J. Nerv. Ment. Dis.*, 132:17–21, 1961.
22a. Geldard, F. A.:   Adventures in tactile literacy. *Am. Psychologist*, 12:115–124, 1957.
23. Gernandt, R. E.:   Vestibular mechanisms.   Ch. XXII in *Neurophysiology* Section I, Vol. I of *Handbook of Physiology.*   Am. Physiol. Soc., Washington, 849, 1959.

24. GRAYBIEL, A., CLARK, B., and ZARIELLO, J. J.:   Observations on human subjects living in a "slow rotation room" for periods of two days. *Arch. Neurol., 3*:55–73, 1960.

25. HABER, H.:   Manned flight at the borders of space.   *J. Am. Rocket Soc., 22*:3–269, 1952.

26. HALL, R. J., BROWN, H. T., PAYNE, T. A., and ROGERS, J. G.:   *Detection Stereotopy.*   Rep. SD 60-119, Hughes Aircraft Co., Fullerton, Calif., December, 1960.

27. HAVILAND, R. P.:   A concept of space travel and operations.   *Visual Problems of the Armed Forces.*   Armed Forces–NRC Committee on Vision, March 30–31, 1961.   Ed. by M. A. Whitcomb, pp. 37–48.

28. ITTLESON, W. H.: .*Visual Space Perception.*   New York, Springer, 1960.

29. JOHNSON, F. S.:   The solar constant.   *J. Meteorology, 11*:431, 1954.

30. JONES, E. R., and HANN, W. H.:   Vision and the Mercury capsule. *Visual Problems of the Armed Forces.*   Armed Forces–NRC Committee on Vision, March 30–31, 1961.   Ed. by M. A. Whitcomb. pp. 49–65.

31. JOYCE, W., and MALLETT, F.:   *Navigation Techniques and Displays for Interplanetary Space Flight.*   Ohio State Univ. Found., Columbus, Ohio: December, 1959, Rep. No. 813.

32. KILPATRICK, F. P.:   Two processes in perceptual learning.   *J. Exper. Psychol., 47*:362–370, 1954.

33. KONECCI, E. B., and TRAPP, R.:   Calculations of the radiobiologic risk factors in nuclear powered space vehicles.   *Aerospace Med., 30*:487–506, 1959.

34. LANSBERG, M. P.:   The function of the vestibular sense and the construction of a satellite.   *Aeromed. Acta, 4*:183–190, 1955.

35. MARGARIA, R., and GUALTIEROTTI, T.:   Body susceptibility to high accelerations and to zero gravity condition.   *Advances in Aeronautical Sciences.*   New York, Pergamon Press, 1961.   pp. 1081–1103.

36. McDONALD, T. C.:   Changing concepts in aviation medicine.   *J. Aviat. Med., 26*:463, 1955.

37. MICKELWAIT, A. B., TOMKINS, E. H., and PARK, R. A.:   Interplanetary navigation.   *Sc. Am., 202*:64–73, 1960.

38. MILLER, J. W., and LUDVIGH, E.:   The perception of movement persistence in the Granzfeld.   *J. Opt. Soc. Am., 51*:57–60, 1961.

39. PIRIE, A.:   Recovery from and protection against radiation damage to the lens.   In *The Structure of the Eye.*   Ed. by Smelser, G. K. Academic Press, 1961, New York and London.

40. SCHAEFER, H. J.:   *Further Evaluation of Tissue Depth Doses in Proton Radiation Fields in Space.*   Nav. School Aviat. Med., Pensacola, Fla., Proj. No. MR 005.13-1002, Subtask No. 1, Rept. No. 17, 1960.

41. STRUGHOLD, H.:   The human eye in space.   *Astronautica Acta, 5*, 1960.

42. STUMPE, A. R.:   Health hazards of new aircraft and rocket propellents. *J. Aviat. Med.*, 29:650–659, 1958.
43. SWARTZ, W. F., OBERMAYER, R. W., and MUEHLER, F. A.:   *Some Theoretical Limits of Man-periscope Visual Performance in an Orbital Reconnaissance Vehicle.* Baltimore, The Martin Co., 1959, Engrg. Rept. No. 10978.
44. TEUBER, H. L., and BENDER, M. B.:   Neuroophthalmology: The oculomotor system. *Prog. Neurol. Psychiat.*, 6:148–178, 1951.
45. TOOLIN, R. B., and STAKUTIS, V. J.:   Visual albedo and total solar illumination as a function of altitude. *Bull. Am. Meteorol. Soc.*, 39:543, 1959.
46. WHITE, W. J.:   *Variations in Absolute Visual Thresholds During Acceleration Stress.* WADC Technical Rept. 60-34, Wright-Patterson AFB, Ohio, April, 1960.
47. WHITE, W. J.:   Visual performance under gravitational stress.   Ch. 11 in *Gravitational Stress in Aerospace Medicine*, ed. by Gauer and Zuidema.   Boston, Little, Brown and Co., 1961.
48. WHITE, W. J., and JORVE, W. R.:   *The Effects of Gravitational Stress upon Visual Acuity.*   WADC Technical Report 56-247, Wright-Patterson AFB, Ohio, November, 1958.
49. WHITE, W. J., and RILEY, M. B.:   *The Effects of Positive Acceleration on the Relation Between Illumination and Instrument Reading.* WADC Tech. Rept. 58-332, Wright-Patterson AFB, Ohio, November, 1958.
50. WHITESIDE, T. C. D.:   The Problem of Vision in Flight at High Altitude. London, Butterworth's Scientific Publications, 1957.
51. WOODWORTH, R. S.:   *Experimental Psychology.* New York, Holt, 1938.

8

ISOLATION AND DISORIENTATION

RANDALL M. CHAMBERS, PH.D.

This chapter reviews and summarizes research on isolation and disorientation as it relates to problems encountered by man during space travel. An attempt is made to identify critical problem areas, to describe significant variables and phenomena, and to systematize the extensive subjective data and inconsistent reports which abound in the scientific literature. In the scientific and historical literature, there are over a thousand reports which describe and discuss isolation, disorientation and closely related conditions which have been experienced by explorers, prisoners, patients, pilots, astronauts and volunteers in experiments and flight simulation studies. Since the environment which man encounters during space flight is physiologically hostile, it is necessary that he be confined at all times within a protective capsule, sealed cabin, pressure suit or similar life support system. He must have his own oxygen supply, atmospheric pressure system, environmental control system, food, water, physical restraints and acceleration protection devices. These requirements for physical protection are instrumental in producing the problematic conditions of isolation and disorientation. Even when all instrumentation systems are operating within the spacecraft, the ability of the astronaut to sense gravity, pressure, motion, light, sound and time cues may be unreliable because of disorientation along some of these parameters. This chapter first considers some of the specific problem areas within the general topic of isolation, and then considers problem areas within the topic of disorientation.

Finally, some of the primary procedures for protecting man against the effects of isolation and disorientation during space travel are discussed.

I. ISOLATION

The term *isolation* is used to refer to a large variety of conditions which have the common denominator of separating a person from the significant parts of the environment to which he is accustomed.[7, 17, 37, 75, 100] The parts of one's environment from which the person is isolated may vary in significance for any given person, and they may involve varying degrees of severity, permanence and permeability.[15, 27, 58, 67] Also, they may involve various kinds of barriers, active or passive, internal or external, threatening or non-threatening.[12, 24, 43, 82, 95] During space flight, the astronaut must be confined in a protective capsule or spacecraft, isolated from other people and society. This may result in physical, psychological, emotional or social separation from the astronaut's long-accustomed environment. Since there are many reports which suggest that isolation is one of the primary problems in long-term space travel,[13, 19, 60, 63, 64, 82, 91, 92, 96, 97, 117] investigators have been concerned that prolonged isolation may affect physiological functioning and psychological performance, unless adequate protection is provided. In the sections to follow, this possibility is considered, and problems and research relating to isolation during space flight are reviewed. Inasmuch as isolation is primarily a condition of separation, and confinement is a condition of physical restriction, these two conditions frequently occur together. An astronaut in his spacecraft is both isolated and confined. In most experimental studies, changes in physiology and performance are frequently considered as resulting from the combined effects of isolation and confinement. These two terms, isolation and confinement, are frequently used interchangeably. In this chapter, the term isolation refers to conditions which separate a person from the significant parts of his environment, and terms such as confinement, sensory deprivation, sensory input overload, and earth separation are used to categorize specific isolation problem areas.

1. Methods and Variables in Isolation Research

A review of the scientific literature indicates that there are essentially three basic methods for producing isolation. Although each method has its own characteristics and procedures, these have been used in many different combinations and variations because each refers to a different category of variables. Thus, for any given condition of isolation, there are a set of variables which pertain to the amount of physical confinement. Also, there are a set of variables which refer to the amount and variety of sensory stimulation which the subject is allowed to receive. Finally, there is a set of variables which deals with the amount of separation from other people and objects upon which the isolated person has dependency for the satisfaction of his desires, comforts and needs. The methods used in isolation research deal with these sets of variables, and may be summarized as follows: a) confining the person to a small limited space or container, b) altering the sensory and perceptual stimulation which the person receives so that the stimulation is drastically changed in terms of quantity, quality or variability, and c) separating the person from other people, objects or information upon which he is dependent.

The first method, confinement to a limited space, refers to the restraint of freedom of movement. Freedom of movement is necessarily limited, for example, when a crew of three test pilots is enclosed in a space cabin simulator for 15 days, or an astronaut wearing an inflated pressure suit is secured within his form-fitting contour couch for 24 hr. The second method, altering the sensory and perceptual stimulation, refers to the manipulation of stimuli available to the person, or the manipulation of the person's own ability to sense and perceive available stimuli, to the extent that the effective stimulation is greatly reduced (sensory deprivation), greatly increased (sensory input overload), or greatly changed in pattern or variability (perceptual patterning). The third method, separation from people, objects, or information upon which the person is dependent or attached, refers to separating the person from his normally valued stimuli, such as occurs during geographic isolation, earth separation or social isolation. It is important to emphasize that the factors associated with isolation are very elu- sive, regardless of the methods used in studying them. The effects of isolation are difficult to measure objectively and reliably. The significant stimulus events, responses, and mechanisms of action are obscure. Their effects are frequently subtle, inconsistent in severity, irregular in occurrence, changeable in quality and highly dependent upon complex variables such as sensory and perceptual sensitivity, personality structure, emotional stability, suggestion and prior experience. Phenomena which occur as a result of iso- lation are disrupted by the presence of an observer or by scientific apparatus, thus making their study very difficult.

Early experiments demonstrated that animals reared in isolation and deprived of their normal sensory cues showed: a) defective sensory development, b) perceptual abnormalities, c) absence of startle and blink reflexes, d) emotional instability, e) inability to respond appropriately to other animals, and f) many peculiar social behavior patterns. Similarly, extreme changes in human behavior have been observed in people who have been isolated for prolonged periods of time, as reported by explorers and ship- wrecked sailors, prisoners in solitary confinement and in concen- tration camps, hospitalized patients, isolated small groups at the Arctic and Antarctic, and curious scientists and philosophers who have isolated themselves in caves and dungeons for prolonged periods of time.[12, 37, 43, 95, 99, 100] The primary symptoms which have been reported are: a) perceptual distortions, b) vivid im- agery and visual illusions, c) bizarre hallucinations, d) dramatic changes in attitude and temperament, e) marked changes in moti- vation, f) extensive emotional reactions and g) deterioration in ability to remember, think and reason.

More recent laboratory experimentation has concentrated on the problem of measuring the effects of isolation by confining a person within a small space, separating him from other people and objects upon which he is dependent, and then systematically altering the sensory and perceptual stimulation which is presented to the isolated person. The term *sensory alteration* is frequently used to describe the general range of conditions which produce changes in the functioning of sensory modalities during isolation. Recent laboratory experiments have reported that even for relatively short periods of time, isolation under these conditions disturbs normal, healthy, well-nourished human subjects. Bexton et al.[7] and Heron et al.[67] demonstrated that following exposure to reduced sensory stimulation during isolation, human subjects showed deficits in visual performance as well as symptoms of emotional irritability and confusion. Vernon et al.[107, 108] demonstrated marked effects of isolation on visual hallucinations and on the performance of certain perceptual and motor skills. Mitchell[82] reported that pilots could not maintain accurate time estimation skills during isolation periods of two days in length. Lilly[74] and Lilly et al.[75] showed that the reduction of sensory inputs during isolation and perceptual disorientation leads to psychotic states in normal, healthy men. Doane et al.[31] found a marked persistence of perceptual effects of four days of isolation, even after the isolation period was terminated. Actually, sensory alteration includes a spectrum of conditions ranging from extreme sensory deprivation to sensory overload. Sensory deprivation refers to a condition in which the amount of sensory input is less than that which is required for normal physiological and psychological functioning, whereas sensory overload refers to a condition in which the isolated person receives so much sensory stimulation that normal functioning is impaired. For example, one of the experimental procedures for achieving extreme sensory deprivation is to require the subject to lie isolated for prolonged periods of time with his body encased in a tightly-fitted restrictive container, devoid of all visual, auditory and motion stimulation. On the other hand, a procedure for achieving extreme sensory overload is to require the subject to sense and respond to stimuli which occur in quantities and frequencies too great to permit satisfactory perception and response.

Whereas isolation is frequently regarded as pertaining to one person isolated from other people and familiar objects, there are many cases in which small groups have been isolated. The condition of isolation of small groups has been vividly described by Byrd (1938, page 16), for example, in which he indicated that even the little things of life have the power to drive disciplined men to the edge of insanity. Since these early observations, studies on the behavior of small isolated groups[29, 91, 92, 95, 111] have shown personality, motivational and attitudinal changes in individuals, as well as marked changes in group social structure. Within small isolated groups, it has been found that there are three periods of adjustment: a) the heightened anxiety during the very initial period of isolation, b) the period of adjustment involved in "settling down" to the prolonged period of isolation, and c) the anticipation which occurs when the crew is preparing to terminate the isolation period.

A review of the methods and variables used in isolation research indicates that there are many categories of isolation, and the categorization of isolation exposures is primarily dependent upon the portion of one's normal environment from which he is separated. Thus, *perceptual isolation*[43, 68, 108] refers to separation from one's normal sensory and perceptual environment. *Social isolation*[29, 85, 92] refers to separation from other people and from society, whereas *cultural isolation*[95] refers to separation from one's own culture, such as being in the midst of an alien cultural environment. *Loneliness, aloneness and solitude*[75] are sometimes used to describe the psychological feeling of being separated from other people. *Psychological detachment*[19, 97, 98] is also used to describe the psychological subjective aspects of being isolated. *Earth separation*[89, 98] or *break-off*,[24, 41, 96, 97] refers to the feeling of being isolated from the earth, as sometimes occurs when flying at an extremely high altitude with respect to earth. *Geographic isolation*,[12, 72, 95] however refers to being at some far-away remote location. *Sensory alteration, perceptual alteration,*[31, 44, 70] *sensory deprivation,*[13, 30, 73, 99, 100] *sleep deprivation,*[76, 84] *fascination,*[26] and *sensory overload*[81] refer to isolation conditions in which a person is exposed to marked changes in the quantity and variety of sensory inputs. These are discussed in detail in later sections of this chapter. In isolation research, the type of isolation being studied frequently designates the primary variables being manipulated.

Any of the above categories of isolation, as experienced by normal healthy men, produces complex symptoms. These are mostly subjective, although some performance symptoms also occur. Time itself is capable of modifying all of the responses to isolation. The imposition of additional stresses, such as hunger, thirst, physical discomforts, injury or threat, greatly intensifies subjective responses to isolation. The symptoms which occur appear to be largely dependent upon the interaction of isolation with other concurrent stresses. However, the degree and rate of development of symptoms appears to be directly related to the intensity, complexity and duration of the individual isolation exposure. Through laboratory experimentation, space equivalence studies, flight simulations and the telemetering of physiological and psychological data during in-flight space operations, it has been possible to study some of the primary variables and their combinations. Some of the most important variables may be summarized as follows:

a) Type (category) of isolation exposure.
b) Size and shape of the confinement chamber.
c) Degree of restriction of movement.
d) Duration of confinement.
e) Social environment, including number of crew members.
f) Voice and visual contact with ground station personnel.
g) Physical condition of the isolated person.
h) Amount of sensory deprivation and/or sensory overload.
i) Intensities of sensory stimuli.
j) Response requirements and their relationship to mission success.
k) Variability and redundancy of sensory stimuli and response requirements.
l) Work-rest ratios, fatigue and boredom.
m) Interactions with physical stresses, such as lack of food, water or air.
n) Interactions with psychological stresses. such as fear, anxiety, aggravation.
o) Interactions with extreme environmental stresses, such as high temperature, noxious gases, vibrations, high accelerations and noise.
p) Motivation and interest.
q) Crew structure and social organization.
r) Personality, temperament and emotional stability.
s) Prior experience and training.

A detailed review of many of the reports concerning isolation and closely related topics indicates that the psychological variables are generally more influential than the physiological ones in altering the severity of any given isolation exposure. If there are tasks which keep the isolated person occupied and in contact with other people via voice or television, for example, many of the phenomena which ordinarily occur during isolation may be avoided.

There is a very close temporal correspondence between the absence of an externally initiated task and the onset of performance decrement. In the space flights accomplished to date by the Mercury astronauts,[120, 121, 123, 124] and the Vostok Cosmonauts, no severe effects of isolation have been reported. It is believed that the voice communications with ground personnel, visual contact with earth and other planets, use of visual instrument displays, carefully planned work schedules, and extensive prior training, minimized the effects of isolation. In these flights, the duration of the isolation was relatively short compared with many of the experimental studies which have been conducted to date. Also, during the space flights themselves, there were so many interactions with other conditions of space travel that the accurate evaluation of subtle isolation effects per se was not possible.

2. Results of Isolation and Confinement Studies

The most frequent means of producing isolation is that of physical confinement. The term confinement is usually used to refer to a large category of conditions which restrict the move-ment of an individual or individuals within specific physical limits.[17, 66, 85] Confinement during space flight is a necessary condition in order to protect the astronaut from the physiologically hostile space environment. In order to study the effects of confinement, the general approach has been to put human subjects in small restrictive containers, such as space cabin simulators, sealed pressure chambers, isolation booths, water tanks, pressure suits, balloon gondolas, aircraft compartments and spacecraft. The physiological and psychological responses are then measured during experimental lengths of confinement time.

Laboratory experiments on the effects of prolonged confinement have reported decrements in psychomotor skill performance, memory, judgment and learning ability. In some of these experiments involving over 20 hr of continuous work during confinement, dramatic and bizarre sensory aberrations, hallucinations, motivational and emotional changes have been reported. In studies reported by Hauty and his associates,[64-66, 103] men were required to sit in an aircraft-type seat isolated and confined within a space cabin simulator and attend a small perceptual field of work. The degree of physical confinement was approximately 46 cu ft. Constant atmospheric pressure, with appropriate oxygen tension levels, and experimental control of the diurnal cycling of work and sleep, with commitments to schedules of attentive and meaningful task requirements, were provided. When subjects were required to attend intensively to their work for as long as 36 hr, perceptual aberrations, such as vivid visual images and hallucinations resulted. Primary tasks were to monitor indicators and take corrective action whenever the indicators departed from their null positions. However, spatial discrimination, perceptual judgment, vigilance and problem solving have been studied in these experiments, using confinement times which have ranged from 30 hr to seven days. In one experiment, Hauty[65] verified that proficiency cannot be maintained much beyond 20 hr during conditions of continuous performance without rest. It has been generally assumed that aberrant behavior during confinement does not begin to occur in most subjects until at least 12 hr of attention is required. In an experiment in which this time was more than doubled (30 hr), the pilots thought that the instruments assumed strange appearances, and they experienced false perceptions, proprioceptive illusions and imaginary sounds. However, the pilots recognized these as being false, and they were also aware that they were deleterious to performance of their tasks.

Monotonous and unvarying environments, prolonged commitments to exacting duties and requirements for continued monitoring and alertness in the event of malfunctioning equipment, are characteristics of confinement which pose a constant threat to any prolonged space flight. These conditions lead to boredom and fatigue, which are considered to be among the most serious problems in maintaining performance reliability during manned flight.[64] Steinkamp *et al.*[103] showed that four pilots maintained their proficiency when using a working schedule of 4 hr on and 4 hr off, as contrasted with pilots who worked for longer periods. Skill in vigilance and monitoring has been found to be very susceptible to fatigue effects,[63] and fatigue has been found to be largely dependent upon task characteristics such as speed and load stress. Confinement always includes some limitations of sensory stimuli and psychomotor responses, and the restraints which are placed on the pilot limit his normal kinesthetic, tactual, proprioceptive, visual and auditory inputs. The resulting stimulus and response restrictions are instrumental in producing many of the decrements which occur during confinement.[19, 23, 63, 64, 92, 98] Studies by Ormiston and Finkelstein,[86] Ormiston,[85] Holt and Goldberger[68, 70] and Adams[1] have demonstrated that boredom and fatigue may be greatly minimized by the inclusion of appropriate work-rest schedules, realistic flight tasks, and communications tasks. These studies have involved confinement times from 8 hr to seven days. Chiles and Adams[23] have pointed out that diurnal variations, or physiological cycling during confinement also produces some of the problems for manned space flight. From birth on, each person develops and maintains a 24-hr rhythm of sleep and wakefulness. Along with this rhythm is a concomitant fluctuation of alertness and efficiency of performance, as well as in body temperature and several other physiological parameters. For any prolonged flight extending over many days, information on physiological cycling must be applied to the handling of problems of space travel. Data are needed concerning cycle lengths longer than the 24 hr day, and experimentation is needed on cycles of activity which are longer than 24-hr duty cycles.

Personality and emotional patterns during prolonged confinement have been very difficult to measure objectively, although subjective reports and subtle behaviors by confined subjects indicate that irritability and hostility do occur. For example, a subject who was confined in a space-cabin simulator for a period of seven days[64] gradually became increasingly irritable, until he finally became openly hostile. Also, whereas the subject began his confinement with an efficient system of work, housekeeping, eating, toiletry, recreation and sleep, his behavior deteriorated to the minimal essentials for working, eating and sleeping as time progressed. Ormiston[86] using a battery of personality tests in an attempt to measure the amount of correlation between personality and other reactions to confinement, confined sixty subjects sitting singly for 8 hr in an aircraft seat located in a 5 by $8^{1}/_{2}$ ft lighted cubicle. He was not able to measure any significant personality changes. Subtle but obvious discomforts and aggravations occur during long-term confinement in water during the simulation of weightlessness. Beckman *et al.*,[4] Benson *et al.*,[6] Chambers *et al.*,[21] and Graveline *et al.*[45] have subjected human subjects to prolonged water immersion ranging from 12 hr to seven days. Discomfort, malfunction of equipment, confinement, and fatigue produced temporary hostilities and emotional aberrations in some subjects.

The problem of aggravation has been demonstrated many times during periods in which the Mercury astronauts and other volunteer subjects were exposed to as much as 12 hr confinement for testing and training in the human centrifuge. In these simulation studies, the astronauts and volunteer subjects were sometimes strapped in contour couches, confined within their pressure suits, placed within the gondola of the centrifuge, and presented with realistic pre-flight tasks, monitoring requirements and communications. After 1 to 2 hr prelaunch wait, they went through accelerations expected on the Atlas rocket, and spent approximately $4^1/_2$ hr in simulated orbital flight. This was followed by re-entry acceleration and egress, or sometimes, repeated centrifuge practice runs.[16-20] Variables other than acceleration itself were more stressing. Pressure points, muscle cramps and pains due to the pilot's restraint system, uncomfortable temperature and closing system, failure of the urinary bag, discomfort due to the biomedical sensors or specific flight gear, or unexplained delays or equipment malfunction, have created conditions reported to be extremely aggravating and sometimes disturbing. However, extensive personality, biochemical, performance and physiological tests conducted before, during and after these exposures, have not shown any significant personality or emotional effects. Since these are observed overtly, but not measured by means of quantitative tests, it is generally concluded that the tests are not themselves sensitive enough to measure the subtle personality effects, even if they do occur.

A similar problem exists with respect to measuring the effects of confinement on higher mental abilities. There is little quantitative evidence regarding the direct effects of confinement on higher mental abilities, except for those which appear to result secondarily from fatigue, boredom or anxiety. Many scientists have called attention to the severity of this problem, as suggested from studies conducted in high altitude balloons,[41, 89, 90, 97, 98, 119] space cabin simulators,[34, 37, 64, 69, 77] space platform simulations,[25, 27, 52, 56] weightlessness simulations,[4, 6, 21, 45] and during space flight.[122-124] Ormiston and Finkelstein[86] confined twenty subjects individually in a small capsule for 48 hr in order to measure the effects of confinement on intellectual functioning. They found no significant decrements on ability to solve arithmetic problems, verbal analogies, same-opposite word meanings or logical reasoning problems. Similarly, there were no significant effects on digit memory and ability to learn nonsense syllables. Mitchell[82] found significant effects of two-day confinement periods on time estimation ability, however.

The high altitude balloon flights have yielded valuable data regarding the effects of prolonged confinement during exposure to hazardous conditions. To date, there have been 18 manned balloon flights. In the 1957 Manhigh II balloon flight, the gondola, which carried Colonel David Simons,[98] was aloft for 32 hr, and it reached over 100,000 ft altitude. In the 1958 Strato-Lab #3, Commander Ross and Commander Lewis[89] achieved an altitude of 82,000 ft and were aloft for 34 hr and 40 min. Lt. McClure, in Manhigh III, was aloft for 12 hr, part of which was at an altitude of over 100,000 ft. This flight, which was conducted in 1958[119] had been preceded by extensive ground based simulations. In 1961, Ross and Prather reached 114,000 ft. in Strato-Lab #5. In these flights there have been a number of differences reported between the ground-based chamber runs and the actual flights. During the balloon flights the pilots experienced a much greater challenge to be alert, to detect new phenomena and to make observations. They were extremely busy, and experienced a sense of pressure and urgency at all times. They were also acutely aware that they were isolated from other people. Whereas during their ground-based control tests, they were frequently restless and impatient, bored, sleepy and aware that they were within immediate assistance and aid, if needed. Comparisons between static ground-based tests and high altitude balloon flights have lead some to conclude that isolation at high altitude, associated with a feeling of earth separation poses major problems for prolonged space flight.[41, 89-91, 96-98, 119]

Available evidence indicates that there are several types of degradation which occur to performance during prolonged isolation and confinement. These are concerned primarily with skill performance proficiency, and they may be measured quantitatively.[17, 18, 20, 33, 63, 66, 81, 107, 116] During prolonged performance one of the primary characteristics as time progresses is an increasing unevenness and irregularity, sometimes called *lapses*. These are temporary decrements which occur for short periods of time during a prolonged time interval. They are possibly related to "microsleeps." Another characteristic of performance during prolonged confinement is that of *approximation*. Although the task does not increase in difficulty level, the subject's behavior becomes less precise, but remains minimally adequate to meet the required criterion of performance proficiency. The subject appears to approximate his performance rather than perform with the accuracy with which he is capable. A third characteristic is *stereotyping* of responses. Regardless of the stimulus situation, the subject has a tendency to make similar responses to all stimuli, and all stimuli appear to have an equivalent value to the subject, in that he performs the same way to all of them. This condition is related to an *increased range of indifference*, or a tendency for the subject to perceive the stimuli as appearing less different than they would under normal work conditions. Another characteristic of performance during prolonged confinement is a systematic *filtering* of certain categories of stimuli, according to some subjective priority scheme. The subject appears to purposely select some stimuli, and omit others, in performing his task. Related to this is the tendency for *response omission*, or the apparent purposeful omission, reduction or cessation of portions of the total task to be performed. *Queuing*, or delaying making certain responses which should be made during peak loads, and relaying them at later times when the work-load is reduced, is a seventh characteristic of performance decrement during confinement. Other characteristics which are typical of performance during confinement, and during other conditions also, are: increased latency of response, increased error amplitudes, and errors in retrieving and processing information. It should be noted that all of the above error characteristics are likely to pass unnoticed during a prolonged isolation and confinement situation, unless special provisions are made for measuring and recording them. They are highly variable, difficult to measure and very sensitive to changes in the test conditions.

It should be emphasized that the condition of confinement itself does not necessarily involve adverse or harmful effects upon man. Men who have been carefully selected and trained may endure short periods of confinement without measurable physiological or psychological effects. This has been shown for the American astronauts as well as for the Soviet cosmonauts, who have made space flights to date. Commander Shepard, for example, was confined a total of 4 hr and 29 min in his Freedom 7 Mercury Capsule on the day of his Mercury-Redstone suborbital flight. Of this time, 15 min and 22 sec were spent in flight.[120] No significant effects were shown for Shepard's flight, nor for Major Grissom's similar Mercury-Redstone suborbital flight.[120, 121] Colonel John H. Glenn, Jr., was confined a total of 8 hr and 36 min in his Friendship 7 Capsule the day of his Mercury-Atlas orbital flight,[123] 4 hr and 55 min of which occurred during flight. Similar confinement conditions have been received by Commander Carpenter and Commander Schirra, who performed Mercury orbital flights. No adverse effects of the confinement or of the isolation were reported.[123, 124] Preliminary information from the four single manned Soviet Vostok space flights have also suggested that there were no adverse effects of confinement and isolation during space flights, even for longer periods of time. Whether flights lasting longer than four days will result in adverse physiological and psychological effects is unknown. Most of the data pertaining to the possible effects of prolonged space flight beyond four days duration have been obtained from studies conducted in space cabin simulators within laboratory environments.

Data from ground based space cabin simulators must be regarded with caution when attempting to generalize to space flight
conditions.[17, 21, 56, 63, 85, 111, 123]   There are major differences between laboratory confinement conditions and those of space flight.
The men who have been selected for participation in simulation
studies have not been as carefully selected, nor as well trained, as
have the men who have been selected for space flight missions.
Finally, the astronauts themselves have not been available to serve
as subjects in simulation studies and experiments involving prolonged isolation.   It is generally assumed that the men selected for
space flight will be less susceptible to adverse effects of prolonged
confinement and isolation than the men who have served in simulation experiments.   Consequently, given appropriate selection
and training prior to flight, and appropriate work-rest schedules,
protective equipment, communications, and activities during
flight, an astronaut would not be expected to encounter the effects
of isolation which have been reported for isolation simulations and
experiments.[15, 30, 43, 64, 67, 74, 92, 103, 107, 108, 119]

For prolonged space flights, involving isolation and confinement for time periods longer than those accomplished to date
by the American and Soviet astronauts and cosmonauts, it is
planned that crews, rather than individuals flying singly, will
make these attempts.   Some of the problems involving the isolation of small groups and crews are reviewed in the next section.

3. Isolation of Small Groups and Crews

Results of recent research suggest that appropriately selected
and well trained crews of astronauts will be able to tolerate, compensate for and overcome the psychological problems which may
otherwise arise during an extended multi-manned flight into
space.   This assumes that the crews are provided with appropriate protection from the hostile space environment, and that
they have ample food and water, adequate gaseous atmosphere,
exercises and activities and performance tasks which are essential
to the success of the mission.   In Project Gemini, crews of two
astronauts will be confined for time periods up to seven days
during prolonged orbital flying around the earth, and in Project

Apollo, crews of three astronauts will be confined for time periods up to possibly 15 days during space flight in the vicinity of the moon. Simulations of prolonged space flight exceeding these time periods for isolation and confinement have been successfully completed at the USAF School of Aviation Medicine, at the USAF Aerospace Medical Laboratory, at the USN School of Aviation Medicine and at several industrial laboratories.

In recent studies at the USAF School of Aviation Medicine, for example, men in groups of two were confined for 17 days and for 30 days in a two man space cabin simulator.[34, 77, 83, 88] The 30-day flight simulation was at an altitude pressure of 18,000 ft with 40 per cent oxygen and 60 per cent nitrogen atmosphere. The 17-day flight was at an altitude pressure of 33,000 ft with essentially 100 per cent oxygen atmosphere. The subjects performed on an operator control system which consisted of 14 tasks designed to measure monitoring, vigilance and information processing skills. In addition, objective and projective psychological tests were administered to the subjects before and after confinement. During the period of confinement, a gradual increase in average response time occurred, and there were indications of reduced motivation levels among the pilots. Although there was relatively little boredom during the confinement period (due to the inclusion of scheduled work-rest cycles, realistic activities and tasks, and communications throughout), and crew morale was high throughout, there were some feelings of resentment and disharmony, and some evidence that individual personality characteristics affected crew interactions. There was no evidence of gross perceptual aberrations. There were no physiological or psychological problems which were considered to be serious enough to impair the success of simulated space flight.

Other studies[1, 23, 36, 37, 43, 44, 69, 70, 85, 95] have shown somewhat similar findings. Recently, six men were confined[11, 61, 62] in approximately 450 cu ft of space in an altitude chamber which maintained atmospheric pressure at approximately 10,000 ft. Two experiments, one for 6 days confinement, and one for 8 days confinement, were conducted. A comprehensive battery of personality tests was administered before and after confinement.

During confinement, tasks such as time estimation, multiple solution problem solving and auditory tracking, were administered. No permanent personality effects were observed in these studies. No effects directly attributable to confinement were observed. In the 8-day confinement study, an emergency situation was introduced on the fifth day. This resulted in significant changes in heart rate, respiration rate, forehead skin temperature, plantar electrical skin conductance and urinary norepinephrine excretion. However, it was concluded that these changes were due to the anxiety provoking stimuli, rather than to confinement and isolation per se. Marked hostility and aggression on the part of the crew members appeared on the sixth and seventh days of confinement, and some effects were noted on social interaction and psychomotor performance. However, the anxiety and the emergency simulation produced these effects.

The presence of danger or hazard during confinement greatly enhances performance and emotional changes. Ross and Lewis[90] while at high altitude in a balloon gondola, refer to extreme aggravation, resulting from the prolonged confinement. They describe it as bordering on personally-directed disgust, resulting from the litter which rapidly accumulated on the cabin floor because of inadequate provision for storage. Simons[97] indicated similar problems while confined at high altitude in a balloon capsule. For example, he felt almost too tired and uncomfortable to make an effort required to put on a thermal suit. This was difficult because of the restricted motion within the 3 ft diam instrument-packed capsule in which he was isolated. The situation was aggravated by the inherent restrictiveness of the partial pressure suit and was complicated further by the necessity of always moving slowly and gently in order to avoid sending mechanical shocks to the brittle balloon which supported the gondola in flight.

That long-term confinement can be tolerated by men in small groups was recently demonstrated by Adams and Chiles[1] who confined B-52 combat-ready crews for 15 days, using several work-rest schedules in the operation of the flight requirements. Their study showed that with proper control of selection and motivational factors, crews would work effectively for periods of at least two weeks and possibly longer, using a four-on and a two-off work-rest schedule. In submarine operations, such as during the transpolar cruise of the submarine Nautilus,[72] it has been demonstrated that men can endure prolonged hazard and confinement provided that appropriate work-rest schedules and activities are provided. In one of the early studies within submarines, Kinsey[72] reported that ideal temperature, humidity, oxygen and carbon dioxide mixtures, fresh water, excellent food, reading and music, games and tournaments and incentive awards were very important. These studies have demonstrated that habituation and conditioning prior to embarkation, as well as providing ties with familiar events and surroundings, are helpful in alleviating the effects of prolonged isolation and confinement. Ruff[91] has suggested that space crews should be provided with as much duplication of earth experience and surroundings as is possible during space flights. The importance of these principles is illustrated in the next two sections in which extreme sensory deprivation and sensory overload are presented to isolated subjects, and in which severe effects on men are observed.

4. Sensory Deprivation

Isolation and confinement problem areas have been largely concerned with the effects of changed environmental stimulation on physiology and behavior. A problem area of major importance is that of *sensory deprivation*. Sensory deprivation consists of a reduction of the totality of stimulation available to the isolated individual, as by reducing the variability, variety or intensity of either specific or nonspecific arousal stimuli. It may vary quantitatively and qualitatively along several continua. It is a phenomenon of isolation to the extent that the individual is separated from his normal environmental cues and sources of information. Sensory deprivation refers to a condition in which the amount of sensory input is less than that which is required for normal physiological and psychological functioning. It does not mean the complete absence of sensory information, merely an insufficient quantity and variety.

There are four major methods which have been used to reduce environmental input to an isolated person: a) absolute reduction of the amount, intensity and variety of sensory stimulation, b) reduced patterning of sensory input, c) the imposition of structure or monotony on the sensory environment without reducing the amount of stimulation and d) reduction of the sensory conduction within the body. These methods have been thoroughly reviewed.[13, 17, 30, 43, 73, 74, 99, 107 and 115]

The method of absolute reduction of sensory stimulation is typified in experiments by Lilly[74] and Lilly and Shurley.[75] They placed each subject in a 34.5°C water-tank located in a sound-proof isolation chamber. Each subject was immersed nude except for a blacked-out form-fitted face mask from which he breathed. This produced a marked reduction in the amount and variety of stimulation available to the isolated subject, by attenuating external physical stimuli at a low level, and accomplishing isothermicity and buoyancy. The second method, the method of reduced patterning of sensory input to a sensory modality, is exemplified by the "ganzfeld" procedure, in which isolated subjects wore eye-cups over the eye, producing a homogeneous visual field.[37, 43, 44, 108] Examples of imposing structure or monotony of the sensory environment are illustrated by Bexton *et al.*[7] in which subjects wearing translucent goggles, cardboard arm-cuffs, and gloves were each placed in small sound-proof cubicles in an attempt to decrease the variation in tactual and visual stimulation. Solomon [(100)] and Heron *et al.*[67] have conducted similar studies. Whereas the above three methods involve manipulation of the external stimulation to the subject, the fourth method involves reduction of sensory conduction *within* the body. To do this, certain drugs such as seryl, mescaline, and LSD-25 have been used.[44, 100] Through the use of drugs such as these, an attempt is made to reduce the sensory conduction within the body without changing the external stimulus conditions.

The early development of the concept of sensory deprivation took place at McGill University, with the publication of a report by Bexton *et al.*[7] on the effects of decreased variation in the sensory environment on twenty-two isolated male college students. These students, wearing translucent goggles, and cardboard cuffs and gloves, were isolated for two days in a partially sound-proof test cubicle. Disturbances in vision, usually lasting not more than 2 min at a time and consisting mostly of difficulty in focusing and in maintaining visual acuity, were among the symptoms produced. The subjects were restless, unable to concentrate on a topic for very long, experiencing "blank" periods, fatigue, confusion, headaches and mild nausea.

Later experiments conducted in anechoic chambers showed that even 3 hr confinement could produce severe symptoms.[110] In a study of 12 college students, experimental sensory deprivation produced a breakdown in adaptive behavior, panic and attempts to escape. Cameron *et al.*,[13] who studied rigorous and sustained reduction in sensory input for periods up to 16 days, found that individuals who are customarily self-contained and self-dependent were capable of withstanding the effects of sensory deprivation better than were highly sociable and dependent persons. Wexler *et al.*[114] exposed 17 male volunteers to sensory deprivation through the use of a tank-type respirator for periods up to 36 hr. All subjects showed impairment in ability to concentrate, distortions in time judgment, pseudosomatic delusions, illusions, hallucinations and intense anxiety reactions.

Several investigations have reported gross distortion of visual perception after sensory deprivation.[31, 37, 43, 67, 73, 108] The wearing of translucent eye cups, thereby producing a limited form of sensory deprivation, has been observed to bring about vivid imagery. In these experiments, two eye-cups consisting of halved ping-pong balls or some similar material, were glued over the subject's eyes. The effects of this have been exhaustively studied for periods of time ranging from 40 min to 8 hr,[44] and visual imagery has been observed in both extremes. Freedman,[36] in a study of perceptual lag, showed that serious distortions in speed of visual perception developed within $1/2$ hr.

Human subjects, when exposed to an environment in which visual, auditory, tactile and kinesthetic sensations are greatly reduced, experience a large variety of personality and emotional disturbances, ranging from chronic anxiety and oppression to illusory experiences and fantasies. Subjects become very irritable, show exaggerated responses to stimuli, and report many types of hallucinations. Relationships of objects within the visual field appear to change, and kinesthetic sensations are distorted. Even for short periods of time, sensory deprivation may produce inaccuracies in tactual and spatial orientation. After 24 hr, illusions of illumination, color, geometry and animation are frequent. Effects on intellectual abilities have been difficult to measure, although subjects report deterioration in learning ability and ability to solve problems. Marked motivational changes are also noted. Physiologically, changes in autonomic indices have generally paralleled behavioral manifestations of anxiety and fear. In animals which have been exposed to extreme sensory deprivation, marked effects on weight and physical resistance to disease have been demonstrated.

The fundamental determinants of these effects are unclear, largely due to the lack of appropriate measurement devices. Cameron *et al.*[13] have shown that individuals tend to take active measures to protect themselves against the disturbing effects of the reduction of sensory input. Four types of defense mechanisms are frequently observed: a) maintaining sensory input by drawing upon one's inner world of memory, imagination and creative thinking, b) maintaining sensory input by purposeless movements and muscular activity, c) increasing the sensory sensitivity and perceptiveness in all sensory modalities, and d) developing intense anxiety, aggression, or fear, to the extent that it is necessary to remove the individual from the sensory deprivation exposure. Lilly and Shurley[75] have concluded that the nervous system has sources of "new information" from "within," and that these are experienced as though they were from "without." The sensory deprived person may utilize these "new sources of information" in an integrative and constructive way. It is not the mere quantitative reduction of sensory input which is the major factor in the behavioral aberrations evidenced in sensory deprivation situations, but also the quality and the meaningful nature of these inputs. Davis *et al.*[30] observed that random visual stimulation was not sufficient to prevent the occurrence of aberrations, and concluded that meaningful contact from the outside world is essential for normal functioning. None of the experiments has succeeded in defining the parameters of stimulation during sensory deprivation. It is the absence of meaningful stimulation which produces the effects, and this has been extremely difficult to measure quantitatively. The utilization of physiological apparatus itself introduces problems of methodology and experimental design which obscures the measurement of the phenomena.

The primary aspect of sensory deprivation which poses a problem during space flight is the narrowing of the variability and variety of sensory stimulation available to the astronaut. During space flight, the interior of the spacecraft may become repetitious, undifferentiated, monotonous and boring. Mental alertness depends to a large extent on having a variety of sensory stimuli, and when the level of stimulation is drastically reduced, a loss of mental efficiency occurs. Providing some variety in the nature of the tasks to be performed and also some variety in the stimulation provided by cockpit instruments and ground communications will minimize this. To date, the space flights of the Mercury Astronauts have revealed no problems concerning sensory deprivation.[102, 120, 121, 123, 124] However, longer flights in the future may be expected to produce sensory deprivation problems unless adequate protective measures are assured. Ruff[92] indicates that the mere awareness of the ways in which isolation during a prolonged space flight may interfere with the gratification of human needs may itself be an effect of major significance. These needs may concern drive satisfaction, such as hunger, thirst, survival, sex or the need for the presence of other people. According to Ruff,[92] if these needs are not gratified, or if the space traveler is uncertain that they will be gratified, the reactions may be ones of frustration, apprehension, anxiety and performance decrement.

5. Sensory Input Overload

The possibility of excessive sensory stimulation during isolation poses problems to the astronaut under conditions of prolonged space flight. During certain critical maneuvers, the astronaut may be overloaded with the necessity of monitoring, selecting and responding to excessive information presented on his instrument panel, periscope, spacecraft window, environmental control system panel and earphones. Sometimes the terms "high workload stress" and "speed-stress" are used to describe the conditions resulting from sensory overload.[63] The astronaut may become overloaded with the necessity of perceiving and responding. He may be unable to process and utilize information as quickly and efficiently as may be required during critical maneuvers or emergency operations in space. Overload could be a serious hazard, for it results not only in performance decrement, but also in personality and emotional impairment. Sensory overload to the astronaut would result in consequent physiological and performance impairment,[17, 33, 66, 80, 81] for during exposure to this condition, he may be unable to process information adequately, and consequently unable to perform psychomotor and monitoring tasks appropriately.

For the astronaut confronted with the necessity of maneuvering his vehicle, there are doubtless certain rates of sensory input transmission which are most efficient. Some of the most thorough work on sensory overload has been done by Miller,[80, 81] using an information overload testing apparatus. He found that the maximum channel capacity of individual subjects was between six and seven bits of information per second. These rates change as a function of the number of components in each channel of information, the number of persons involved, and the condition of the person. For situations involving a high task load, the operator is limited by a built-in ceiling in his ability to integrate and organize and respond to a sequence of events. This limit is somewhat constant, and performance impairment begins to occur as soon as the operator's maximum capacity is reached.[63] This decrement is sometimes expressed as fatigue, drowsiness, anxiety and general reduction in the precision of performance. The effects of information overload may be expressed in many ways, some of which have been discussed in Section 2, Isolation and Confinement studies, of this chapter. One of the most important of these is *omission*, in which the pilot does not utilize all of the information which is available to him. Another is that of *filtering*, in which the pilot selects certain categories of sensory input and information, even though he should use all categories. The effects of information overload (or sensory input overload) may also be seen in the process of *approximation*, in which the pilot gives an approximate guess, rather than a precise response. Sometimes, the pilot delays responses during peak loads, with the hope of catching up on them during lulls. This has frequently been called *queuing*.[81] Finally, the pilot may simply *escape*, which involves leaving the situation entirely, or, effectively stopping the flow of sensory input.

These overt behaviors are sometimes used as expressions of information overload. They pose special problems when the subject is required to maintain prolonged concentration and attention. During prolonged flight, the astronaut may be required to detect many signals which have very low attention value, some of which may occur infrequently over a long period of time. In a review of over 80 experimental papers, it was found that vigilance generally dropped within the first half hour. Then it stabilizes within a few hours, and then becomes very unreliable. The astronaut, confined in his spacecraft for long periods of time, must remain vigilant and active. His ability to resist the associated performance decrements which occur during sensory input overload will depend heavily on the training which he has received,[102, 122] how well he has been selected,[117] and upon his endurance within specific flight missions in which he may encounter the information overload problem.

6. Sleep Deprivation

Closely related to the problem of sensory deprivation and sensory overload during prolonged isolation and confinement is the problem of *sleep deprivation*. When produced experimentally, sleep deprivation is sometimes called prolonged wakefulness. Sleep deprivation, if prolonged, is characterized by extensive physiological and psychological changes, some of which are disorientation, misperceptions, and performance impairments. The condition of sleep deprivation poses a potentially serious problem to the astronaut during prolonged space flight. Although the space flights accomplished to date by the Mercury Astronauts have not been long enough to present sleep deprivation problems,[120, 121, 123, 124] the astronauts who fly in Project Gemini and Project Apollo will encompass sufficient time periods so as to encounter some of the problems of sleep deprivation and possibly insomnia. During prolonged confinement in the Strato-Lab and the Manhigh balloon flights, the problems associated with prolonged wakefulness have already been encountered. [89, 90, 97, 98, 119] Normal mission profiles to distant planets, as well as space flight during malfunctioning and emergency conditions, may require extensive monitoring, vigilance, and wakefulness.

In addition to the application of *tortura insomniae* during the 19th Century, the psychopathological effects of prolonged wakefulness have been studied intensively on confined normal healthy adults during World War II, the Korean conflict, sleep marathon contests, flight simulation studies and laboratory experiments. As early as 1896, the first laboratory observations of the dramatic effects of sleep deprivation during confinement were reported.[87] The effects of sleep deprivation on performance and physiology are gradual and specific. The performance decrements, visual phenomena, disorientation and perceptual distortions which occur during sleep deprivation up through five days are of major scientific interest today.

Studies of prolonged sleep deprivation on normal human subjects have shown some consistent results. Psychomotor performance, as on a rotary pursuit task or a reversed digit writing task, shows decrement after 24 hr. Attention span shortens, and some visual illusions of pattern change and movement occur. The performance deficits have been interpreted within a framework of "lapses" in which a lapse is defined as a "microsleep," lasting from 2 to 3 sec, and accompanied by a brief decline in EEG alpha amplitude and a temporary cutting off of external input. Lapses occur briefly and frequently, and they are disruptive to vigilance and any other ongoing behavior which requires concentration.[113] By the 72nd hr of sleep deprivation, immediate memory and ability to reverse digits drops severely. The loss of peripheral vision and the loss of fine movements of the eyes results in a marked tendency to stare. Visual sensations may include diplopia, illusions and impressions of fog, mist and visual imagery. Task performance decrement continues progressively, although well learned semi-automatic performance is possible for short periods. Attention to external sensory input requires greater sympathetic arousal and mobilization of energy resources, for energy sources appear to be no longer readily available to the sleep deprived subject. By the fourth day of sleep deprivation, relatively severe memory losses occur, and there is a marked stereotyping of motor responses. Misconceptions, disorientation and hallucinations are frequent. Subjects sometimes report feelings of numbness and detachment. The experience of the "hat illusion," or "pressure band effect," is commonly reported by these subjects. There are tingling sensations of the skin, humming and ringing noises in the ears, and decreased sensitivity to discrete stimuli. Stationary objects appear to have rhythmical movements at times, and visual imagery of complex geometric designs occur frequently. At the end of the fifth day, psychotic symptoms appear, gross mental aberrations occur, and prolonged disorientation in terms of time, place, person and one's self is commonly reported. [15, 76, 84, 87, 113, 116] In nearly all of the reported experiments, the "fifth day turning point" has been accompanied by significant biochemical and physiological changes. After the termination of the sleep deprivation period, psychological and physiological after-effects may be present from 7 to 10 days. Even after five days of recovery time, the subtle psychological effects may be undiscerned by the casual observer and indeed by the subject himself.

Calm and regular sleep is essential for maintaining efficient physiological and psychological functioning, especially during prolonged isolation and confinement. Among the most striking effects of sleep deprivation are the misconceptions, disorientations, visual hallucinations and performance decrements. Even after 24 hr of prolonged wakefulness, subtle effects on one's performance and perceptual orientation occur. If these were to occur during space flight, the astronaut would probably be unaware of them and would be unable to remember them clearly. There are many reports that suggest precautions which must be made to

insure sufficient sleep for the astronaut during prolonged flight.
1, 12, 19, 23, 33, 34, 63, 66, 89, 98, 116, 122

7. The "Break-off" Phenomenon—the Feeling of Earth Separation

The term "break-off" has been used frequently to describe a feeling of earth separation sometimes experienced by men confined and isolated at high altitude. The term appears in various ways and connotations, but the most descriptive definition is that given by Clark and Graybiel[24] (p. 121) as "a feeling of physical separation from the earth when piloting an aircraft at high altitude." The break-off phenomenon has been uniquely associated with isolation at high altitude, as illustrated further in the Glossary of the 1958 *Air University Quarterly Review*, page 148: "The occurrence during high altitude flight of the feeling of being totally separated and detached from the earth and human society." Men who have reported "break-off" have characterized it as a feeling of identification with other objects and concepts in space. Some pilots react to this perceived detachment with exhilaration and feelings of omnipotence. Others react with expressions of loneliness and depression. Some pilots report no awareness of the phenomenon or of its symptoms; whereas others report that the phenomenon comes and goes, depending on the conditions of the flight.[24, 41, 89, 96–98] Consequently, whether "break-off" is truly unique to altitude is still a matter of speculation.

The most consistent data regarding this phenomenon has been obtained from subjective reports of pilots during prolonged balloon flights. Ross,[89] Ross and Lewis,[90] and Simons,[97] who have experienced high altitude balloon flights and a number of control tests at sea level in sealed cabins, report that the phenomenon is truly unique to high altitude. They indicate that break-off will be difficult, if not impossible, to simulate at sea level conditions. Ross[89] described the experience as follows (p. 331): "Again . . . the psychological reactions of earth separation was experienced. . . . It was a sense of being physically, and almost spiritually, completely detached from earth. It was not fear, nor depression, but probably more akin to exhilaration and of wanting to fly on." Earlier, Ross and Lewis[90] described the experience as a strange sensation of separation from the earth, a sense of remoteness, a feeling of isolation that was always present. Radio contact with colleagues many miles below did nothing to destroy this feeling. In their reports, these authors, as well as Simons[97, 98] have frequently emphasized the sensation of complete detachment from the earth.

Whereas Ross and Lewis experienced this as a crew of two in the Strato-Lab flights, Simons, in his Manhigh II balloon flight[98] wrote a similar account (p. 147): ". . . I experienced a separation of emotional ties and interests from the earth below and felt an identification with the void of space above . . ." Reports similar to these have been written by McClure[119] who ascended to 99,000 ft, and by Ross and Prather who rose to 114,000 ft.

Pilots of jet aircraft have also reported the break off phenomenon.[5, 24, 41, 96] Bennett[5] reported that this usually occurs when the pilot is flying straight and level, when he is relatively inactive, when he has only slight changes in his instrument readings when he has a relatively constant view outside, and when he receives steady and monotonous auditory stimulation. Bennett reports that the pilots have subjective feelings of being completely isolated in space, of being in a dream-like state of unreality, of feeling as if going off to sleep although not sleepy. These feelings are attributed to the isolation of the pilot from his normal level of change in perceptual field. Clark and Graybiel[24] report that break-off could be abolished in jet pilots by a return to a lower altitude, by joining up with another plane, or by voluntarily becoming interested in some problem or activity associated with the flight.

Some of the primary precipitating factors are reported to be: a) flying at high altitude, b) flying alone, c) flying with minimum activity required, d) flying for prolonged periods of time, and e) flying with minimum stimulus change.[5, 24, 41, 89, 90, 96-98, 119]

It should be emphasized, however, that the break-off phenomenon has not been reported by Walker and White, each of whom have flown a number of high altitude X-15 flights, nor by Shepard or by Grissom, who flew 15 min suborbital space flights. Neither Glenn nor Carpenter, who orbited the earth for approximately $4^1/_2$ hr, nor Schirra, who orbited the earth for approximately 9 hr, have reported break-off or the feeling of earth separation. Consequently, the significance of the break-off phenomenon is difficult to ascertain, in view of the conflicting evidence which has been presented for space flights, balloon flights and jet aircraft flights.

Whether break-off, or the feeling of earth separation, is a real phenomenon, or whether it is some unique psychological experience, will doubtless remain a mystery for years to come, unless some method other than subjective reporting can be devised for studying its presence or absence or characteristics. In comparative studies in which the same pilots were exposed to prolonged isolation in the same equipment at altitude as on the ground, the effect has been reported by some pilots as being present only at altitude. However, this holds only for some studies involving balloons and aircraft, since none of the spacecraft pilots and astronauts have reported this effect. Similarly, since the men who have flown balloons and jet aircraft while experiencing break-off are different men from those who have been isolated in the Arctic and Antarctic regions, in submarines, and in bathyscaphs in the deep sea, it has not been possible to draw any direct comparisons with respect to break-off and other possible types of isolation experiences. Finally, the possibility exists that the isolated pilot and his crew are highly suggestible to ideas and expectations, some of which may be considered as feelings of break-off and earth separation. Whereas these feelings have been the subject of much discussion and interest in the scientific literature, the possibility that they may occur during prolonged isolation in space does not pose any known significant problems at this time.

8. Fascination and "Freezing"

Fascination is a term used in aviation to describe a state of narrowed attention associated with excessive concentration on one portion of a task to the extent that the pilot fails to respond to other clearly defined portions required in executing the complete piloting task.[3, 26] It is associated with the problem of isolation and confinement, and is especially problematic in situations involving the operation of complex equipment. The pilot fails to respond to certain clearly defined stimulus situations, in spite of the facts that: a) all of the necessary cues are present, b) the pilot is fully aware of these cues, c) he knows the proper responses and procedures, and d) he is experienced in air operations.   A majority of pilots suffer from fascination at one time or another.[3, 26]   It appears to be a condition of heightened attention, accompanied by blocking and by compulsion types of behavior. It is a kind of disorientation in which the pilot perceives a stimulus, but fails to respond.   Since the phenomenon is most likely to occur at times when the consequences are most exciting and the most dangerous, it may take on special significance during prolonged isolation in the hazardous environments of space travel.

Clark *et al.*[26] studied the occurrence of fascination in 725 flight students and instructors.   They found that approximately 90 per cent of this sample had experienced the phenomenon.   Sometimes called fixation, fascination is a term well known to students and their flight instructors.[26]   However, to date, there have been no reports dealing directly with fascination as experienced by astronauts or cosmonauts during space flight.

Fascination does not have a single clear-cut well-defined etiology.   It does involve excessive concentration, prolonged attention, waiting, monitoring and time-sharing during conditions of isolation and work-load stress.   The state of narrowed attention and excessive concentration results in an apparent loss of voluntary control, and an inability to react.   There are four major types of situations in which fascination may occur during confinement in flight.   One is the situation in which the pilot becomes completely engrossed in some aspects of the task and completely disregards other critical tasks.   Another situation is that in which the pilot becomes preoccupied with irrelevant factors which are not directly related to flying, and consequently fails to respond.   A third situation is that in which the pilot clearly preceives the total situation, but takes a detached attitude, and merely observes as a spectator rather than as a participant.   The fourth situation is one in which the pilot may feel magnetic attraction to the task, described as a feeling of being compulsively and helplessly drawn to a particular instrument or target.   In some respect, fascination as experienced by the pilot is similar to the hypnotic effect experienced by the Eskimo seal hunter who, isolated and sitting motionless in his kayak for prolonged periods of time, becomes entirely immobile, appears hypnotized, and, even when an appropriate condition for harpooning presents itself, he is unable to move his arms at the critical moment.

Fascination has been related to a variety of specific variables, such as tenseness, mental blocks, day-dreaming, misinterpreted perceptions and difficulty in shifting attention. It has also been compared with "freezing,"[78] a term which describes the inability to respond during exposure to danger. During "freezing," the pilot is unable to manipulate his controls or to act at all. Another related phenomenon of possible similar origin is "voodoo death." Cannon[14] has reviewed cases of "voodoo death" which occurred during isolation, and has associated these sudden, unaccountable deaths with an attitude of hopelessness. Richter[88] has theorized that "voodoo death" is due to overactivity of the parasympathetic branch of the automomic nervous system.

It is difficult to evaluate the significance of fascination, "freezing," and "voodoo death" during prolonged isolation and confinement conditions. Mebane[78] contends that emotional factors are seldom openly expressed, and consequently they are very difficult to detect. It does appear that as space travel becomes longer and more complex, and as the astronaut is given more direct and immediate control of his spacecraft and its trajectory, the problems of fascination and freezing during prolonged isolation may prove difficult to solve. Whereas there are no reports of these phenom‧ena occurring during American or Soviet space flights accomplished to date, the absence of specific quantitative data does not negate the necessity for providing protection against possible effects of longer exposures.

II. DISORIENTATION

Disorientation refers to a number of psychophysiological conditions in which a person's perceived sensations and frames of reference are at variance with reality in terms of time, position, location, motion or acceleration. Disorientation implies false perceptions, incorrectly sensed cues, and inappropriate responses to sensory stimuli. The conditions of isolation are very conducive to disorientation, since these may at times involve: a) elimination of certain sensory cues, b) gross distortion of the ways in which sensory cues are presented, and c) gross distortion of ability to perceive cues accurately. Disorientation usually describes a condition of false perceptions which occur by means of the temporal, visual, auditory, kinesthetic, proprioceptive or vestibular senses. However, as has been reviewed earlier in this chapter, the term is sometimes used to describe general states of confusion and emotional instability. During space flight, the astronaut is primarily dependent on his visual and auditory senses for maintaining his orientation. There are also vestibular, kinesthetic and proprioceptive sensations which occur during portions of space flight, and these also act to provide orientation information. In the following sections, problems of disorientation in time, location, position, and motion are reviewed as they relate to space flight, and the results of recent experiments are discussed.

1. Time Disorientation

Time is defined as measured duration. Time disorientation implies an inaccuracy or false perception regarding the duration of time which has elapsed, or the rate at which time is elapsing at any given instant. Orientation in time is an important problem area for manned space travel, since the pilot of a spacecraft must use time measures, concepts and perceptions in piloting his craft. So far as the astronaut is concerned, there are essentially four kinds of time to be considered: clock time (capsule or elapsed time), geographic time, physiologic time and psychologic time. During space travel, the various discrepancies between clock time, geographic time, physiologic time and psychologic time are major factors in producing time disorientation.

Both clock time and geographic time maintain constant units of measurement. However, physiologic time and psychologic time are composed of units which may vary in duration as a function of many different kinds of activities and stresses. Clock time refers to the number of seconds, minutes or hours which have elapsed since lift-off, as indicated on the astronaut's instrument panel. It presents a continuous record of time in flight. Geographic time refers more to the time at any given geographical region, and is referenced to specific geographical zones and boundaries. Physiologic time is sometimes called the "metabolic clock," and it behaves according to a previously conditioned series of diurnal sequences. (See Chapter 9). The physiological time cycle, which has resulted largely from this conditioning procedure, consists of several different organization levels: the body as a whole, the different organs and tissues within the body, and the production of different hormones.[59] Man on earth has become habituated to a somewhat standard day-night cycle which is approximately 24 hr in length. He is sensitive to light-dark cycles, and some of his physiological systems function according to various circadian rhythms which have been conditioned throughout his life span. Psychologic time refers more to the psychologically perceived, or estimated time measures. Psychologic time refers to the man's accustomed work-rest cycle and other behavior. The awareness of time passage, or the ability of a person to estimate the passage of time, is also largely conditioned by prior experience.

The pilot must maintain orientation in physiologic, psychologic, geographic and clock time. While orbiting through space at 18,000 mph or faster, the astronaut must be able to respond properly to signals in order to avoid catastrophe or to avoid getting off course.[82] He must make accurate time estimations for short periods of time, as well as maintain orientation during prolonged time intervals. Some of the most thorough work which has been done on time perception during isolation and confinement has been by Mitchell[82] who studied thirty-four Air Force pilots who were isolated individually. Their ability to estimate passages of time ranging from 1 sec to 48 hr was studied. During periods of isolation in complete darkness in an anechoic chamber, the shortest time interval was overestimated; 5 sec was judged accurately, while 6, 30, 60 and 120 min were significantly underestimated. Some subjects become very disoriented in time. That prolonged confinement extending to eight days duration distorts ability to judge the passage of time has been demonstrated by

Burns and Gifford,[11] Hanna and Gaito,[61] Mitchell,[82] Ross[89] and others.[100]   However, studies involving shorter periods of time, such as 8 hr confinement (Ormiston,[85]) and 12 hr confinement (Chambers *et al.*,[21]), have not demonstrated any significant effects on time perception.

Studies have suggested that the level of the pilot's activity may greatly influence his ability to make accurate time judgments. If the activity level is greatly reduced as compared with the normal response level, the performance of precise timing tasks may be impaired. Similarly, it has been shown that acceleration forces impair time perception skills,[17, 35] thus suggesting that the pilot's timing ability during launch and re-entry accelerations may be distorted. Other factors which affect time perception are: a) the number of stimulus events to which the pilot is responding, b) the degree of confinement, c) one's physiological state, d) the presence of fear, anxiety or aggravation, and e) body temperature.[32]

Much has been written in the scientific literature concerning the physiological day-night cycle, since this influences one's alternate sleep and wakefulness, activity habits and work schedules, and many physiological systems within the body. During space flight, and the consequent possible absence of the normal cues associated with the day-night cycle, some difficulty may be encountered in performing in a predictable reliable way. Another problem lies in the fact that shifts in proficiency which normally occur as a function of this cycle may not be acceptable for space flight requirements involving prolonged confinement.[64, 103]   Finally, unless some of the day-night cycle cues are provided, subtle time perception changes may occur which may impair the ability to perform skills requiring the use of the time sense. At an altitude of 100 miles, a manned satellite orbiting the earth passes through 18 light dark cycles, while man on earth passes through one light-dark cycle. In free space well beyond, many variations in the day-night cycle occur. During these events "incomplete time adaptation" may occur,[104] since the astronaut's physiological cycle, of "metabolic clock" behaves as though it were still in the area just left. Physiological adaptation to new time cycles occurs very slowly. The phenomena of incomplete time adaptation may be expected to pose problems to the somewhat established internal physiological rhythms of body temperature, hunger, digestion, general activity level, metabolic rates and circadian rhythms.[32, 59]

The importance of accurate time estimation and the ability to perform precise time estimation tasks cannot be overemphasized. The detection, activation and monitoring of emergency escape and ejection systems in spacecraft require very rapid and precise timing performance by the astronaut and his crew. Slight disorientation in terms of time perception could mean the difference between success and failure of an escape maneuver.

2. Visual Disorientation

During space flight, the astronaut is expected to make visual astronomical observations for purposes of accumulating scientific data, and for the purposes of navigation, reconnaissance and maintaining vehicle attitude. He will make visual references to the horizon and to external objects, and, during rendezvous, docking, re-entry and landing, he will use not only visual cues from his instrument panel, but also those from his periscope and spacecraft window. Visual orientation is essential in performing space maneuvers, and any disorientation in this sense modality would endanger any space flight.

Visual disorientation has already been discussed as one of the primary effects of prolonged isolation, during the special conditions of: a) confinement, b) sensory deprivation, c) sensory input overload, or d) sleep deprivation. Under the topic of visual disorientation, one cannot discount the problems of visual imagery, visual illusions and visual hallucinations which occur without a stimulus.[3, 7, 29, 30, 37, 43, 67, 73, 84, 100, 108] Freedman and Greenblatt,[37] Goldberger and Holt,[43, 44] and Vernon *et al.*[108] observed that during visual "ganzfeld" conditions (conditions in which the subject wears translucent eye-cups and thereby has a homogeneous visual field) from 40 min to 8 hr or longer, visual images appear in most subjects, even though there are no visual stimuli, and consequently visual disorientation results.

In addition to the visual disorientation which occurs in the absence of stimulation, there are other kinds of visual disorientation which occur because of the complexity of the visual stimuli which the astronaut must use. The visual world as seen from extremely high altitude is different from that which man experiences on earth. Examples of phenomena which account for this difference are: extremely sharp contrast illumination, frequent extremes in brightness and darkness, absence of normal size and distance cues, empty-space myopia and the absence of standard points of reference. Glenn[42] reported that during earth-orbit and looking toward the horizon, the view is completely different than when flying at high altitude in an airplane. However, he demonstrated the possibility of using the earth's horizon to manually pilot vehicle attitude, and found that he could maintain orientation during space flight. He indicated that he did tend to rely much more completely on vision, however, than he does when gravity cues are present, as in flying an airplane. Astronaut Carpenter[124] saw four distinct cloud layers during some phases of his orbital flight. Even in a high altitude balloon, the visual world appears much different than when viewed from the earth.[98] For example, at 102,000 ft, Simons noted what appeared to be three horizons. Simons,[97, 98] Ross,[89] and McClure[119] have commented on the beauty of the earth as seen from high altitude balloons. Generally speaking, the visual world as seen from spacecraft is a pleasant and rewarding experience also,[89, 98, 120, 121] provided that appropriate visual protective equipment for extreme brightness and glare and for contrast, is provided. Astronauts Shepard,[120] Grissom,[121] Glenn,[123] and Carpenter[124] have viewed the earth from over 100 miles altitude, at various velocities ranging from 5000 to 17,500 mph, and have each commented on the beautiful views. However, since windows of spacecraft will be small and widely spaced, and since visual navigation has been shown to be feasible from spacecraft,[123, 124] maintaining visual orientation is considered to be essential.

One possible difficulty in visual orientation is that produced by empty-space myopia.[9, 10] This condition refers to an increase in the refractive power of the human eye. The condition is somewhat similar to "night myopia," which is produced when the eye views during total darkness.

Theories regarding space myopia have been concerned with increased accommodation, representing a relaxation of the accommodative mechanisms to a resting level which is different from the maximally inhibited accommodative state normally found under photopic viewing of objects. Other theories have suggested: a) an involuntary positive stimulation of the ciliary muscle, or, b) an increased spherical aberration, due to increased dilation of the pupil. When at rest on earth, the eyes tend to accommodate for standard distances, so that objects found beyond these distances are out of focus and are not readily perceived. Within the earth's atmosphere, as during ordinary low altitude flying, for example, this condition causes no severe problem since the eyes can readily accommodate to distant scenery by progressive accommodation to a series of objects.[10] However, when traveling in space, the astronaut may not have a progression of objects in front of him and with his eyes at the normal resting accommodation, he may have difficulty in determining whether his eyes are focusing at a point or at infinity. Objects even as close as a few hundred feet may be missed visually. The absence of normal cues of distance and size also complicates the accommodation and convergence performance of the eyes. These problems have not been emphasized in the space flights accomplished to date.[120, 121, 123, 124] However, during prolonged space flight, space myopia may pose problems in maintaining visual orientation.

During launch and re-entry, vision is impaired temporarily by acceleration.[18, 20] The absolute thresholds of foveal and peripheral vision are a function of the combined accelerations and illumination factors. Positive acceleration levels of 4G approximately triple foveal thresholds. Sustained transverse accelerations over 5G produce tearing of the eyes, difficulty in moving the eyes and some loss of peripheral vision. Visual acuity is significantly reduced, and brightness contrast requirements increase.[18] Ability to read instrumental dials, to respond quickly to visual stimuli and to maintain visual acuity is also impaired by vibrations which may occur during launch and re-entry.

During the portion of space flight involving weightlessness, the otolith organs, which are primarily responsible for the perception of position and motion of the whole body, do not function to sense either position or motion. The proprioceptive and kinesthetic senses also remain undisturbed and do no provide reliable signals. Thus, in order that the astronaut may get orientation information concerning his position and movement in space during weightlessness, he must rely almost entirely on his visual sense.[9, 56, 105, 122] There is physiologically no gravitational reference point, and consequently, the astronaut is dependent upon his visual sense for maintaining orientation. Even the perception of the horizontal, for example, may be difficult at times during space flight, for his postural determinant mechanisms will be inactive.[51, 105]

Since there is an absence of vestibular, kinesthetic and proprioceptive cues with respect to earth during weightlessness, there are long-terms periods in which there is no "up or down." Individual elements of the astronaut's display panel within the spacecraft should have recognizable characteristics which are independent of the gravitational vertical with respect to up and down, in order that they may be interpreted for any position. Using the periscope, for example, the astronaut will be using the horizon in all directions, and it will be important to be oriented properly so that man can make roll references as well as pitch and yaw references. The problem during this phase is essentially one of orientation in space. The astronaut's visual display panel should be designed so that it may be interpreted entirely on the basis of dimensions within the total display, and independent of the gravitational vertical to which the observer is normally accustomed.

3. Labyrinthine Sensitivity

For providing the sensations and perceptions necessary for maintaining continuous position orientation and motion orientation in space, the astronaut has three primary systems of sensory input: a) the visual system, b) the labyrinthine system (the vestibular apparatus of the inner ear) and c) the extralabyrinthine system (peripheral pressure, muscle, and posture senses). As indicated in the previous section, the vestibular apparatus of the inner ear and the pressure, muscle, and posture senses of the extralabyrinthine system are inaccurate or inactive during some phases of space flight. In order to maintain orientation in position and motion in space, the astronaut must select and use those senses which are most accurate and reliable during any particular portion of his flight. Discussions of the mechanisms of action of the labyrinthine and extralabyrinthine systems are presented in order to summarize some of the disorientation problems which are encountered.

The labyrinthine system (vestibular apparatus) has two distinctly different orientation functions: a) one concerned with sensing the position of the head in space, and b) one concerned with sensing any change in the rate of motion. The former is mediated primarily by the otolith organs, and the latter is mediated primarily by the crista ampullares and associated cupula of the semicircular canals.[40]

Within the inner ear are three semi-circular canals, each of which is named according to its relative position in the head: the horizontal, the superior vertical and the posterior vertical canal. These canals are filled with endolymph, and they are placed approximately at right angles to each other, one for each major plane of the body. The semi-circular canals open into a larger common chamber, the *utricle,* by means of five apertures one of which is common to the superior and posterior canals. At one end of each canal, near its junction with the utricle, is a swelling known as the *ampulla.* The sensory epithelium in the ampullae of the semi-circular canals is collected into transverse crest-like elevations, the *cristae ampullares,* which are firmly attached to their bony foundations, but which protrude toward the lumen and are free to swing at their other ends. These are the receptor organs of the canals.[40,56] The cristae ampullares contain sensory hairs which project into a gelatinous mass, the cupula. The cupula acts as a spring-loaded over-critically damped torsion pendulum. The receptor organs of the utricle, called the *maculae,* are covered by a gelatinous substance which contains argonite, concentrations of calcium carbonate. These are called the *otoliths,* and have a specific gravity which ranges from 2.93 to 2.95,[40] thus being denser than that of the surrounding endolymph. The otoliths have various grades of fineness, and are situated in their own particular areas of the receptor surface. Although there is undoubtedly some intimate coordination between the activities of the receptors in the cristae ampullares of the semi-circular canals and the otolith organs in the utricle, the two sets of end organs are different in structure and appear to be stimulated by somewat different kinds of acceleration.

The gelatinous pad containing the otoliths and underlying hair cells in the utricle serve as a type of transducer for converting linear accelerations into neural impulses. When the head is oriented in different positions relative to the direction of gravity, the otoliths are displaced and their hair cells at their base signal this displacement. It is generally assumed that displacement of the otoliths with respect to the macula and attendant stimulations of hair cells will be maximum when the head is an upright position, and less when the subject is lying on his side. A change in threshold occurs with a change in head position. There have been many attempts to measure the threshold of the utricles for changes in resultant linear accelerations. Using the oculogravic illusion as a means of measuring thresholds, values as low as 0.000344G have been reported for subjects in the sitting position and 0.00203G for subjects lying on their sides. However, data based on tilt-table studies have reported thresholds as high as 0.010G and higher.

When the head is exposed to angular accelerations in the vertical, transverse or anteroposterior axis, the cristae ampullares and associated cupulae are stimulated by increases or decreases in velocity of rotation. The semi-circular canal-endolymph-cupula system responds very efficiently to angular accelerations, e.g., to the inertial torque resulting from tangential accelerations of different magnitude around the circumference of the canal.

Excessive stimulation of the labyrinthine canals by angular accelerations influences the position of the eyes. Reflex eye movements, referred to as *oculovestibular nystagmus*, occur. As the body moves, the eye muscles compensate in order that they may remain fixed on any object. As the body turns, the eyes swing slowly in the opposite direction in order to maintain their fixation. Having turned as far as possible, they swing back quickly in the opposite direction to fix on a new object which in turn they follow by a slow deviation. Thus there is both a slow movement and a quick movement in oculovestibular nystagmus. The movement of nystagmus may be in either the horizontal, frontal or sagittal plane. If this rotation is accomplished with the eyes closed, postrotatory nystagmus will be observed. In addition, excessive stimulation produces psychomotor disturbances such as past-pointing. It is believed that postrotatory nystagmus is due to the retardation of endolymph which causes a deviation of the cupula, this time in the opposite direction. This postrotatory nystagmus occurs and lasts as long as is necessary for the cupula to return to its original starting position through its elastic recoil.

Angular accelerations of the head or whole body comprise the usual stimulus to the semi-circular canal system. This system is usually brief in duration, and the cupula displacement effected by the angular accelerations is restored to its resting position, in part by the deceleration. Normally, the after-effects of small and brief body or head movements are either inconsequential or absent, since the vestibular reactions are not disturbing under conditions which approximate these normal motions. They are highly consistent and predictable. However, unusual body and head movements which are not normally encountered in locomotion may provide misinformation, illusions and disturbing effects. Examples of such movements may consist of the following: a) prolonged angular acceleration, b) angular acceleration followed by a constant velocity, rather than a deceleration, and c) stimulation which produces excessive Coriolis accelerations in the canal system.

To explain the physical changes in the canals that result in the stimulation of the receptor cells, several different theories have been formulated. The hydrodynamic theory suggests that the elastic cupular ridge is swayed by the flow of endolymph. Any change in speed or rotation causes a movement of the endolymph and consequent deflection of the cupula and the hairs of the sensory cells. Owing to inertia, the endolymph of the involved pair of canals lags behind the progress of the wall of its containing tube and therefore executes a movement opposite to the direction of turning. Some investigators hesitate to accept the hydrodynamic theory because of the capillary nature of the canals and the viscosity of the endolymph, and suggest the hydrostatic and pressure theories as alternates.

For sensitivity to linear acceleration, it is theorized that the otoliths respond to the differential pull of gravity upon them. The fact that the otoliths within the utricle are primarily responsible for static position sense is well established, although the mode of action is uncertain. The effective stimulus is the pull of gravity, the sensory cells being differentially stimulated in different positions. When the stimulation of the utricle maculae on both sides are equalized, the sensation is that of the normal position. Any disturbance of the equilibrium necessarily exerts a different pull of gravity upon the receptor structures, and the otoliths change their relative orientation with respect to the underlying macular surface. Other theorists report that the gliding of the otoliths and bending of the hairs of the sensory cells caused by changes of the position of the head are the effective stimulus events.

4. Extralabyrinthine Sensitivity

The perception of posture, position and movement of the limbs of the body is accomplished primarily by the extralabyrinthine (peripheral) system. This system consists primarily of the pressure sense, the muscle sense and the posture sense. Each of these senses consists largely of mechanoreceptors which are found in the skin, skeletal muscle and in the connective tissue.[39, 40] During exposure to the acceleration stresses of launch and re-entry, and the weightlessness condition of orbit and interplanetary flight, and miscellaneous transition maneuvers in space, the extralabyrinthine system provides the primary cues for orientation of position and movement of the surfaces and limbs of the body.

The nerve endings for the *pressure* (touch) *sense* of the skin are the nervous plexuses around the hair follicles and the Meissner corpuscles in the skin. These sensory nerve endings respond to changes in pressure and weight resulting from mechanical deformations of the skin. During space flight, the pressure sense produces contact cues with the seat, control devices, and restraint equipment. During high G exposures, these cues assist in maintaining orientation with respect to acceleration forces.

The receptors of the *muscle sense* are the muscle spindles which are found in some of the body muscles. These provide orientation cues with respect to tension of the muscles, as may be produced by active and passive muscle movements, body weight and acceleration forced during launch and re-entry.[105]

The *posture sense* consists primarily of the Pacinian corpuscles which are scattered throughout the tissues beneath the skin, and in the connective tissues surrounding and penetrating the muscles. These respond primarily to tension among the various body parts, and are related to the postural reflexes. They are stimulated mechanically when the muscles change their form during active and passive movement. Taken together, the posture sense, the muscle sense and the pressure sense constitute a functional system which senses and controls the position and movements of body parts, and also influence to some limited extent the position and movement orientation of the whole body.

The nerve endings of these senses react primarily to mechanical forces, and are consequently called mechanoreceptors. During exposure to acceleration forces, there are sensations of external contact over the surface of the body, and within the body, which are perceptible. Sometimes the astronaut's sensations and interpretations regarding the direction and magnitude of accelerations are likely to be incorrect.[16, 22, 27, 94] Acceleration forces applied from foot to head $(-a_z)$ produce sensations such as increased pressure at the buttocks, heaviness of the head and body, downward pull of the diaphragm and pressure in the lower parts of the body. Sensations during applied transverse back to chest accelerations $(+a_x)$ are pressure on the chest, substernal pain, pressure around the eyes, and pressure along the back, and dorsal part of the head, neck and legs. Sensations during applied transverse chest to back accelerations $(-a_x)$ are fullness and possible pain in the face and eyes, anterior parts of the trunk, legs and ankles.

During weightlessness, the exteroceptive function of the mechanoreceptors is eliminated. However, the proprioceptive function is not. Consequently, there is little disturbance of the precision of performance in maintaining orientation of the hands, arms and legs. Available data from space flights which involved weightlessness for times ranging from 5 min to 66 hr indicate that extensive prior training and knowledge of results during flight operations provided sufficient protection to enable the astronauts to orient their arms, legs and fingers. However, the use of certain instruments and the performance of certain tasks required several trials during flight in order that the exact amounts of muscular effort and coordination could be applied. The importance of traction, and of being secured to some stationary object such as the astronaut's contour couch, was demonstrated. Performance tasks may be performed proficiently with the eyes open. However, when the eyes are closed, performance impairment occurs unless there are other sensory cues for orientation. Weightlessness studies conducted in zero-G trajectory airplanes have emphasized the problem of orientation during the transition period from high gravity, such as from acceleration to weightlessness, or from weightlessness to acceleration. Experiments have shown that disorientation and loss of motor coordination occur during these brief transitional stages, even when the shift from gravity to no gravity, and back again, is small.[39, 120, 121]

Attempts have been made to study some of the effects of prolonged weightlessness on orientation by using water immersion techniques.[4, 6, 9, 21, 45] The pressure from the supporting water is evenly distributed over almost the entire surface of the body; consequently sensations from the pressoreceptors of the skin remain below the threshold of perception, although gravity continues to act upon the whole body. Similarly, tension sensations from the muscles of the legs are absent during buoyancy if there is no foothold. Brown[8] reported that subjects could not make accurate orientation judgments while immersed. Chambers *et al.*[21] found that subjects restrained in water to *the neck level* for 12 hr consistently "overshot" a target when required to position their arms and fingers. Benson *et al.*[6] found similar results for subjects totally immersed for 18 hr. Similar results were reported by Gerathewohl *et al.*[39] and von Beckh[109] who asked subjects to thrust a stylus during zero flights, and to draw crosses in prearranged squares. In all cases, however, practice and knowledge of results improved positioning accuracy.

It must be emphasized that the linear and angular acceleration environment is itself insufficient to predict the sensory and perceptual experience of orientation and adjustment in three-dimensional space. There are a great variety of manifestations and nervous impulses which are generated in the labyrinthine and extralabyrinthine structures, and these have far-reaching effects. They reach the central control centers, the autonomic centers, the reticular formation with its integrative and monitoring functions, the subcortical and cortical areas which influence perception and emotion. The pattern of stimulation for orientation in position and motion is more effective than mere stimulus strength. The vestibular, ocular and extralabyrinthine systems interact to serve as determiners of perceptual orientation and psychomotor adjustment to linear and angular accelerations.[38, 40, 46, 56]

5. Illusions of Position and Motion

Illusions of position and motion pose problems of orientation during space travel. These illusions may be defined as false or incorrect perceptions of one's position and motion. Unless adequate protection and controls are provided, significant problems exist when there is an absence of necessary perceptual frames of reference, when sensory cues are perceived incorrectly, or when there are unpredictable movements of the spacecraft or of other objects with which the astronaut may be in contact. Examples of illusions are described by Astronaut John Glenn[42] in his Friendship VII Mercury Capsule during his earth-orbital space flight. When the sustainer engine cutoff occurred and acceleration suddenly dropped to zero, he experienced a sensation of being tumbled forward. During prior training on the human centrifuge, Glenn had experienced the sensation of apparent tumbling forward during sudden deceleration. Glenn also reported that during the firing of his retrorockets during re-entry preparations in his Friendship VII Mercury Capsule, he perceived the false sensation that he was suddenly accelerating in the reverse direction. Similar illusions have been reported by Astronauts Shepard, Grissom,

Carpenter and Schirra. In this section, some of the illusions and false perceptions of major interest to space travel are summarized.

A category of illusions which are of major importance are the oculogyral illusions. These describe a type of disorientation which results from vestibular stimulation produced by angular accelerations. The illusion has been defined as an apparent movement of objects in the visual field having its genesis in stimulation of the sensory receptors in the semicircular canals.[53] The illusion is frequently described as the sensation that the visual field is spinning about the body axis.[54] Oculogyral illusions vary greatly, depending upon the circumstances under which the stimulation of the labyrinthine canals occur. They may occur when the horizontal semi-circular canals are stimulated by the onset and cessation of angular acceleration, as when the head is fixed in position on a rotating device, such as the human centrifuge. They may also occur after the cessation of rotation, if a subject previously adapted to rotation, rotates his head in the frontal plane. The former case is sometimes called the acceleration oculogyral illusion, to distinguish it from the latter case, which is sometimes called the post-adaptation oculogyral illusion. There are many types of oculogyral illusions, all of which are essentially false sensations of rotation of visually observed objects. Schafer[94] lists three types of oculogyral illusions encountered in flying airplanes. Gray and Crosbie[47] list 18 sensations which represent variations in the oculogyral illusion.

If a person fixes his eyes on a lighted target which turns as he turns, the target at first appears to turn as the subject turns. Then it may appear displaced during rotation. When real rotation stops, it may continue to move for a short time. Following angular acceleration, the motion which the observer perceives is in the direction of turn. Shortly after the subject has attained a constant angular velocity, he experiences no further visual motion. However, deceleration reverses the apparent direction of visual movement. After coming to stand-still and the cessation of motion, apparent motion may be revived, but this time in the opposite direction. In darkness, a weak stimulation of the labyrinth causes apparent motion which may persist after all other sensations of the rotation have disappeared. The illusion occurs following rotation of an object whether or not there is rotation of the subject relative to the seen objects and whether or not there is motion of these objects relative to one another.

The total experience is complex. The sensations of angular speed and displacement may seem discordant, the plane of apparent bodily rotation may shift, and motion sickness and disturbing autonomic reactions may occur. Geldard[38] indicates that the visual effects are closely correlated with nystagmic responses, and considers them to be delicate indicators of labyrinthine stimulation. However, the oculogyral illusion is regarded as being a more sensitive indicator. The oculogyral illusion begins to appear with accelerations or decelerations of as little as 0.12 degree/sec.[2] On devices such as the human centrifuge, the oculogyral illusion appears differently when observed at large and small radii of turn. As the speed of the centrifuge increases, the subjects seem to see the objects they are observing as traveling in a long curved path with its center of curvature in the same direction as the center of the centrifuge. As the centrifuge is slowed, the spinning almost always seems to be around an axis which passes through the body of the subject. By increasing the linear accelerations in steps, and by holding the angular accelerations constant, the duration of the oculogyral illusion decreases as the linear acceleration increases.

When a person who is subjected to passive rotation in one plane turns his head in another plane, his subjective feeling is that of rotating in a plane approximately orthogonal to the other two. In a rotating room, for example, the rotation of the subject's head out of the plane of rotation of the room produces the effect frequently described as the Coriolis illusion. Maximum Coriolis effects usually occur when the head makes secondary rotations about an axis perpendicular to the primary axis of the rotation. They result from vestibular stimulation and are generated whenever an object on a rotating device, such as a centrifuge, moves in a direction which is not parallel to the axis of rotation. During flight, if a pilot inadvertently turns his head during the peak acceleration phase of a fast "pull-out" from a dive or a close turn, his semi-circular canals may be stimulated to the extent that he becomes disoriented. It is generally assumed that Coriolis effects are produced by Coriolis accelerations which stimulate the semi-circular canals. However, mathematical analyses have shown that torques may be generated by Coriolis accelerations which also stimulate the otolith organs.[48]

Guedry and Montague[57] who have studied the vestibular Coriolis reaction extensively, indicate that the magnitude and direction of the nystagmic reactions and subjective aspects are predictable. Subjects in their experiments used a control stick to indicate the apparent dives and climbs produced by vestibular stimulation, and developed a method to measure the magnitude of compensatory adjustment. The threshold of detection of Coriolis acceleration in terms of the Coriolis illusion appears to be between 0.0982 and 0.1946 rad/sec, according to Gray *et al.*[48] Clark and Hardy[27] have reported a threshold for the illusion when the head is at an angular velocity of 0.06 rad/sec in a plane perpendicular to the plane of centrifuge rotation.

Coriolis accelerations are very important because of the possibility that space stations may be rotating in order to utilize centrifugal acceleration as a form of artificial gravity, and the fact that motion sickness has been associated with head motions within rotating systems.

Vertigo is a commonly experienced illusion. It is a false sensation of rotation, or whirling around, in which the observer feels as if the surroundings are revolving about him, or, sometimes, as if he is revolving about his surroundings.[3] After exposure to successive high-G transverse runs on the centrifuge, some subjects report vertigo as long as 48 hr following exposures. Pilots have reported vertigo up to 40 days following high-G acceleration exposures on the centrifuge.

Another interesting illusion is the oculogravic illusion. This is an apparent tilting or displacement movement which results from the stimulation of the otolith apparatus in the utricle of the inner ear. During acceleration, a target may appear to be displaced upwards. The degree of displacement corresponds to the angle between the resultant force and normal force of gravity. Conversely, during deceleration, the target may appear to move downwards. Schafer[94] lists four types of oculogravic illusions encountered during flying airplanes. Sometimes a person, rather than the visual field itself, appears to be tilted. The manner in which stimulation of the otoliths produces these sensations is not well understood.

On the centrifuge, the oculogravic illusion originates from the resultant of centrifugal accelerations, tangential acceleration and the acceleration of gravity. For example, during the onset of transverse acceleration, a person may experience a sensation of tilting backwards, or, if the subject is seated erect, and is exposed to a gradual increase in the rate of rotation, he may perceive that his chair is tilted. A luminous line observed in darkness would appear to tilt in the same direction. The inclusion of the visual stimulus during any given test improves the ability to detect the illusion. If the subject views a luminous horizontal line while facing the direction of motion, he will perceive an apparent rotation of the luminous line about its center, and in the same direction of the perceived bodily tilt. If the centrifuge is rotating counterclockwise, the luminous line will appear to rotate clockwise.[49] Similarly, *down* may appear to move from beneath the subject's body to one side, and he therefore observes himself as lying on his side. If the subject is asked to set the luminous line to the horizontal, he may be expected to rotate it clockwise from the true horizontal to make it appear subjectively horizontal.

Present evidence indicates that the minimum angle of rotation of the direction of resultant acceleration through the body which can be perceived as an oculogravic illusion is approximately 1.5 deg when the subject is in the erect position and 8.9 deg when the subject is lying on his side. It has been difficult to obtain thresholds when subjects are in the inverted position, however, and tentatively it is concluded that the otolith organ functions best when the head is upright, and that it is very inaccurate when the head is inverted.[51, 112]

The oculo-agravic illusion is another interesting false perception. This occurs during sub-gravity and zero-gravity. A luminous target seen in the dark appears to be displaced in an upward direction during sub-gravity. An induced after-image moves downward during acceleration and upward during the onset of weightlessness.

Another faulty perception of movement of an object fixed in the visual field is the autokinetic illusion. This occurs when other visual references are absent or inadequate. Without a frame of reference, an illuminated object viewed in total darkness may appear to move in various random patterns. During flying, a pilot may be greatly confused because he cannot tell when a particular object viewed in the visual field is actually moving, or whether it merely appears to move. If he cannot distinguish real movement from apparent movement, he may become greatly confused.

In addition to the illusions outlined above, there are several false reactions which occur, mostly during blind flight, which produce disorientation problems. These have been described by Armstrong[3] and may be summarized as follows: sensations of climbing while turning; sensations of diving during recovery from a turn; sensations of diving beyond the vertical; illusions of turning; unperceived banks; sensations of opposite tilt in a skid; overestimating the degree of bank; and the sensation of being tilted following gradual recovery from a roll.

It is important to note that illusions and disorientation are brought about by an interaction of the vestibular, ocular, and proprioceptive systems. The subject attempts to adjust perceptually and physiologically to combinations of linear and angular accelerations, and also he attempts to adapt his overt performance responses to these sensations.

The perception of the horizontal, for example, may be difficult at times during space flight. When a man is upright, during conditions of normal gravity, he can view a line in an otherwise uniform field and can set it to the horizontal or vertical with precision. In addition to visual cues, however, he also uses postural determinant mechanisms, such as the otolith organs of the inner ear. This accuracy declines when the man is tilted away from the vertical. Similarly, if rather than tilting the man with respect to the acceleration field, the acceleration field is changed with respect to the man, a similar distortion in ability to set a line to the horizontal or vertical occurs. When the head is on the side, or inverted, setting the horizontal or upright is extremely difficult. With the head in the inverted position, extreme variability occurs among subjects and errors are extremely large.[51] In aircraft during turns and in special rotating devices, visual and postural cues may become discrepant and the observer's perceived horizontal or vertical may show gross deviations from a gravitational vertical. The direction and magnitude of the gravitational force acting on the body affects the visual perception of the horizontal or the vertical. Antecedent visual frames of reference are contributing factors in the perception of illusion. During periods of prolonged rotation, gradual and continuous changes occur in the frame of reference from the original cues to the new gravitation cues.

Major significance is given to illusions of motion and position because of the possibility that rotating space vehicles and space platforms may be used in space travel.[27, 52, 53, 56] If a human within a rotating capsule of sufficient velocity tilts his head only a few times relative to the axis of rotation, he may experience apparent rotations which may be confusing, nauseous or accompanied by symptoms of motion sickness. These angular accelerations may be at times relatively great in magnitude, occur simultaneously about two or more axes, and be either impulse or periodic in form. Biologically, these can produce high-level, simultaneous stimulation of two or more sets of the semi-circular canals for sustained intervals. The vestibular performance characteristics in response to high-level, periodic angular accelerations are of special concern in the possible development of proposed space platforms.

6. Motion Sickness

Motion sickness is frequently associated with severe disorientation. Motion sickness readily occurs in human subjects who are disoriented in motion and position. It is a somewhat general term, and includes a large class of related sicknesses, such as sea sickness, car sickness, swing sickness, air sickness and canal sickness. Whereas the exact causes and mechanisms are somewhat controversial, it is generally agreed that the labyrinthine system and the

ocular system are specifically involved, and that the extralabyrinthine system, autonomic and central nervous systems are also
involved.[56, 101] Nausea, pallor, vertigo, sweating, prostration and
vomiting are some of the primary symptoms. Early workers generally assumed that linear accelerations, rather than angular accelerations, cause motion sickness. Sea sickness, for example, is not
accompanied by nystagmus, and consequently it was assumed
that the sickness must be a function of linear acceleration. Also,
since persons with reduced labyrinthine activity exhibited a low
incidence of sea sickness, it was assumed by many that the primary
factor was the stimulation of the otolith organs by linear acceleration. However, angular accelerations of ships at sea are not necessarily below the threshold for semi-circular canal stimulation,
which appears to be approximately 3–4°/ sec², as measured by
nystagmus, and 0.5–1.0°/sec², as measured by the oculogyral illusions as an index of semi-circular canal stimulation. Studies conducted in elevators have shown that when amplitudes between
1–9 ft are presented at varying frequencies, motion sickness
occurs more frequently for large waves than for small ones.
Similarly, lower accelerations of around 0.25G were more effective
than higher ones of around 0.65G. It has been reported that
intervals of approximately 1.1 sec are more effective than shorter
or longer ones. Later studies, however, demonstrated that head
movements and changing visual stimulation during these exposures were significant factors. Also, using gliders, airplanes and
swings, it has been demonstrated that head motions, and consequently angular accelerations, are critical in the development of
motion sickness. Although there are some cases in which linear
accelerations alone seem to result in motion sickness, it is generally
assumed that the associated angular accelerations are largely
responsible.

During exposure to a continuously rotating platform or room,
nodding the head or certain whole body movements, produces
angular accelerations which result in Coriolis accelerations at
right angles to the direction of the nod. This stimulates the
semi-circular canals in such a way so as to produce a condition
which has been called *canal sickness* by Graybiel *et al.*[52] The

term *canal sickness* is used to designate a specific type which results from unusual stimulation of the semi-circular canals. The head movements which result from rotations about an axis in the neck involve only short radii of turn, whereas the linear components of Coriolis accelerations are negligible. The linear Coriolis acceleration is assumed to be below the threshold for stimulating the otolith organs. It is assumed that the Coriolis accelerations affect only the semi-circular canals and consequently the sickness that results from the rotating room or rotating platform exercise is a canal sickness. Guedry and Montague[57] and Gray[46] have attempted to relate observations of visual Coriolis illusion to the equation of motion. The relative contributions of different accelerations, however, are not certain. Frequent symptoms are visual and postural illusions, nystagmus, sweating, apathy, somnolence, nausea and vomiting.

Motion sickness, including canal sickness, may be prevented by either of three general approaches: drugs, habituation and selection of persons immune to motion sickness. Although anti-motion sickness drugs are effective, the side effects of the drugs themselves tend to limit their usage for space flight. Much research data is needed on "time-to-sickness" parameters, individual differences and definitions of the limits of motion to which habituation may occur. In-flight studies are needed on the effects of angular movements in pitch, roll and yaw during weightlessness.

III. SELECTION, TRAINING AND HUMAN ENGINEERING

The etiology and preventive measures for illusions and other types of disorientation, as well as the effects of prolonged isolation and confinement, are complex. Study has demonstrated the importance of selection, training and human engineering in preparing man to sustain exposure to these conditions. Once the stimuli, responses and basic physiological and psychological mechanisms are understood, techniques of selection, training and human engineering may be used to increase man's ability to tolerate these conditions and to perform as a reliable and functioning unit within any particular spacecraft system.

1. Selection

Individuals differ greatly in their ability to tolerate prolonged isolation and confinement. Consequently, astronauts who are to sustain these conditions during space flight must be very carefully selected. Men differ greatly in their ability to perform tasks under conditions of sensory deprivation or sensory input overload. Some pilots show unusual symptoms such as breakoff, fascination, freezing and various emotional responses, whereas others do not. Ability to maintain orientation in time, position and motion is an area of vast individual differences. Susceptibility to motion sickness and canal sickness varies greatly. For example, deaf persons do not have oculogravic illusions when subjected to the accelerations which produce these illusions in men with normal labyrinthine functioning.[118] Marked individual differences also exist in the rates of adaptation to the effects of disorientation. An extreme example of this is reported by Crampton and Schwam,[28] who reported that in the cat, a series of 12 acceleration-deceleration trials typically reduced nystagmus by 80 per cent, whereas in the turtle, repeated testing showed little, if any, reduction in vestibular nystagmus.

One of the major tasks with respect to preparing man to tolerate conditions of isolation and disorientation is to select candidates who have some initial ability to tolerate these conditions. Many of the procedures developed in selecting the seven Mercury astronauts (Wilson,[117]) show promise. The astronaut selection and evaluation programs developed by the Lovelace Foundation, the U. S. Air Force, the U. S. Navy and the National Aeronautics and Space Administration are leading to new knowledge on individual differences, and the development and validation of new tests and related selection procedures.

2. Adaptation and Training

Research has demonstrated the value of adaptation and training as providing some protective measures against the effects of isolation and disorientation. For example, adaptation to the oculogyral illusion was demonstrated by Graybiel *et al.*[53] in an experiment in which four healthy males were confined in a small rotating room for 64 hr. Major habituation to the unusual sensory input was demonstrated by some subjects. From a point of view of manning orbital satellites which may rotate from 2 to 10 rpm, the study suggested that the oculogyral illusions and associated reactions may decline or be completely eliminated during prolonged exposure to rotation. In a related study, Clark and Graybiel[25] studied the psychological performance of six subjects during adaptation to a rotating room during a period of two days. Rotations varied from 1.71 to 10.0 rpm. Although a detrimental effect was produced on the motivation of the subjects, the subjects were able to maintain their performance levels on psychological tasks. Guedry and Montague[57] and Graybiel *et al.*[53] have demonstrated that the vestibular Coriolis reaction diminishes within adaptation trials. It has been found that compensatory reactions also occur. Kennedy *et al.*[71] have observed adaptation patterns in three groups of subjects to the oculogyral illusions, to motion sickness and to canal sickness who were exposed to a constant rotation of 1 rpm.

In preparation for space flight, training should include exposure to the unique and complex aspects of the visual world to which the astronaut will be exposed. Practice should be provided in making visual references to the horizon and to external objects performing vehicle orientation in pitch, roll and yaw flight attitude. Similarly, practice in making size and distance judgments, as well as practice in using the periscope and instrument panel to correct for the various unusual and misleading exterior visual references should be provided. Similarly, thorough training in compensating for misleading cues from the vestibular and proprioceptive mechanisms should be provided. Obviously, extensive training in sustaining prolonged periods of confinement and isolation, in the absence of needed cues, or the presence of excessive cues and task requirements, is necessary. Misleading perceptions of the duration, direction and plane of whole-body movements are very likely to provide several problems in orientation and navigation. Training devices proved useful to date include the human centrifuge, the multiaxis spin test inertial facility, the rotating room and the frictionless platform.[18, 102, 122] To date, the seven Mercury astronauts have received training on at least 20 different training devices which provide familiarization with the effects of acceleration and disorientation.

3. Human Engineering

The third major tool in providing protection against the effects of isolation and disorientation is that of human engineering. Human engineering, starting from basic data on sensory capabilities and response characteristics of man in specific mission profile situations, attempts to provide maximum compatibility between man and his equipment, in order to minimize decrement and maximize human reliability. In isolation and confinement situations, this involves providing the appropriate balance between automatic and manned operated systems, appropriate cues and work-rest schedules, information feedback and the most appropriate displays and controls for the astronaut to use in sustaining the duration of the isolation. Human engineering also attempts to provide appropriate sensory cues, compensation networks and piloting equipment, so as to minimize disorientation, or else to assist the astronaut in being aware of disorienting situations and facilitating his ability to adapt to them.

The effectiveness of man in space may depend to a large extent upon the success of physiologists and psychologists to mitigate or prevent the degradative effects of confinement and isolation. Techniques have been developed which offer promise for increasing the reliability of the human operator for prolonged periods of time.[19, 33, 63, 65] One major approach is that of improving the design of the equipment and the man-machine system itself. By simplifying the task, by reducing the amount of input information overload, and by using feedback augmentation on certain performance tasks, reliability of the human operator may be improved. Other approaches involve the human pilot himself. Overtraining in specific primary and subordinate tasks greatly improves his performance reliability. The development of appropriate work-rest cycles, the use of information feedback techniques, orientation aids, improved information displays, and programmed variations of stimuli, are some of the practical approaches which have been developed for assisting man during prolonged confinement.

A final approach which offers promise is the use of energizer drugs which may enhance performance at selected lull periods.

IV. SUMMARY AND CONCLUSIONS

This chapter reviews research on isolation and disorientation as it relates to problems encountered by man during space travel. The term isolation is used to refer to a large variety of conditions which have the common denominator of separating a person from the significant parts of the environment to which he is accustomed. Disorientation refers to false sensations, incorrectly sensed cues, misperceptions, and inappropriate responses to stimuli which result in perceptual frames of reference which are at variance with reality. The conditions of isolation are very conducive to disorientation, since these may at times involve: a) elimination of certain sensory cues, b) gross distortion of the ways in which sensory cues are presented and c) distortion of ability to sense and perceive cues accurately. Methods and variables used in isolation research are reviewed, and problems encountered in confining a person to a small limited space are considered. These are compared with problems produced by the alteration of the available sensory and perceptual stimulation, and the separation of the person, or small groups of persons, from other people and objects upon which dependency exists. The effects of greatly reducing the amount and variability of effective stimulation (sensory deprivation) and the effects of greatly increasing the amount of sensory stimulation (sensory input overload) are compared. Controversial interacting problem areas, such as sleep deprivation, fascination and freezing, and the feeling of earth separation are also considered. It is indicated that the categorization of isolation exposures is primarily dependent upon the portion of one's normal environment from which he is separated. Through laboratory experimentation, space equivalency studies, flight simulations, and the telemetering of physiological and psychological data during in-flight space operations, it has been possible to study some of the primary variables and their combinations. Special problem areas, such as time disorientation and visual disorientation, are evaluated in terms of astronaut performance requirements during prolonged space flight. In considering the problems of disorientation in position and motion, the roles of the visual system, the labyrinthine system (vestibular apparatus) of the inner ear, and the extralabyrinthine system (peripheral pressure, muscle and posture senses) are summarized. Illusions of position and motion are described, and their involvement in space flight operations are discussed.

Despite all of the technical literature which emphasizes the possible hazardous effects of isolation and disorientation on the astronaut during prolonged space flight, it seems reasonable to conclude that the astronauts and their crews will not suffer from the potentially detrimental effects of isolation and disorientation provided that: a) the astronaut and his crew are appropriately selected and trained, b) they are provided with piloting and related tasks which keep them occupied during critical portions of the flight and c) they are provided with a continuous capability for maintaining contact with the essential aspects of the environment. It is emphasized that once the stimuli, responses, and basic physiological and psychological mechanisms are understood for specific space flight missions, techniques of selection, adaptation and training, and human engineering may be used to increase man's ability to tolerate the stressful conditions and to perform as a reliable unit within any spacecraft system. The effectiveness of man in space flight during prolonged confinement and exposure to disorientation may depend to a large extent upon the success of physiologists and psychologists to mitigate the potentially degradative effects on perceptual, motor and intellectual performance.

REFERENCES

1. ADAMS, O. S., and W. D. CHILES: *Human Performance as a Function of the Work-Rest Ratio During Prolonged Confinement.* Aerospace Medical Laboratory, Wright-Patterson Air Force Base, Ohio. *ASD TRR 61-720*, November, 1961.
2. AMBLER, R. K., J. R. BERKSHIRE, and W. F. O'CONNOR: *The identification of potential astronauts.* U. S. Naval School of Aviation Medicine, Pensacola, Florida. *Res. Rept. No. 33*, June, 1961.

3. ARMSTRONG, H. D.: Vertigo and Related States. Pp. 225–237, In, H. G. Armstrong (Ed). *AeroSpace Medicine.* Baltimore, Williams & Wilkins Co., 1961.

4. BECKMAN, E. L., K. R. COBURN, R. M. CHAMBERS, R. E. DEFOREST, W. S. AUGERSON, and V. G. BENSON: Physiologic changes observed in human subjects during zero-G simulation by immersion in water up to neck level. *Aerospace Med.,* 32:1031–1041, 1961.

5. BENNETT, H.: Sensory deprivation in aviation. Pp. 161–173, In, Solomon, *et al.* (Eds). *Sensory Deprivation.* Cambridge, Harvard Univ. Press, 1961.

6. BENSON, V. G., E. L. BECKMAN, K. R. COBURN, and R. M. CHAMBERS: Effects of weightlessness as simulated by total body immersion upon response to positive acceleration. *Aerospace Med.,* 33:198–203, 1962.

7. BEXTON, W. H., W. HERON, and T. H. SCOTT: Effects of decreased variations in sensory environment. *Canad. J. Psychol.,* 8:70–76, 1954.

8. BROWN, J. L.: Orientation to the Vertical during water immersion. *Aerospace Med.,* 32:209–217, 1961.

9. BROWN, J. L., W. BEVAN, W. SENDERS, and R. TRUMBULL: *Report of the Working Group on Sensory and Perceptual Problems Related to Space Flight.* Natl. Acad. Sci. Natl. Research Council, Publ. No. 872, 1961.

10. BROWN, R. H.: Empty-field myopia and visibility of objects at high altitudes. *Am. J. Psychol.,* 70:376–385, 1957.

11. BURNS, N. M., and E. C. GIFFORD: *Environmental Requirements of Sealed Cabins for Space and Orbital Flights.* Naval Air Material Center, Philadelphia. Rept. No. *NAMC-ACEL-414,* 1960.

12. BYRD, R. E.: *Alone.* New York: Putnam's Sons, 1938.

13. CAMERON, D. E., L. LEVY, T. BAN, and L. RUBENSTEIN: Sensory deprivation: Effects upon the functioning human in space systems. In, *Psychophysiological Aspects of Space Flight.* B. E. Flaherty, (Ed.) pp. 225–237. New York, Columbia University Press, 1961.

14. CANNON, W. B.: Voodoo death. *Psychosomatic Med.,* 19:182–190, 1957.

15. CAPPON, D. and R. BANKS: Studies in perceptual distortion. *AMA Arch. Gen. Psychiat.,* 2:346–349, 1960.

16. CHAMBERS, R. M.: *Control Performance Under Acceleration with Side-Arm Attitude Controllers.* Aviation Medical Acceleration Laboratory U. S. Naval Air Development Center, Johnsville, Pa. *Rept. No. NADC-MA-6110,* November, 1961.

17. CHAMBERS, R. M.: *Problems and Research in Space Psychology.* Aviation Medical Acceleration Laboratory, U. S. Naval Air Development Center, Johnsville, Pa. *Rept. No. NADC-MA-6145,* April, 1962.

18. CHAMBERS, R. M.: Human operator performance in acceleration environments. Chapter 7, in Burns, N. M., R. M. Chambers, and E. Hendler (Eds). *Unusual Environments and Human Behavior.* New York, The Free Press, 1963.

19. CHAMBERS, R. M., and R. FRIED: Psychological aspects of space flight. Pp. 173–256, In, Brown, J. H. U. (Ed). *The Physiology of Man in Space.* New York, The Academic Press, 1962.

20. CHAMBERS, R. M., and L. HITCHOCK: Effects of high G conditions on pilot performance. Pp. 204–227, In, *Proceedings of the IAS-NASA National Meeting on Manned Space Flight.* Inst. of Aerospace Sciences, New York, May, 1962.

21. CHAMBERS, R. M., D. A. MORWAY, E. I. BECKMAN, R. DeFOREST, and K. R. COBURN: *Effects of Water Immersion on Performance Proficiency.* Aviation Medical Acceleration Laboratory, U. S. Naval Air Development Center, Johnsville, Pa. *Rept. No. NADC-MA-6133,* August, 1961.

22. CHAMBERS, R. M., and J. G. NELSON. Pilot Performance capabilities during centrifuge simulations of boost and reentry. *Amer. Rocket Society J., 31:*1534–1541, 1961.

23. CHILES, W. D., and O. S. ADAMS: *Human Performance and Work-Rest Schedule.* Aerospace Medical Laboratory, Wright-Patterson Air Force Base, Ohio. *Rept. No. ASD TR 61-270,* July, 1961.

24. CLARK, B., and A. GRAYBIEL: The break-off phenomenon. A feeling of separation from the earth experienced by pilots at high altitude. *J. Aviat. Med., 28:*121–126, 1957.

25. CLARK, B., and A. GRAYBIEL: Human performance during adaptation to stress in the Pensacola slow rotating room. *Aerospace Med., 32:*93–106, 1961.

26. CLARK, B., M. A. NICHOLSON, and A. GRAYBIEL: Fascination: A cause of pilot error. *J. Aviat. Med., 24:*429–440, 1953.

27. CLARK, C. C., and J. D. HARDY: *Gravity Problems in Manned Space Stations.* Aviation Medical Acceleration Laboratory, U. S. Naval Air Development Center, Johnsville, Pa. *Rept. No. NADC-MA-6033,* March, 1961.

28. CRAMPTON, G. H., and W. J. SCHWAM: Turtle vestibular responses to angular acceleration with comparative data from cat and man. *J. Comp. & Physiol. Psychol., 55:*315–321, 1962.

29. DAVIS, J. M., W. F. McCOURT, J. COURTNEY, and P. SOLOMON: Sensory deprivation: The role of social isolation. *Arch. Gen. Psychiat., 5:*84–90, 1961.

30. DAVIS, J. M., W. F. McCOURT, and P. SOLOMON: Effect of visual stimulation on hallucinations and other mental experiences during sensory deprivation. *Am. J. Psychiat., 116:*889–892, 1960.

31. Doane, B. K., W. Mahatoo, W. Heron, and T. H. Scott: Changes in perceptual function after isolation. *Canad. J. Psychol., 13*:210–219, 1959.
32. Fischer, R., F. Griffin, and L. Liss: Biological aspects of time in relation to (model) psychosis. *N. Y. Acad. Sci., 96*:44–65, 1962.
33. Fitts, P. M.: Skill maintenance under adverse conditions. Pp. 309–322, In, B. E. Flaherty (Ed). *Psychophysiological Aspects of Space Flight*. New York, Columbia University Press, 1961.
34. Flinn, D. E., J. T. Monroe, E. H. Cramer, and D. H. Hagen: Observations in the SAM two-man space cabin simulator. IV. Behavioral factors in selection and performance. *Aerospace Med., 32*: 610–615, 1961.
35. Frankenhaeuser, M.: Effects of prolonged gravitational stress on performance. *Acta Psychologica, 14*:92–108, 1958.
36. Freedman, S. J.: *Sensory Deprivation and Perceptual Lag*. Aerospace Medical Laboratory, Wright-Patterson Air Force Base, Ohio. *Rept. WADD TR 60-745*, December, 1960.
37. Freedman, S. J., and M. Greenblatt: *Studies in Human Isolation*. Aero-Medical Laboratory, Wright Air Development Center, Wright-Patterson Air Force Base, Ohio. *Rept. No. 59-226*, September, 1959.
38. Geldard, F. A.: *The Human Senses*. New York, John Wiley & Sons, Inc., 1953.
39. Gerathewohl, S. J., H. Strughold, and H. D. Stallings: Sensomotor performance during weightlessness: eye-hand coordination. *J. Aviat. Med., 28*:7–12, 1957.
40. Gernandt, B. E.: Vestibular mechanisms. Pp. 549–564, In, *Handbook of Physiology, Section 1: Neurophysiology, Volume I*. J. Field, (Ed.) Amer. Physiol. Society, Baltimore, Waverly Press, Inc., 1959.
41. Giffen, M. B.: Break-off: A phase of spatial disorientation. *Armed Forces Medical Journal, 10*:1299–1303, 1959.
42. Glenn, J. H., Jr.: Pilot's flight report. Pp. 296–309, In, *Proceedings of the IAS-NASA National Meeting on Manned Space Flight*, Institute of Aerospace Sciences, New York, May, 1962.
43. Goldberger, L., and R. R. Holt: Experimental interference with reality contact (perceptual isolation): Method and group results. *J. Nerv. Ment. Dis., 127*:99–112, 1958.
44. Goldberger, L., and R. R. Holt: *Studies on the effects of perceptual alteration*. Aerospace Medical Laboratory, Wright-Patterson Air Force Base, Ohio. *Rept. No. ASD TR 61-416*, August, 1961.
45. Graveline, D. E., B. Balkem, R. E. McKenzie, and B. Hartman. Psychobiologic effects of water-immersion-induced hypodynamics. *Aerospace Med., 32*:387–400, 1961.

46. Gray, R. F.: Functional relationships between semicircular canals and otolith organs. *Aerospace Med., 31*:413–418, 1961.

47. Gray, R. F., and R. J. Crosbie: *Variation in Duration of Oculogyral Illusions as a Function of the Radius of Turn.* Aviation Medical Acceleration Laboratory, U. S. Naval Air Development Center, Johnsville, Pa. *Rept. No. NADC-MA-5806,* May 1958.

48. Gray, R. F., R. J. Crosbie, R. A. Hall, J. A. Weaver, and C. C. Clark: *The presence or absence of visual coriolis illusions at various combined angular velocities.* Aviation Medical Acceleration Laboratory, U. S. Naval Air Development Center, Johnsville, Pa. *Rept. No. NADC-MA-6131,* June, 1961.

49. Graybiel, A.: The Oculogravic Illusion. *Arch. Opthal., N. Y., 8*:605–615, 1952.

50. Graybiel, A.: The importance of the otolith organs in man based upon a specific test for utricular function. *Ann. Otol., 65*:470, 1956.

51. Graybiel, A., and B. Clark: Perception of the horizontal or vertical with head upright, on the side, and inverted under static conditions, and during exposure to centripetal force. *Aerospace Med., 33*:147–155, 1962.

52. Graybiel, A., B. Clark, and J. J. Zarriello: Observations on human subjects living in a "slow rotation room" for periods of two days. *Arch. Neurol., 3*:55–73, 1960.

53. Graybiel, A., F. E. Guedry, W. Johnson, and R. Kennedy: Adaptation to bizarre stimulation of the semicircular canals as indicated by the oculogyral illusion. *Aerospace Med., 32*:321–327, 1961.

54. Graybiel, A., and D. I. Hupp: The oculogyral illusion: a form of apparent motion which may be observed following stimulation of the semicircular canals. *J. Aviat. Med., 17*:3–27, 1946.

55. Guedry, F. E., and N. Beberman: *Adaptation Effects in Vestibular Reactions.* U. S. Army Medical Research Laboratory, Fort Knox, Ky. *Rept. No. 293,* January, 1957.

56. Guedry, F. E., and A. Graybiel. *Rotation Devices other than Centrifuges and Motion Simulators.* National Academy of Sciences–National Research Council, Publication No. 902, Washington, D. C., 1961.

57. Guedry, F. E., and E. K. Montague: Quantitative evaluation of the vestibular Coriolis reaction. *Aerospace Med., 32*:487–500, 1961.

58. Hagen, D. H.: *Crew Interaction During a Thirty-Day Simulated Space Flight.* USAF School of Aerospace Medicine, Brooks AFB, Texas. *Rept. No. 61-66,* June, 1961.

59. Halberg, F.: Circadian rhythms: A basis of human engineering for aerospace. Pp. 166–193, In Flaherty, B. E. (Ed.) *Psychophysiological Aspects of Space Flight.* New York, Columbia University Press, 1961.

60. HANNA, T. D.: A physiologic study of human subjects confined in a simulated space vehicle. *Aerospace Med., 33*:175–182, 1962.
61. HANNA, T. D., and J. GAITO: Performance and habitability aspects of extended confinement in sealed cabins. *Aerospace Med., 31*:399, 1960.
62. HARDY, J. D., and C. C. CLARK: The development of dynamic flight simulation. *Aero/Space Engineering, 18*:48–52, 1959.
63. HARTMAN, B. O.: Time and load factors in astronaut proficiency. Pp. 278–303, In, Flaherty, B. E. (Ed.), *Psychophysiological Aspects of Space Flight*. New York, Columbia University Press, 1961.
64. HAUTY, G. T. Human performance in the space travel environment. *Air University Quarterly Rev., 10*:89–97, 1958.
65. HAUTY, G. T.: Maximum effort-minimum support simulated space flights. *Aero/Space Engineering, 19*:44–47, 1960.
66. HAUTY, G. T., and R. B. PAYNE: Fatigue, confinement, and proficiency decrement. *Am. J. Psychiat., 116*:385–391, 1959.
67. HERON, W., K. DOANE, and T. H. SCOTT: Visual disturbances after prolonged isolation. *Canad. J. Psychol., 10*:13–18, 1956.
68. HOLT, R., and L. GOLDBERGER: *Personological correlates of reactions to perceptual isolation*. Wright Air Development Center, Wright-Patterson Air Force Base, Ohio, *WADC Rept. No. 59-735*, November, 1959.
69. HOLT, R. R., and L. GOLDBERGER: *Research on the effects of isolation on cognitive functioning*. Wright Air Development Division, Wright-Patterson Air Force Base, *WADD Rept. No. 60-260*, March, 1960.
70. HOLT, R. R., and L. GOLDBERGER: Assessment of individual resistance to sensory alteration. Pp. 248–262, In, Flaherty, B. E. (Ed) *Psychophysiological Aspects of Space Flight*. New York, Columbia University Press, 1961.
71. KENNEDY, R. S., and A. GRAYBIEL: Symptomatology during prolonged exposure in a constantly rotating environment at a velocity of one revolution per minute. *Aerospace Med., 33*:817–825, 1962.
72. KINSEY, J. L.: Psychologic aspects of the "Nautilus" transpolar cruise. *Armed Forces Med. J., 10*:451–462, 1959.
73. LEIDERMAN, P. H., J. MENDELSON, D. WEXLER, and P. SOLOMON: Sensory deprivation: clinical aspects. *AMA Arch. Internal Med., 101*:389–396, 1958.
74. LILLY, J. C.: Mental effects of reduction of ordinary levels of physical stimuli on intact, healthy persons. *Psychiat. Res. Rept., 5*:1–28, 1956.
75. LILLY, J. C., and J. T. SHURLEY: Experiments in solitude, in maximum achievable isolation with water suspension, of intact healthy persons. Pp. 238–247, In, Flaherty, B. E. (Ed.) *Psychophysiological Aspects of Space Flight*. New York, Columbia University Press, 1961.

76. LUBY, E. D., J. L. GRISELL, C. E. FROHMAN, H. LEES, B. D. COHEN, and J. S. GOTTLIEB: Biochemical, psychological, and behavioral responses to sleep deprivation. *Ann. N. Y. Acad. Sciences,* 96:71–79, 1962.
77. McKENZIE, R. E., B. O. HARTMAN, and B. E. WELCH: Observations in the SAM two-man space cabin simulator. III. System Operator Performance Factors. *Aerospace Med.,* 32:603–610, 1961.
78. MEBANE, J. C.: Neuropsychiatry in aviation. Pp. 443–466, In, Armstrong, H. G. (Ed.) *Aerospace Medicine.* Baltimore, Williams & Wilkins, 1961.
79. MENDELSON, J., P. KUBZANSKY, P. H. LEIDERMAN, D. WEXLER, C. DuToIT, and P. SOLOMON: Catechol Amine excretion and behavior during sensory deprivation. *AMA Arch. Gen. Psychiat.,* 2:147–155, 1960.
80. MILLER, J. G.: Input overload and psychopathology. *Amer. J. Psychiat.,* 116:695, 1960.
81. MILLER, J. G.: Sensory overloading. Pp. 215–224, In, Flaherty, B. E. (Ed.) *Psychophysiological Aspects of Space Flight.* New York, Columbia Univ. Press, 1961.
82. MITCHELL, M. B.: *Time Disorientation and Estimation in Isolation.* Aeronautical Systems Division, Wright-Patterson Air Force Base, Ohio. *Rept. No. ASD-TDR-62-277,* April, 1962.
83. MORGAN, T. E., F. ULVEDAL, and B. E. WELCH: Observations in the SAM two-man space cabin simulator. II. Biomedical Aspects. *Aerospace Med.,* 32:591–602, 1961.
84. MORRIS, G. O., H. L. WILLIAMS, and A. LUBIN: Misperception and disorientation during sleep deprivation. *AMA Arch. Gen. Psychiat.,* 2:247, 1960.
85. ORMISTON, D. W.: *A methodological study of confinement.* Aerospace Medical Laboratory, Wright-Patterson Air Force Base, Ohio. *Rept. No. WADD TR 61-258,* March, 1961.
86. ORMISTON, D. W., and B. FINKELSTEIN: *The Effects of Confinement on Intellectual and Perceptual Functioning.* Aerospace Medical Laboratory, Wright-Patterson Air Force Base, Ohio. *Rept. No. ASD TR 61-577,* October, 1961.
87. PATRICK, G. T., and J. A. GILBERT: On effects of loss of sleep. *Psychol. Rev.,* 3:469–483, 1896.
88. RICHTER, C. P.: On the phenomenon of sudden death in animal and man. *Psychosomatic Med.,* 19:191–198, 1957.
89. ROSS, M. D.: Reactions of a balloon crew in a controlled environment. *J. Aviat. Med.,* 30:326–333, 1959.
90. ROSS, M. D., and M. L. LEWIS: The Strato-Lab balloon system for high altitude research. *J. Aviat. Med.,* 29:375–385. 1958.

91. RUFF, G. E.: Man in space: isolation. *Astronautics,* 4:22–23; 110–111, 1959.
92. RUFF, G. E.: Psychological effects of space flight. *Aerospace Med.,* 32:639–642, 1961.
93. RUFF, G. E., and E. Z. LEVY: Psychiatric evaluation of candidates for space flight. *Am. J. Psychiat.,* 116:385–391, 1959.
94. SCHAFER, G. E.: Sensory illusions in flying. *J. Aviat. Med.,* 22:207–211, 1951.
95. SELLS, S. B.: *Military Small Group Performance under Isolation and Stress. III. Environmental Stress and Behavior Ecology. Tech. Rept. No. 61-21,* Artic Aeromedical Laboratory, Fort Wainwright, Alaska, October, 1961.
96. SELLS, S. B., and C. A. BERRY: *Human Factors in Jet and Space Travel.* New York, Ronald Press, 1961.
97. SIMONS, D. G.: Pilot reactions during "Manhigh II" balloon flights. *J. Aviat. Med.,* 29:1–14, 1958.
98. SIMONS, D. G.: *Manhigh II: USAF Manned Balloon Flight into the Stratosphere.* Air Force Missile Development Center, Holloman Air Force Base, N. M. *Tech. Rept. No. AFMDC-TR-28,* June, 1959.
99. SOLOMON, P., P. E. KUBZANSKY, P. H. LEIDERMAN, J. H. MENDELSON, R. TRUMBULL, and D. WEXLER: *Sensory Deprivation.* Cambridge, Harvard Univ. Press, 1961.
100. SOLOMON, P., P. H. LEIDERMAN, J. MENDELSON, and D. WEXLER: Sensory Deprivation: A Review. *Am. J. Psychiat.,* 114:357–363, 1957.
101. STEELE, J. E.: *Motion Sickness and Spatial Perception.* Aerospace Medical Laboratory, Wright-Patterson Air Force Base, Ohio. *Rept. No. ASD TR 61-530,* November, 1961.
102. SLAYTON, D. K.: Pilot training and preflight preparation. Pp. 53–60. In, *Proceedings of a Conference on Results of the First U. S. Manned Suborbital Space Flight.* Washington, D. C.: U. S. Govt. Printing Office, June, 1961.
103. STEINKAMP, G. R., W. R. HAWKINS, G. T. HAUTY, R. B. BURWELL, and J. E. WARD: Human experimentation in the space cabin simulator. USAF School of Aviation Medicine, Brooks Air Force Base, Texas. *Rept. No. 59-101,* August, 1959.
104. STRUGHOLD, H.: Physiologic day-night cycle after long distance flights. *International Rec. of Med. and Gen. Practice Clinics,* 168:576–579, 1955.
105. STRUGHOLD, H.: Sensory-physiological aspects of the space flight situation. Pp. 56–65, In, Flaherty, B. E. (Ed.) *Psychophysiological Aspects of Space Flight.* New York, Columbia University Press, 1961.

106. VERNON, J., and T. E. McGILL: The effect of sensory deprivation upon rote learning. *Am. J. Psychol., 70*:637, 1957.

107. VERNON, J. A., T. E. McGILL, W. I. GULLICK, D. K. CANDLAND: Effect of sensory deprivation on some perceptual and motor skills. *Percept. & Motor Skills, 9*:91–97, 1959.

108. VERNON, J. A., T. E. McGILL, and H. SCHIFFMAN. Visual hallucinations during perceptual isolation. *Canad. J. Psychol., 12*:31–34, 1958.

109. VON BECKH, H. J. Human reactions during flight to acceleration preceded by or followed by weightlessness. *Aerospace Med., 30*:391–409, 1959.

110. VOSBURG, R., N. FRASER, and J. GUEHL: Imagery sequence in sensory deprivation. *Arch. Gen. Psychiat., 2*:356–357, 1960.

111. WALTERS, R. H., and G. B. HENNING: Isolation, confinement and related stress situations—some cautions. *Aerospace Med., 32*:431–434, 1961.

112. WEAVER, J. A., and R. F. GRAY: *The Perception of Oculogravic Illusions by Inverted Subjects.* Aviation Medical Acceleration Laboratory, U. S. Naval Air Development Center, Johnsville, Pa. *Rept. No. NADC-MA-6207,* July, 1962.

113. WEST, L. J., H. H. HANSZEN, B. K. LESTER, F. S. CORNELISOON, JR.: The psychosis of sleep deprivation. *Ann. N. Y. Acad. Sciences, 96*: 66–70, 1962.

114. WEXLER, D., J. MENDELSON, H. LEIDERMAN, and P. SOLOMON: Sensory deprivation. A technique for studying psychiatric aspects of stress. *AMA Arch. Neurol. & Psychiat., 79*:225–233, 1958.

115. WHEATON, J. L. *Fact and fancy in sensory deprivation studies.* Air University School of Aviation Medicine, Brooks Air Force Base, Texas. *Rept. No. 5-59,* August, 1959.

116. WILLIAMS, J. L., A. LUBIN, and J. J. GOODNOW: Impaired performance with acute sleep loss. *Psychol. Monogr., 73*:(No.484), 1959.

117. WILSON, C. L. (Ed.): *Project Mercury Candidate Evaluation Program.* Wright Air Development Center, Wright-Patterson Air Force Base, Ohio. *Rept. No. WADC-TR-59-505,* December, 1959.

118. WOELLNER, R. C., and A. GRAYBIEL: *The Loss of Counter-rolling of the Eyes in Three Persons Presumably without Functional Otolith Organs.* Naval School of Aviation Medicine, Pensacola, Fla. *Rept. No. 50. December,* 1959.

119. *Manhigh III. USAF Manned Balloon Flight Into the Stratosphere.* Air Force Missile Development Center, Holloman Air Force Base, New Mexico. *Rept. No. AFMDC-TR-60-16,* April, 1961.

120. *Proceedings of a Conference on Results of the First U. S. Manned Suborbital Space Flight.* U. S. National Aeronautics and Space Administration—National Institutes of Health, and National Academy of Sciences. Washington 25, D. C.: U. S. Government Printing Office, June 6, 1961.

121. *Results of the Second U. S. Manned Suborbital Space Flight July 21, 1961.* National Aeronautics and Space Administration, Manned Spacecraft Center, U. S. Government Printing Office, Washington 25, D. C., 1961.

122. *The Training of Astronauts. Report of a Working Group Conference.* Armed Forces-National Research Council Committee on Bio-astronautics. Publication No. 873. National Academy of Sciences—National Research Council, Washington, D. C., 1961.

123. *Results of the First United States Manned Orbital Space Flight, February 20, 1962.* Manned Spacecraft Center, National Aeronautics and Space Administration, U. S. Government Printing Office, Washington 25, D. C., 1962.

124. *Results of the Second United States Manned Orbital Space Flight, May 24, 1962.* Manned Spacecraft Center, National Aeronautics and Space Administration. U. S. Government Printing Office, Washington, D. C., 1962.

9

PHYSIOLOGIC RHYTHMS

Franz Halberg, M.D.

I. CIRCADIAN (ABOUT 24-HR) RHYTHMS

1) Scope, Generality, Reproducibility: The alternation of sleep and wakefulness and of rest and activity are obvious human rhythms with periods of about 24 hr. Many other body functions at different levels of organization in man, Figure 1, or experimental animal, Figure 2, also show rhythms with similar periods. These can be *reproducibly* described under defined conditions of observation and sampling, as soon as we realize that we are here usually dealing with statistical physiologic phenomena. In other words, these rhythms must be described by an appropriate num- ber of observations on a given individual. Alternatively, one or a few observations may serve the same purpose, if they are made on a sufficiently large number of comparable individuals. With this qualification, Figures 1 and 2 illustrate the scope in experi- mental medicine of rhythms that can all be described by the ad- jective "circadian"—derived from the Latin *circa*-about and *dies*-day.

2) Deviations from an Exact 24-hr Period: The term "circa- dian" can be applied to physiologic periods of exactly 24-hr length as well as to periods that, individually or on the average, are slightly yet consistently shorter or longer than 24 hr—by minutes or by a few hours.

For instance, circadian may be used to describe the period of either of the two curves shown in Figure 3. One of these, the solid line, is of average 24-hr length; the other, the dashed line, has a mean period of about 23 hr and 20 min.

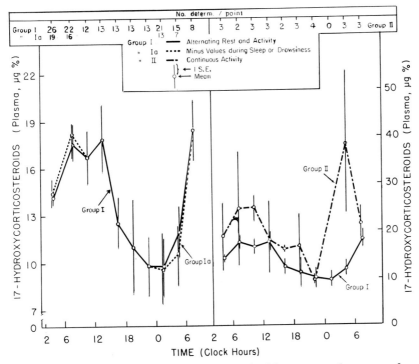

Fig. 1a. Time-course of adrenal cycle in healthy mature human males. Group I subjects, on a schedule of diurnal activity and nocturnal rest and sleep (N = 13). Group II subjects active by day and by night, without sleep (N = 3). Group I curve is the same in both halves of Figure; ordinates show different scales for the plasma 17-hydroxycorticoid value. The human adrenal cortical cycle persists at least for two days under conditions of continuous "over-all" activity with an increase in over-all hormone level and in "amplitude" and a shortening of cycle length.[1,2]

It is methodologically important (Figure 4) to recognize circadian periods that differ from exactly 24 hr, since, e.g., the peak of a given rhythmic function with such a period will occur at a different time each day.[4] Thus, if the period is shorter than 24 hr, the peak will occur earlier each day, dotted line in Figure 3, while it will occur later each day if the circadian period is longer than 24 hr.

An average period of rhythm, consistently and significantly different from 24 hr by minutes or a few hours, has theoretical

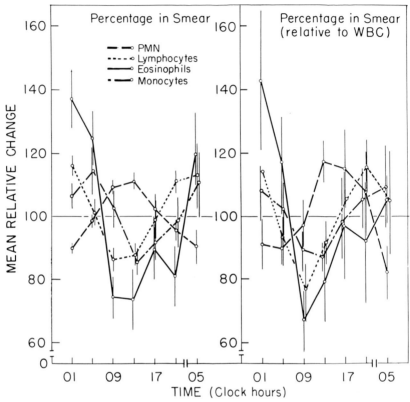

Fig. 1b. Formed elements in blood from 15 human subjects studied concomitantly on a standardized routine providing for diurnal activity and meals (06-2130) and nocturnal rest. Data expressed as % of series man. Vertical bars represent one standard error of the mean. Note internal timing (differences in phase).

implications as well. We know of no exact environmental counterparts to such periods, which can be called free-running ones, by analogy to a free-running oscillator.

Circadian functions, more often than not, are actually interacting periodically among themselves as well as with external factors. Their physiologic periodicity, as such—or, for sure, the ability of a given function under appropriate conditions to show a frequency of about one cycle/day—is as much, or more, characteristic of organisms or of their subdivisions as it is character-

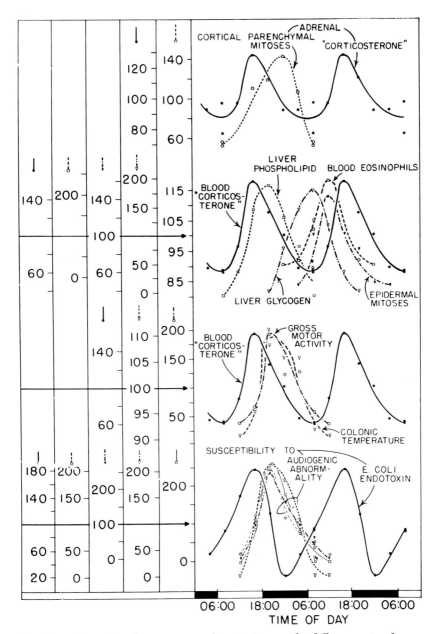

Fig. 2a. Circadian frequency-synchronization with differences-in-phase—
positive, negative, or zero. Results of light-synchronized periodicity analysis
on mice. Ordinates are relative changes, expressed as per cent of series mean.
(See printed text on figure.)

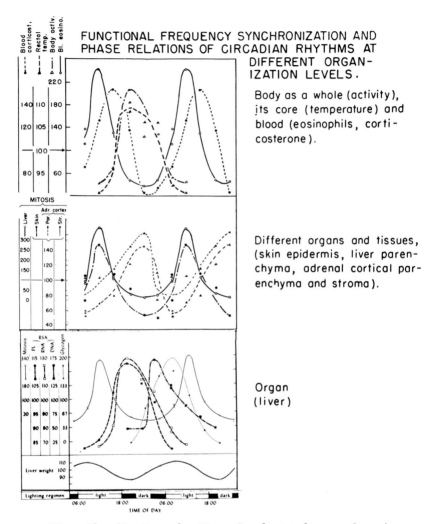

FUNCTIONAL FREQUENCY SYNCHRONIZATION AND PHASE RELATIONS OF CIRCADIAN RHYTHMS AT DIFFERENT ORGANIZATION LEVELS.

Body as a whole (activity), its core (temperature) and blood (eosinophils, corticosterone).

Different organs and tissues, (skin epidermis, liver parenchyma, adrenal cortical parenchyma and stroma).

Organ (liver)

Figure 2b. (See Legend to Figure 2 and printed text on figure.)

istic of a given system's response to factors topographically external to it. In other words, the integrative periodicity, e.g., of circadian organisms, is to a significant extent the system's own "action"; it is intimately related to those many external factors which can elicit "reaction" but not solely dependent upon such influences.

In current usage, diurnal is still in use as a synonym for circadian. This practice can be questioned since diurnal has two meanings, referring as it does to part of the day as well as to the entire day. The well-established uses of diurnal for distinguishing events limited mainly to day-time from those limited to other parts of the 24-hr period, as in diurnal (vs nocturnal) filariasis or epilepsy, or in "diurnality" (vs "nocturnality") of activity patterns, constitute weighty arguments for restricting this adjective to designate the day-time only. Moreover, diurnal does not convey the notion that physiologic periods can consistently differ in length from exactly 24 hr. Finally, reference to "diurnal variations" usually evokes the association of certain physiologic events with some particular time of day, without further qualification. This image must be removed, since circadian rhythms with non-24-hr periods show a peak at different times of day on consecutive days, Figure 3, and even 24-hr synchronized circadian rhythms can be phase-shifted so that the peak occurs at any clock hour of one's choice.

3) Synchronizer: Figure 5 shows that the peaks of circadian rhythms can indeed be shifted by changes in routine. An environmental cycle or routine may be called the synchronizer of a given circadian physiologic rhythm if two requirements are met: First, the rhythm can adapt its circadian period to the particular environmental cycle length. Second, the timing[4] of the rhythm can be changed by phase-shifts of the environmental cycle. The peak of a rhythm can thus be made to coincide with a desired clock hour. Therefore, indications of external timing—i.e., timing as to local clock hour—are meaningful only if the synchronizer schedule is also indicated.

Internal timing—i.e., the time relation of two or more circadian rhythms to each other—can change following a shift of the dominant synchronizer, since the time necessary for a shift of rhythm can vary with the plasticity of the organism's particular rhythm analyzed. The interdependence of superficially related periodic physiological functions can thus be analyzed by means of "phase-shifting" through study of shift-times. Just as one separates different compounds by their rate of travel in paper-

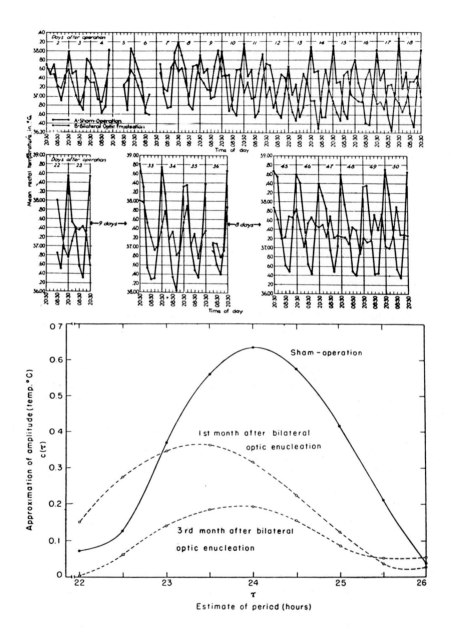

Fig. 3. Effect of blinding upon rectal temperature rhythm in the mouse. Top: Mean rectal temperatures during 50 days following blinding. The temperature rhythm of blinded mice leads in phase that of sham-operated mice. Bottom: Periodograms suggest the slight but clear shortening of cycle length during the first month after blinding. A tendency toward return to a 24-hour synchronized circadian rhythm may be seen during the third month after blinding, from the periodogram. These periodograms, on mean temperatures of blinded mice, show a decrease in amplitude, which is not present in periodograms of individual blinded mice. The decrease in amplitude results from differences in free-running period among individual blinded mice. These data on blinded mice are of interest in several ways. First, they demonstrate a change in period of the circadian temperature rhythm occurring in the absence of fever or hypothermia. Second, the small change in period, involving for the group of blinded mice a period of about 23 hours 20 minutes, can be quantified objectively by a periodogram; and what seems more important, it has repeatedly been reproduced in separate experiments based upon the detection of a predicted temporary "anti-phase" at 3 weeks after blinding. For the methodologic significance of such data see also Figure 4. (See printed text on figure).[3,4]

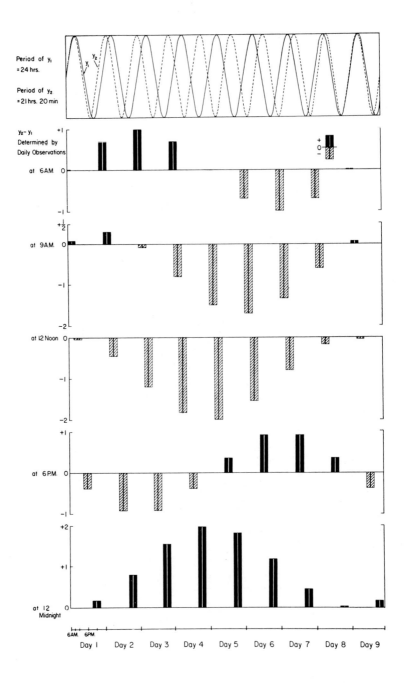

Fig. 4. Circadian system physiology is not merely a study of clock-hour effects. Work at a fixed time of day does not forestall disastrous pitfalls, possibly invalidating much research on rhythmic functions. This is seen from a study of the time-course of an inter-group differ-ence between synchronized controls and desynchronized experimentals —when comparisons are made 24 hr apart, at one *or* the other clock hour. A given physiologic function, y, is assumed to be circadian periodic in both groups compared. y_1 could represent a 24-hr synchro-nized case, while y_2 could differ in period from y_1 by 160 min in time. On the plot, y_1 and y_2 start out in phase at 06, in each case. Note that the difference between the two groups being compared will un-dergo drastically different changes with time, as a function of the particular clock hour chosen for observation.[4]

chromatography, one may dissociate certain rhythmic functions (in time, rather than space) by their rate of travel following inversion of the dominant synchronizer (e.g., lighting).

4) Hormone Effects in the Light of Circadian System Analysis: Figure 6 shows that a hormone effect, such as that of pituitary growth hormone (STH), may be apparent when analyzed in one stage of the circadian system—i.e., circadian system phase— but not in another. STH was administered to one group of mice for three successive days, while control mice received saline injections. One-half of the mice from each group were killed at

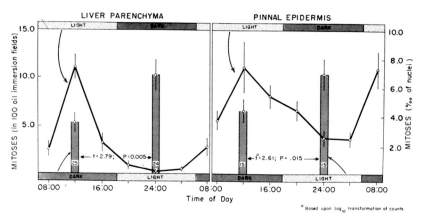

Fig. 5a. Reversal of circadian mitotic rhythms in two tissues following an inversion of lighting regimen. Data on liver mitoses at 8 days after inversion of lighting, those in pinnal mitoses at 23 days thereafter.

noon, the other half at midnight, after maintenance under conditions standardized for periodicity analysis, including light from 0600 to 1800 alternating with darkness. The effect of STH upon hepatic mitoses in these immature mice was statistically significant at the daily time of high mitotic activity but was not seen at the time of low mitotic activity, in comparisons of counts from saline-injected and STH-injected animals.

The effect of another hormone, namely adrenocorticotropic hormone (ACTH), *in vivo* and also *in vitro*, depends predictably upon the state of the adrenal gland at injection time. Figure

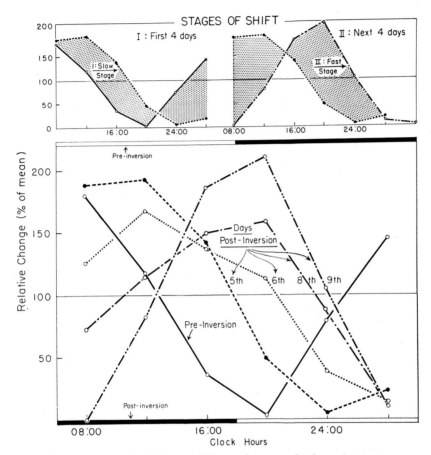

Fig. 5b. Time course of phase shift in glycogen rhythm of intact mouse liver. Expressed as mg of glycogen/gm of liver; the values at times of peak and trough, respectively, were 54.1 ± 3.10 (at ≈ 12:00), and 1.53 ± 0.34 at ≈ 24:00) on the 5th day after lighting inversion, and 55.8 ± 2.77 (at ≈ 20.00) and 0.04 ± 0.11 (at ≈ 08:00) on the 9th day (*P* of difference <0.01).[6]

7 summarizes an experiment involving seven groups each of sixty mice sacrificed every 4 hr. starting 0800 of one day and ending at 0800 of the next. At each point, twelve pools of blood each from five mice were obtained for determination of serum corticosterone. The adrenals of these mice also were removed,

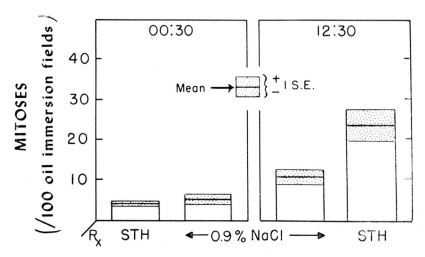

Fig. 6. Hepatic mitotic activity in mice given a three day course of STH (daily at ≈ 16:30) is significantly higher than in controls given saline, if livers are removed at noon on the day following injection (right-hand section of figure). This effect is not apparent in materials removed at midnight (left-hand section). Light from 0600 to 1800 alternating with darkness.[7]

defatted, quartered and corticosterone production was evaluated from incubations without hormone addition or with the addition of 0.04, 0.4 or 4.0 International Units of ACTH. Significant quantitative differences in the effect of ACTH as a function of circadian system phase are readily apparent in Figure 7.[8]

5) Resistance to Injury: A mammal's circadian time structure at the moment of exposure to injury can predictably tip the scale between death and survival—following the administration of agents ranging from physical ones such as noise, Figure 8, to bacterial endotoxins, Figure 9, and even drugs, such as ouabain. For the experiment described in Figure 8, inbred D_8 mice were weaned at 21 ± 2 days of age, immediately singly housed in so-called periodicity rooms, maintained at 24 ± 0.5°C and illuminated by artificial light only. One group of mice was in light from 0600 to 1800, another in light from 1800 to 0600, alternating with 12 hr of darkness in each case. About one-half of the mice

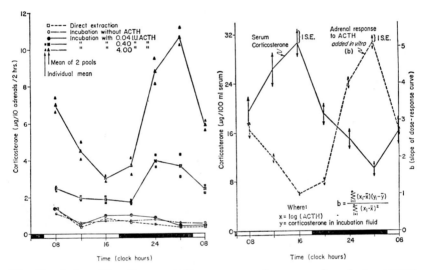

Fig. 7. *Left:* Circadian periodic response of mouse adrenals to ACTH added *in vitro.* Each point represents the means of duplicate flasks per treatment and time. Total of 700 C adrenals incubated. *Right:* Phase relations of circadian rhythms in serum corticosterone and in adrenal responsivity to ACTH *in vitro.* (Broken line) slope of log dose-response relation of quartered adrenals to ACTH added *in vitro*—computed from data on the left. (Solid line) serum corticosterone; mean of 12 pools, each from five mice per time point. Total of 420 C mice.

from each group were exposed to noise between 0700 and 0900, the other half between 2000 and 2200. Following noise exposure a set of abnormal responses may be observed, ranging from "uncontrolled" running to convulsion and, possibly, death. Significant differences for all these types of audiogenic abnormality can be seen in Figure 8, as a function of test time for the animals from both rooms. The spotcheck thus reveals, first, that noise exposure had different effects as a function of circadian system phase (compare per cent abnormality at 0800 and 2100 for the mice in light by day and separately for the mice in light by night). The same figure reveals further that the higher suscepti-

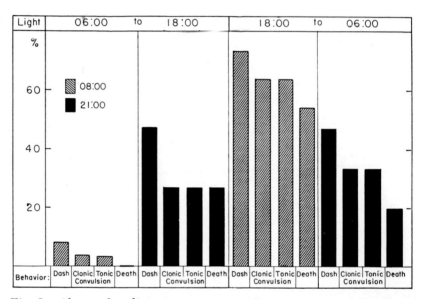

Fig. 8. Abnormal audiogenic responses in D_8 mice, on two schedules of light and darkness, alternating at 12-hr intervals. Note the difference in incidence of abnormality at 08:00 and 21:00, on each lighting regimen. Note also the difference in time of high abnormality, in mice exposed to light from 18:00 to 06:00, as compared with that in mice exposed to light from 06:00 to 18:00. Total tested: 102 mice, about five weeks of age, of both sexes.[9]

bility to noise occurred at a different time in the mice maintained in light by night as compared to those maintained in light by day.

Figure 9 summarizes two seven-time-point experiments. In each, seven groups of inbred *C* mice were injected intraperitoneally at 4-hr intervals with 100 µg of Difco's *E. coli* lipopolysaccharide. The first group was injected at 0800, the following

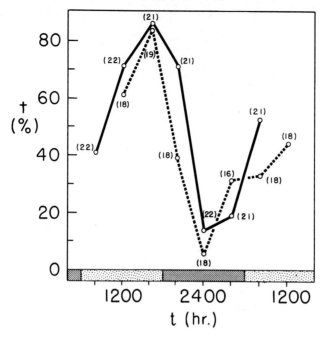

Fig. 9. Susceptibility rhythm to a bacterial endotoxin. A dose compatible with survival of most animals at one time is highly lethal when injected into a separate group of comparable animals at certain other predictable times.[10,11]

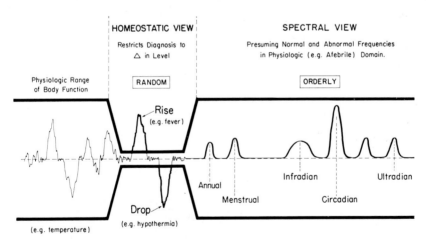

Fig. 10. Comparison of two views of normal body function. The spectral view searches for an approximation of order as indicated by the normal frequency-structure of a physiologic function. A range otherwise neglected as random by the more conventional homeostatic approach can thus be analyzed. Both views, spectral and homeostatic, detect gross abnormality, once certain normal limits are exceeded. However, only the spectral view can serve as a reference standard for changes in frequency that are not associated with gross changes in the level, e.g., of body temperature.[12]

groups at 4-hr intervals until 0800 of the next day. In each experiment, the groups differed from each other only in terms of injection time, the genetic background of the mice and the dose of endotoxin injected being kept comparable. Mortality was evaluated at one week post-injection and revealed significant differences as a function of injection time, as may be seen from Figure 9.

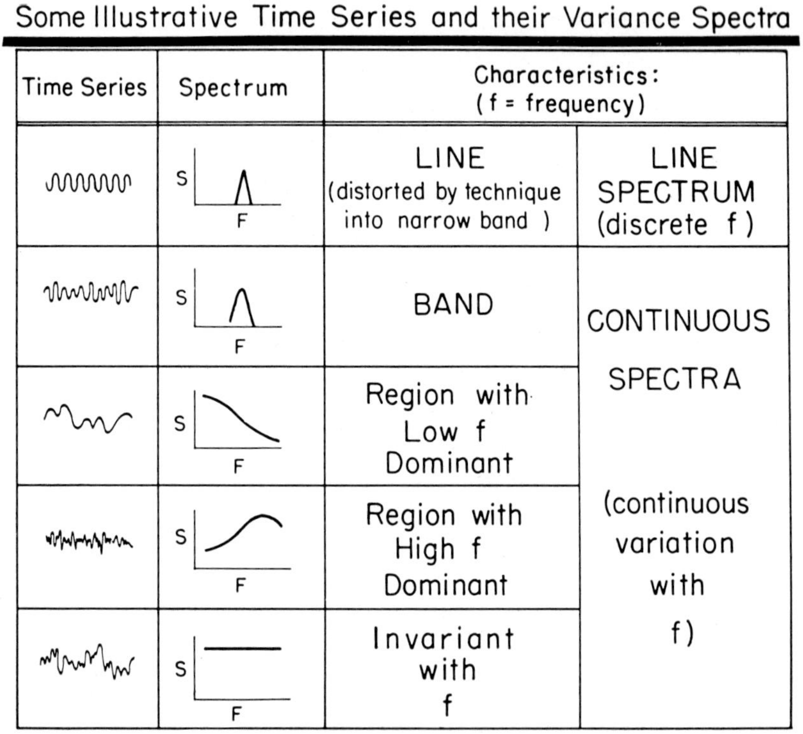

Some Illustrative Time Series and their Variance Spectra

Time Series	Spectrum	Characteristics: (f = frequency)	
◌◌◌◌◌◌	S ⋀ F	LINE (distorted by technique into narrow band)	LINE SPECTRUM (discrete f)
◌◌◌◌	S ⋀ F	BAND	CONTINUOUS SPECTRA
∿∿	S ⌐╲ F	Region with Low f Dominant	
◌◌◌◌	S ╱⌐ F	Region with High f Dominant	(continuous variation with f)
◌◌◌◌	S ──── F	Invariant with f	

Fig. 11.   The frequency content of time series as revealed by their variance spectrum; slightly amplified version of abstract figure, drawn and discussed originally by Mercer.[13–15]

It is pertinent that the toxicity of a number of drugs as well has been shown to depend predictably upon circadian system phase. Furthermore, the times of the peak and trough in susceptibility of mice to various agents are not all the same, and information on such hours of changing resistance is of interest to students of bioassay. Such information on predictable hours of changing resistance underlines the importance of circadian organization to an understanding of factors underlying resistance to injury.

II. VARIANCE SPECTRA

Circadian functional integration and adaptation provide but one component to the broad spectrum of physiologic frequencies.

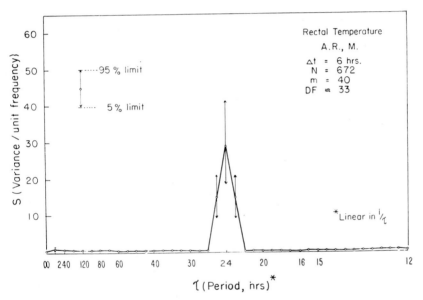

Fig. 12a. Variance spectrum of human rectal temperature showing narrow, banded circadian component; the latter is essentially a line—its widened base is largely the result of the smoothing process used for analysis. Ordinate in $(0.1°F)^2$/cycle/480 hr.[15]

This component and others may be quantified and visualized by variance spectra, according to Tukey, Figure 10. Figures 11–14 summarize halting steps in this direction. In body temperature records obtained under standardized conditions and, what seems important, in the absence of fever or hypothermia, spectral components may serve as a gauge of disease and/or drug effect.[15]

III. PHYSIOLOGIC RHYTHMS AND BIOASTRONAUTICS

Man's exploration of extraterrestrial space has raised or renewed his interest in circadian rhythms. Whether organisms deprived of their natural geophysical environment continue to show circadian rhythms is a question of basic biology that has often been raised in the past, by implication, Figure 15, or

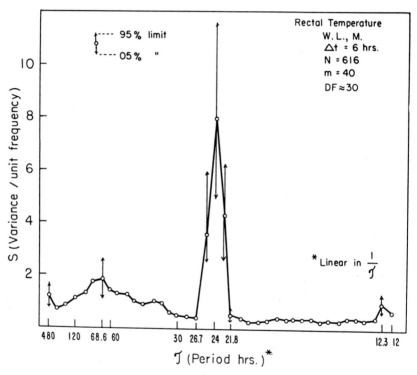

Fig. 12b. Variance spectrum of human rectal temperature revealing significant circadian component plus components with lower frequencies (longer periods). Note width of latter and lesser variance fraction in circadian component of this spectrum, as compared with corresponding value in Figure 12a.
Ordinate in $(0.1°F)^2$/cycle/480 hr.[15]

explicitly. Whether astronauts a) can perform optimally on a non-24-hr work-rest cycle, b) presumably without a 24-hourly periodic geophysical and/or other environmental input, constitutes an applied problem. Information from submarines or simulated space-flights is relevant to a) above, but in the opinion of some authors not necessarily to b).

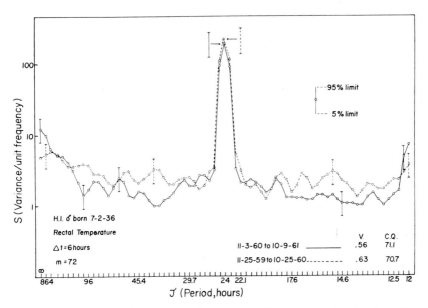

Fig. 13. Variance spectra of two human rectal temperature series from the same subject. Note remarkable agreement of spectral estimates in the circadian domain, from one year to the next. Note further that spectral estimates are plotted on a logarithmic scale against frequency on a linear scale. The graph appears more irregular than is warranted.

In the context of the broader problems of bioastronautics, the student of physiologic rhythms should emphasize that his is a second-order applied problem, although it is a first-order basic problem. We know already that man can withstand relatively short flights into outer space and to assure his survival, *inter alios,* circulatory and respiratory physiologists must continue to take care of the first-order applied problems in the fields of their competence. It seems reasonable to suggest, however, that the longer the flight, the more important the second-order practical problems of physiologic rhythms, or, more broadly, of temporal organization will become. Some of these problems but not all

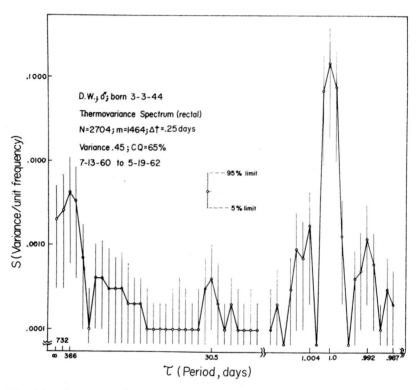

Fig. 14. Summary of 2704 consecutive six-hourly rectal temperature measurements on the same subject. The circadian component is most prominent. A component with a frequency of 1 cycle in about 366 days remains of questionable significance in these limited data.

of them resemble those confronting us in submarines. From fewer astronauts, living as yet under more crowded conditions than do submariners and sent eventually on long missions into outer space, we shall expect, however, top performance in tasks

That period of twenty-four hours,
formed by the regular revolution of our
earth, in which all its inhabitants partake,
is particularly diftinguifhed in the phyfical
œconomy of man.   This regular period
is apparent in all difeafes ; and all the other
fmall periods, fo wonderful in our phyfical hiftory, are by it in reality determined.   It is, as it were, the unity of our
natural chronology.—

CHRISTOPHER WILLIAM HUFELAND, M. D.

PUBLIC LECTURER ON MEDICINE AT JENA.

THE

A R T

OF

PROLONGING LIFE.

L O N D O N:

PRINTED FOR J. BELL, NO. 148, OXFORD-STREET,

M.DCC.XCVII.

Fig. 15.   Reproductions from a book by Hufeland, 2nd English translation, 1797:   top, part of page 201; bottom, title page.[11]

that will warrant the responsibilities and effort associated with incorporating man into a machine system.

Until limitations to payloads are eventually overcome, a very few astronauts, for instance, may have to alternate on duty, eventually for long periods. The demands of a logistically desirable non-24-hr work-rest schedule may then bring about the impaired performance of one man, at least, if not of others. Tests for

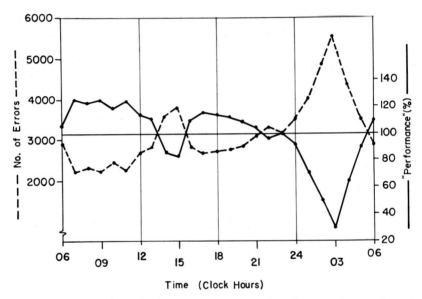

Figure. 16.   Circadian rhythm in performance, based upon the number of errors made in the routine checking of gas meters at different clock hours, 175,000 readings during a period from 1912–1931, reported by Bjerner, B., A. Holm, and A. Swensson, 1948, Om Natt-och Skiftarbete, Statens Offentliga Utredningar, Sweden, and discussed by Lehmann, G., in *Man's Dependence on the Earthly Atmosphere*, New York, Macmillan, 1962.[16]

predicting this behavior and information as to how it comes about—and how it can be corrected—can be sought by gauging physiologic rhythms not only in performance *per se* (Figure 16) but in the periodic mechanisms underlying such rhythms.

Problems of physiologic rhythms thus are pertinent to human engineering for life in aerospace, particularly with respect to astronaut selection and performance. They are so, irrespective of whether this latter time dimension of life on earth is acquired or innate, while information on the latter problem in itself is a first-order contribution to basic biology. Bioastronautics can provide such data and thus fill an important gap in our knowledge.*

REFERENCES CITED

1. HALBERG, F.: Circadian temporal organization and experimental pathology. Ediz. *Minerva Medica,* VII Conferenza Internazionale della Societa per lo Studio dei Ritmi Biologici, Atti, Siena, 1960.
2. HALBERG, F., FRANK, G., HARNER, R., MATTHEWS, J., AAKER, H., GRAVEN, H., and MELBY, J.: The Adrenal Cycle in men on different schedules of motor and mental activity. *Experientia, 17*:282, 1961.
3. HALBERG, F., and VISSCHER, M. B.: *Some Physiologic Effects of Lighting.* Proceedings of the First International Photobiological Congress (4th International Light Congress) Amsterdam (August) 1954, pp. 396–397.
4. HALBERG, F., LOEWENSON, R., WINTER, R., BEARMAN, J. and ADKINS, G. H.: Physiologic circadian systems; differences in period of circadian rhythms or in their component frequencies. *Minn. Acad. Sci., 28*:53–75, 1960.
5. HALBERG, F., BARNUM, C. P., SILBER, R. H., and BITTNER, J. J.: 24-hr rhythms at several levels of integration in mice on different lighting regimens. *Proc. Soc. Exp. Biol. and Med., 97*:897–900, 1958.
6. HALBERG, F., ALBRECHT, P. G., and BARNUM, C. P.: Phase shifting of liver-glycogen rhythm in intact mice. *Am. J. Physiol., 199*:400, 1960.
7. HALBERG, F., and HOWARD, R. B.: 24-hr periodicity and experimental medicine. Examples and interpretations. *Postgraduate Medicine, 24*:349–358, 1958.
8. UNGAR, F., and HALBERG, F.: Circadian rhythm in the in vitro response of mouse adrenal to adrenocorticotropic hormone. *Science, 137*:1058–1060, 1962.
9. HALBERG, F., JACOBSON, E., WADSWORTH, G. and BITTNER, J. J.: Audiogenic abnormality spectra, twenty-four hour periodicity, and lighting *Science, 128*:657–658, 1958.
10. HALBERG, F., JOHNSON, E. A., BROWN, B. W. and BITTNER, J. J.: Susceptibility rhythm to *E. coli* endotoxin and bioassay. *Proc. Soc. Exp. Biol. and Med., 103*:142–144, 1960.

* Acknowledgments: Supported, in part, by grants from the U. S. Public Health Service, 5-K6-GM-13,981; NB-04531-02; C-4359 C4, American Cancer Society (E-155E), Elsa U. Pardee Foundation, Department of Public Welfare, State of Minnesota, and NASA (NsG-517).
Dedicated to the memory of Professor John J. Bittner.

11. HALBERG, F.:   The 24-hr scale: a time dimension of adaptive functional organization. *Perspectives in Biology and Medicine,* 3:491–527, 1960.

12. CIRCADIAN SYSTEMS.   Report of the 39th Ross Conference on Pediatric Research. Ross Laboratories, Columbus, Ohio, 1961, p. 93.

13. MERCER, D. M. A.:   Analytical methods for the study of periodic phenomena obscured by random fluctuations.   In: *Cold Spring Harbor Symposia on Quantitative Biology.*   Long Island Biological Assoc. N. Y. 1960, p. 73.

14. PANOFSKY, H., and HALBERG, F.:   II.   Thermo-variance spectra; simplified computational example and other methodology.   *Experimental Medicine and Surgery,* 19:323–338, 1961.

15. HALBERG, F., and PANOFSKY, H.:   I.   Thermo-variance spectra; method and clinical illustrations.   *Experimental Medicine and Surgery,* 19:284–309, 1961.

16. SCHAEFER, KARL E., ed.:   *Man's Dependence on the Earthly Atmosphere.*   New York, Macmillan, 1962.

ADDED REFERENCES

1. HALBERG, F.:   Circadian rhythms, a basis of human engineering for aerospace.   In: *Psychophysiological Aspects of Space Flight,* B. Flaherty, ed.   Columbia University Press, 1961, pp. 166–194.

2. STRUGHOLD, H.:   Day-night cycling in atmospheric flight, space flight, and on other celestial bodies.   *Annals New York Acad. Sci.,* 98:1109–1115, 1962.

3. HAUTY, G. T.:   Periodic desynchronization in humans under outer space conditions.   *Annals New York Acad. Sci.,* 98:1116–1125, 1962.

4. *Cold Spring Harbor Symposia on Quantitative Biology,* Vol. 25, New York, Long Island Biological Association, 1960.

5. *Photoperiodism and Related Phenomena in Plants and Animals,* R. B. Withrow, ed.   Publ. 55 of the Am. Assoc. Adv. Sci., Washington, D.C., 1959.

6. ASCHOFF, J.:   Comparative physiology: diurnal rhythms.   *Ann. Rev. Physiol.,* 25:581–600, 1963.

7. Circadian (about twenty-four-hour) rhythms in experimental medicine. In: *Proc. Royal Soc. Med.,* 56:253–260, 1963.

8. REINBERG, A., and GHATA, J.:   *Rhythmes et cycles bioligiques.*   Paris, Presses Universitaires de France, 1957.

9. KLEITMAN, N.:   *Sleep and Wakefulness,* Rev. & Enl. Ed. Chicago, Univ. Chicago Press, 1963.

10. BÜNNING, E.:   *.Die Physiologische Uhr,* Zweite Auflage.   Berlin, Springer Verlag, 1963.

11. MENZEL, W.:   *Meschliche Tag-Nacht-Rhythmik und Schichtarbeit.* Basel, Benno Schwabe, 1962.

AUTHOR INDEX

SUBJECT INDEX

Radiometer, 5
Radio-nuclide, 60
Radio-sonde, 6
Rayleigh's Law, 13
Rectal temperature rhythm, 305
Reflectance, 11
Reflective suits, 28
Rem units, 59
Rendezvous, 215
Respiration, 100
Reynold's number, 37
Rhythms, 298
    susceptibility, 313
"Riometer," 56
Roentgen, 58

Salt replacement, 44
Scattering, 13
Selection, 283
Semicircular canal, 204
Sensation of warmth, 21
Sense, 272
Sensory, 209
Sensory deprivation, 227, 248
Sensory input overload, 252
Sensory overload, 236
Seryl, 249
Shielding from direct rays of the sun, 28
Skin, 17
    absorption coefficients, 15
    blood flow, 21
    optical properties of, 11
    reflectivity of, 11
    thermal characteristics of, 16
Sleep deprivation, 236, 254
Social isolation, 236
Solar cosmic storms, 71
Solar prominances, 69
Solar radiation, 10
Space environment—emissivity of, 25
Space radiations—properties of, 65
Space suit—emissivity of, 25
"Specific dynamic effect," 138
Specific heat, 17
Sputnik II, 50

Steady state—development of, 32
Stephan-Boltzman constant, 25
"Stormer-Alfven trajectories," 75
Strato-lab, 242
Stresses—heat or cold, 42
Stroke volume, 184
Sub-gravity, 196
Sun-radiant flux from, 25
Sweat evaporation, 27
Sweating, 38
Sweat-rates, 43
Synchronizer, 303

Tactual sense, 225
Temperature,
    dry bulb, 6
    equivalent black body, 5
    in space travel, 3
    mean radiant, 28
    radiant, 5
    sky and cloud, 5
    yearly, 4
Thermal, 31
    comfort, 42
    conductivities, 30
    conductivity, 17
    environments, 4
    environments, the earth, 4
    equilibrium, 8
    exposure—physiological
    limitations of, 42
    gradient, 33
    inertia for, 17
    sensation, 21
Tilt-table testing, 202
Time disorientation, 262
Time perception, 226
Tolerance times for high wall
    temperatures, 45
Toxic substances, 118
Training, 283

Ultraviolet, 11
Utricle, 269